Advanced Pattern Recognition Technologies with Applications to Biometrics

David Zhang
The Hong Kong Polytechnic University, Hong Kong

Fengxi Song
New Star Research Institute of Applied Technology , China

Yong Xu
ShenZhen Graduate School of Harbin Institute of Technology, China

Zhizhen Liang
City University of Hong Kong, Hong Kong

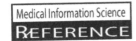

Medical Information Science
REFERENCE

MEDICAL INFORMATION SCIENCE REFERENCE

Hershey · New York

Director of Editorial Content:	Kristin Klinger
Director of Production:	Jennifer Neidig
Managing Editor:	Jamie Snavely
Assistant Managing Editor:	Carole Coulson
Typesetter:	Jennifer Henderson
Cover Design:	Lisa Tosheff
Printed at:	Yurchak Printing Inc.

Published in the United States of America by
Information Science Reference (an imprint of IGI Global)
701 E. Chocolate Avenue, Suite 200
Hershey PA 17033
Tel: 717-533-8845
Fax: 717-533-8661
E-mail: cust@igi-global.com
Web site: http://www.igi-global.com/reference

and in the United Kingdom by
Information Science Reference (an imprint of IGI Global)
3 Henrietta Street
Covent Garden
London WC2E 8LU
Tel: 44 20 7240 0856
Fax: 44 20 7379 0609
Web site: http://www.eurospanbookstore.com

Library of Congress Cataloging-in-Publication Data

Advanced pattern recognition technologies with applications to biometrics / by David Zhang [et al.].

    p. cm.

Includes bibliographical references and index.

 Summary: "This book focuses on two kinds of advanced biometric recognition technologies, biometric data discrimination and multi-biometrics"--Provided by publisher.

 ISBN 978-1-60566-200-8 (hardcover) -- ISBN 978-1-60566-201-5 (ebook)

 1. Biometric identification. I. Zhang, David, 1949-

 TK7882.B56A35 2009

 006.4--dc22

                              2008040444

British Cataloguing in Publication Data
A Cataloguing in Publication record for this book is available from the British Library.

All work contributed to this manuscript is new, previously-unpublished material. The views expressed in this manuscript are those of the authors, but not necessarily of the publisher.

Table of Contents

Section I
Biometric Discriminant Analysis

Section III
Biometric Fusion

Preface

With the increasing concerns on security breaches and transaction fraud, highly reliable and convenient personal verification and identification technologies are more and more requisite in our social activities and national services. Biometrics, which use the distinctive physiological and behavioural characteristics to recognize the identity of an individual, are gaining ever-growing popularity in an extensive array of governmental, military, forensic, and commercial security applications.

The beginning of biometrics can be traced back to centuries ago, from when fingerprint has been used for forensics. Automated biometrics, however, has only 40 years of history. In the early 1960s, the FBI (Federal Bureau of Investigation) began to put more effort in developing automated fingerprint acquisition and identification systems. With the advances in hardware, sensor, pattern recognition, signal and image processing technologies, a number of biometric technologies, such as face, iris, retina, voice, signature, hand geometry, keystroke, ear, and palm print recognition, have been developed, and novel biometrics, such as dental, odor, and skin reflectance, have also been investigated to overcome some of the limitations of current biometric recognition technologies.

Historically, the development of biometric technologies is originated from different disciplines. For example, the beginning of fingerprint recognition research is an interaction of forensics and pattern recognition. Voice recognition technology, on the contrary, came from signal processing, and face recognition started from computer vision. This multi-discipline characteristic, however, makes it very challenging to establish an infrastructural theory framework for developing biometric recognition technologies.

Generally, a biometric system can be regarded as a pattern recognition system, where a feature set is first extracted from the acquired data, and then compared with the stored template set to make a decision on the identity of an individual. A biometric system can be applied to two fields, verification and identification. In verification mode, the decision is whether a person is *who he claims to be?*" In identification mode, the decision is *"whose biometric data is this?"* A biometric system is thus formalized into a two-class or multi-class pattern recognition system.

A biometric system usually includes four major modules: data acquisition, feature extraction, matching, and system database, where feature extraction and matching are two of the most challenging problems in biometric recognition research, and have attracted researchers from different backgrounds: biometrics, computer vision, pattern recognition, signal processing, and neural networks. In this book, we focus on two advanced pattern recognition technologies for biometric recognition, biometric data discrimination and multi-biometrics. Biometric data discrimination technology, which extracts a set of discriminant features by using classical or improved discriminant analysis approaches, is of course one kind of advanced pattern recognition technology. Multi-biometrics, which integrates information from multiple biometric traits to enhance the performance and reliability of the biometric system, is another kind of advanced pattern recognition technology.

The book begins with the topic of biometric data discrimination technologies. Discriminant analysis, which aims at dimensionality reduction while retaining the statistical separation property between distinct classes, is a natural choice for biometric feature extraction. From the late 1980s, many classical discriminant analysis technologies are borrowed and applied to deal with biometric data or features. Among them, principal component analysis (PCA, or K-L transform) and Fisher linear discriminant analysis (LDA) turns out to be effective, in particular for face representation and recognition. Other linear approaches, such as independent component analysis (ICA), canonical correlation analysis (CCA), and partial least squares (PLS), have been investigated and applied to biometric recognition. Recently, non-linear projection analysis technology represented by kernel principal component analysis (KPCA), kernel Fisher discriminant (KFD), and manifold learning, also show great potential in dealing with biometric recognition problems.

Biometric data discriminant analysis is not a simple application of discriminant analysis to biometric data. Biometric data is usually high dimensional and their within-class variations should not be neglected, as the neglect will cause the serious performance degradation of classical discriminant analysis approaches. Various improvements to discriminant analysis techniques have been proposed to make it more suitable for biometric data. Now discriminant analysis has been widely applied to face, ear, fingerprint, gait recognition, and multi-biometrics. Further, the present demand for more reliable biometric recognition technologies is also contributing to the development and improvement on linear/nonlinear discriminant analysis technologies.

The form of biometric data and features is diverse. Biometric data mainly exists in the following three forms: 1D waveform (e.g. voice, signature data), 2D images (e.g. face images, fingerprints, palm prints) or image sequences (i.e., video), and

3D geometric data (such as 3-D facial or hand geometric shapes). Because of the diversity in biometric data and feature forms, it is difficult to develop a universal feature extraction technology which is capable to process all kinds of biometric data.

To deal with the diversity in biometric data forms, a family of tensor discriminant analysis technologies has been investigated. A tensor is a higher order generalization of a vector or a matrix. In fact, a vector is a first-order tensor and a matrix is a tensor of order two. Furthermore speaking, tensors are multilinear mapping over a set of vector spaces. If we have data in three or more dimensions, then we mean to treat them as higher-order tensors. In this way, tensor technologies present a generalized representation and analysis of biometric data discrimination technologies. Nowadays, tensor principal component analysis, tensor discriminant analysis, tensor independent component analysis, and other tensor analysis approaches have been successfully applied to face, palm print, and gait recognition.

In advance of the application of biometric data discrimination technologies, we should determine the appropriate representation of the biometric data. Generally, biometric data discrimination technologies can be performed in either data space or feature space. On the one hand, discrimination technologies can be used to derive the discriminative features directly from the original biometric data. On the other hand, a set of salient features are first extract from biometric data, and discrimination technologies are then performed in the feature space for the second feature extraction. It should be noted that the feature space may be implicit or infinite dimensional for kernel-based methods. In this way, biometric data discrimination technologies provide a general means to integrate different kinds of features for effective biometric feature extraction and matching.

In general, biometric data discrimination technologies share the following characteristics: (1) high dimensionality, which makes direct classification in original data space almost impossible; (2) difference in sample quality, where robust discrimination technologies should be developed to address biometric data with poor quality; (3) small sample size, where the data dimensionality is much higher than the size of the training set, resulting in the singularity and poor estimation of the scatter matrix. Recently, with the efforts of related researchers, progresses have been achieved in solving these problems.

From the late 1990s, the authors of the book have been devoted to biometric data discrimination research, and developed a series of novel and effective discriminant criteria and discriminant algorithms, which cover both vector-based and tensor-based discrimination technologies. The class of new methods includes: (1) Extensions of Fisher's discriminant criterion: we present three classification-oriented extensions of Fisher's discriminant criterion: large margin linear projection (LMLP), minimum norm minimum squared-error, and maximum scatter difference. All these three criteria are classification-oriented and designed to deal with the small sample size problem; (2) Orthogonal discriminant analysis: we investigate two novel orthogonal discriminant analysis methods: Orthogonalized Fisher discriminant (OFD) and Fisher discriminant with Schur decomposition (FDS). Theoretical analysis and experimental results indicate that both OFD and FDS are optimal solutions to multiple Fisher discriminant criterion; (3) Parameterized discriminant analysis: we introduce three parameterized linear discriminant analysis methods. The first is parameterized direct linear discriminant analysis. The second is weighted nullspace linear discriminant analysis, and the third is weighted linear discriminant analysis in the range of within-class scatter matrix; (4) New facial feature extraction methods: we present two novel facial feature extraction methods, multiple maximum scatter difference (MMSD) and discriminant based on coefficients of variances (DCV). MMSD is an extension of binary linear discriminant analysism and DCV is a generalization of the null-space LDA; (5) Tensor PCA: we introduce the algorithms and discuss the properties of a group of tensor PCA methods; (6) Tensor LDA: we investigate the algorithms and discuss the properties of a group of tensor linear discriminant analysis and tensor locality preserving projection methods.

The second topic of the book is multi-biometrics, which combines information from multiple biometric traits to improve the accuracy and reliability of biometric systems. Individual biometric system, the biometric system using a single biometric characteristic, usually suffers from some inherent limitations and can not provide satisfactory recognition performance. For example, manual workers with damaged or dirty hands may not be able to provide high-quality fingerprint images, and thus failure to enrol would happen for single fingerprint recognition system. Multi-biometric systems, which integrate information from multiple biometric traits, provide some effective means to enhance the performance and reliability of the biometric system. In recent years, multi-biometric technologies have received considerable interests in biometric recognition research. Several true multi-modal databases have released for testing multi-biometric recognition algorithms. To facilitate multi-biometric research, the (USA) National Institute of Science and Technology (NIST) presents an open resource of Biometric Scores Set - Release 1 (BSSR1), which includes true multi-model matching scores generated by face and fingerprint recognition algorithms.

To combine information from individual biometric traits, there are three levels of fusion strategies in general, feature level fusion, matching score level fusion, and decision level fusion. In feature level fusion, the data obtained from each sensor is used to compute a feature vector. As the feature extracted from one biometric trait is independent of that extracted from the other, a new feature vector can be constructed using the concatenation rule, the parallelity rule, or the competitive rule for performing multi-biometric based personal authentication. It should be noted that the new feature vector may have a higher dimensionality than the original feature vector generated from each sensor, and feature reduction techniques may be further employed to extract useful features from the set of the new feature vector. In matching score level fusion, each subsystem using one biometric trait of the multi-biometric system provides a matching score indicating the proximity of the feature vector with the template vector. These scores can be combined to assert the veracity of the claimed identity. A number of transformation-based, classifier-based, and density-based score fusion methods have been used to combine scores of multiple scores. In decision level fusion each sensor first acquire one of multiple biometric traits and the resulting feature vectors are individually classified into the two decisions - accept or reject the claimed identity. Then a scheme that exploits the known decisions to make the final decision is used. So far, boolean conjunctions, weighted decision methods, classical inference, Bayesian inference, Dempster–Shafer method, and voting have been proposed to make the final recognition decision. In the field of multi-biometrics, a great number of studies of feature level fusion, matching score level fusion and decision level fusion have been made. Though fusion of multi-biometric are generally recognized as three classes as described above, in real-world applications of multi-biometric system it is possible that the "Fusion Process" may be simultaneously involved in different levels such as in both the matching score level and the decision level.

In recent years, the authors and their collaborators have insisted on research on multi-biometric technologies. Our investigations cover all the three categories of multi-biometric technologies, which include: (1) Feature level fusion: we investigate two novel feature level fusion methods, a pixel level fusion method to combine face and palm print traits, and a feature level fusion method to combine phase and orientation information of palm print images for effective personal recognition; (2) Matching score level fusion: We present a practical application example to study the effectiveness of matching score level fusion in face and palm print recognition; (3) Decision level fusion: We introduce a group decision-making combination approach to combine decisions of multiple face recognition algorithms.

The book is organized into three main sections. As an overview of the book, Chapter I describes the basic concepts necessary for a premier understanding of biometric data discrimination and multi-biometric technologies. Section I explores some advanced biometric data discrimination technologies developed for the small sample size (SSS) problem, where we first provide a brief introduction of linear discriminant analysis and the SSS problem, and then describes our solutions to SSS by developing extensions to Fisher's discriminant criterion and novel improved discriminant analysis approaches. Section II describes several tensor-based biometric data discrimination technologies, including tensor principal component analysis, tensor linear discriminant analysis, and tensor locality preserving projections.

Other recently developed tensor approaches, such as tensor independent component analysis, tensor non-negative matrix factorization, tensor canonical correlation analysis, and tensor partial least squares, are also introduced in this section. Section III deals with the second topic of the book, multi-biometrics. We first introduce the fundamental conception and categories of multi-biometrics technologies, and then describe three kinds of multi-biometric technologies, feature level fusion, matching score level fusion, and decision level fusion by providing several implementation examples.

This book includes fifteen chapters. Chapter I briefly introduces two advanced biometric recognition technologies, biometric data discrimination and multi-biometrics, to enhance the recognition performance of biometric systems. In Section 1.1, we discuss the necessity, importance, and applications of biometric recognition technology. A brief introduction of main biometric recognition technologies are then presented in Section 1.2. In Section 1.3, we describe biometric data discrimination and multi-biometric technologies. Section 1.4 outlines the history of related work and highlights each chapter of this book.

Chapter II is a brief introduction to biometric data discriminant analysis technologies. Section 2.1 describes two kinds of LDA methods: classification-oriented LDA and feature extraction-oriented LDA. Section 2.2 discusses LDA for the small-sample-size problem. Section 2.3 briefly introduces the organization of Section I.

In Chapter III, we present three novel classification-oriented linear discriminant criteria. The first one is the large margin linear projection criterion, which makes full use of the characteristic of the SSS problem. The second one is the minimum norm minimum squared-error (MNMSE), which is a modification of the classical minimum squared-error (MSE) discriminant criterion. The third one is the maximum scatter difference, which is a modification of the Fisher's discriminant criterion.

In Chapter IV, we first give a brief introduction to Fisher's linear discriminant, Foley-Sammon discriminant, orthogonal component discriminant, and application strategies for solving the SSS problem. We then present two novel orthogonal discriminant analysis methods: one is orthogonalized Fisher discriminant; the other is Fisher discriminant with Schur decomposition. At last, we compare the performances of several main orthogonal discriminant analysis methods under various SSS strategies.

Chapter V describes three kinds of weighted LDA methods. The first is parameterized direct linear discriminant analysis. The second is weighted nullspace linear discriminant analysis. The third is weighted LDA in the range space of within-class scatter matrix. At last, we give a summery of the chapter.

Chapter VI introduces two novel facial feature extraction methods. The first is multiple maximum scatter difference (MMSD), which is extension of a binary linear discriminant criterion, that is maximum scatter difference. The second is discriminant analysis based on coefficients of variances (DCV) which can be viewed as a generalization of null space LDA. At last, we give a summery of the chapter.

Chapter VII gives the background for developing tensor-based discrimination technologies. Section 7.2 introduces some basic notations in tensor space. Section 7.3 discusses several tensor decomposition methods. Section 7.4 introduces the tensor rank.

Chapter VIII presents some variants of classical PCA, and discusses the properties of tensor principal component analysis. Section 8.1 gives the background and development of tensor principal component analysis. Section 8.2 introduces tensor principal component analysis. Section 8.3 discusses some potential applications of tensor principal component analysis in biometric systems. We summarize this chapter in Section 8.4.

In Chapter IX, classical LDA and its several variants are introduced. In some sense, the variants of LDA can avoid the singularity problem and achieve computational efficiency. Experimental results on biometric data show the usefulness of LDA and its variants in some cases.

In Chapter X, we describe two subspace analysis technologies: tensor independent component analysis and tensor non-negative matrix factorization, which can be used in many fields like face recognition and other biometric systems. Section 10.1 gives the background and development of two subspace analysis. Section 10.2 introduces tensor independent component analysis. Section 10.3 gives tensor nonnegative factorization. Section 10.4 discusses some potential applications of these two subspace analysis in biometric systems. We summarize this chapter in Section 10.5.

Chapter XI deals with two tensor-based classifiers, tensor canonical correlation analysis and tensor partial least squares, which can be used in many fields such as biometric systems. Section 11.1 briefly surveys the history in developing tensor-based classifiers. Section 11.2 introduces tensor-based classifiers. Section 11.3 gives tensor canonical correlation analysis and tensor partial least squares. We summarize this chapter in Section 11.4.

Chapter XII describes the basic concepts of biometrics and motivation of multi-biometrics. Section 12.2 provides the definitions and notations of biometric and multi-biometric technologies. Section 12.3 presents two feature extraction approaches for biometric images, where one of which is a linear feature extraction approach and the other is a nonlinear feature extraction approach. Section 12.4 briefly indicates some techniques associated with each kind of multi-biometric technologies.

Chapter XIII mainly presents the basic concepts and two examples of feature level fusion methods. As the beginning of this chapter, Section 13.1 provides an introduction to feature level fusion. Section 13.2 briefly surveys current feature level fusion schemes. Section 13.3 shows a feature level fusion example that fuses face and palm print. Section 13.4 shows a feature level fusion example that fuses multiple feature presentations of a single biometric trait. Section 13.5 offers brief comments.

In Chapter XIV, we aims at describing several basic aspects of matching score level fusion. Section 14.1 provides a brief introduction of basic characteristics of matching score fusion. Section 14.2 describes a number of matching score fusion rules. Section 14.3 presents the normalization procedures of raw matching scores. Section 14.4 provides several brief comments on matching score fusion.

Chapter XV deals with the decision fusion rules, the classifier selection approach, and a case study of face recognition based on decision fusion, as well as a summary of multi-biometric technologies. In a multi-biometric system, classifier selection techniques may be associated with the decision fusion as follows: classifier selection is first carried out to select a number of classifiers from all classifier candidates. Then the selected classifiers make their own decisions and the decision fusion rule is used to integrate the multiple decisions to produce the final decision. Section 15.1 provides an introduction to decision level fusion. Section 15.2 presents some simple and popular decision fusion rules such as the AND, OR, RANDOM, and Voting rules, as well as the weighted majority decision rule. Section 15.3 introduces a classifier selection approach based on correlations between classifiers. Section 15.4 presents a case study of group decision-based face recognition. Section 15.5 offers several comments on the three levels of multi-biometric technologies.

Chapter XVI aims at summarizing the book from a holistic viewpoint. Section 16.1 summarizes the contents of the book and indicates the relationship between different chapters in each section. Section 16.2 reveals that how the methods and algorithms described in different sections can be applied to different data forms of biometric traits. Section 16.3 provides comments on the development of multi-biometrics.

In summary, this book is a comprehensive introduction to theoretical analysis, algorithms, and practical applications of two kinds of advanced biometric recognition technologies, biometric data discrimination and multi-biometrics. It would serve as a textbook or as a useful reference for graduate students and related researchers in the fields of computer science, electrical engineering, systems science, and information technology. Researchers and practitioners in industry and R&D laboratories working on security system design, biometrics, computer vision, control, image processing, and pattern recognition would also find much of interest in this book.

In the preparation of this book, David Zhang organizes the contents of the book and is in charge of Chapters I, II, VII, XII and XVI. Fengxi Song handles Chapters III through VI. Zhizhen Liang and Yong Xu write Chapters VII through XI and Chapters XIII through XV, respectively. Finally, David Zhang looks through the whole book and examines all chapters.

Acknowledgment

The authors are full of gratitude to our co-workers and students for their persistent support to our research. Our sincere thank goes to Prof. Zhaoqi Bian of Tsinghua University, Beijing, Prof. Jingyu Yang of Najing University of Science and Technology, Najing, China, and Prof. Pengfei Shi of Shanghai Jiaotong University, Shanghai for their invaluable advice throughout this research. We would like to thank our team members, Dr. Wangmeng Zuo, Prof. Jian Yang, Prof. Xiaoyuan Jing, Dr. Guangming Lu, Prof. Kuanquan Wang, Dr. Xiangqian Wu, Dr. Jingqi Yan, and Prof. Jie Zhou for their hard work and unstinting support. In fact, this book is the collaborative result of their many contributions. We would also like to express our gratitude to our research fellows, Feng Yue, Laura Liu, Dr. Ajay Kumar, Dr. Lei Zhang, Dr. Hongzhi Zhang, Bo Huang, Denis Guo, and Qijun Zhao for their invaluable help and support. Thanks are also due to Martin Kyle, for his help in the preparation of this book. The financial support from the HKSAR Government, the central fund from the Hong Kong Polytechnic University, the NFSC funds (Nos. 60332010, 60602038, and 60402018), and the 863 fund (No. 2006AA01Z193) in China are of course also greatly appreciated. We owe a debt of thanks to Jan Travers and Kristin Roth of IGI Global, for their valuable suggestions and keeping us on schedule for the preparation and publishing of the book.

Chapter I
Overview

ABSTRACT

A biometric system can be regarded as a pattern recognition system. In this chapter, we discuss two advanced pattern recognition technologies for biometric recognition, biometric data discrimination and multi-biometrics, to enhance the recognition performance of biometric systems. In Section 1.1, we discuss the necessity, importance, and applications of biometric recognition technology. A brief introduction of main biometric recognition technologies are presented in Section 1.2. In Section 1.3, we describe two advanced biometric recognition technologies, biometric data discrimination and multi-biometric technologies. Section 1.4 outlines the history of related work and highlights the content of each chapter of this book.

1.1 INTRODUCTION

Reliable personal recognition techniques play a critical role in our everyday and social activities. In access control, authorized users should be allowed for entrance with high accuracy while unauthorized users should be denied. In welfare benefit disbursement, people not only should verify whether the identity of a person is whom he/she claimed to be, but also should avoid the occurrence that one person claims to be another person to receive the welfare benefit twice (double dipping).

Traditionally, there are two categories of personal recognition approaches, token-based and knowledge-based (Miller, 1994). In the token-based approach, the identity of a person is verified according to *what he/she has*. Anyone possessed a certain physical object (token), e.g., keys or ID cards, is authorized to receive the associated service. The knowledge-based approaches authenticate the identity of an individual according to *what he/she knows.* Any individuals with certain secret knowledge, such as passwords and answers to questions, would receive the associated service. Both the token-based and the knowledge-based approaches, however, have some inherent limitations. In the token-based approach, the "token" could be stolen or lost. In the knowledge-based approach, the "secret knowledge" could be guessed, forgotten, or shared.

Biometric recognition is an emerging personal recognition technology developed to overcome the inherent limitations of the traditional personal recognition approaches (Jain, Bolle, & Pankanti, 1999a; Zhang, 2000, 2002, & 2004; Wayman, 2005; Bolle, 2004). The term biometrics, which comes from the Greek words bios (life) and metrikos (measure), refers to a number of technologies to authenticate persons using their physical traits such as fingerprints, iris, retina, speech, face and palm print or behavior traits such as gait, handwritten signature and keystrokes. In other words, biometric recognition recognizes the identity of an individual according to *who he/she is.* Compared with the token-based and the knowledge-based methods, biometric identifiers cannot be easily forged, shared, forgotten, or lost, and thus can provide better security, higher efficiency, and increased user convenience.

Biometric recognition lays the foundation for an extensive array of highly secure authentication and reliable personal verification (or identification) solutions. The first commercial biometric system, Identimat, was developed in 1970s, as part of an employee time clock at Shearson Hamill, a Wall Street investment firm (Miller, 1994). It measured the shape of the hand and the lengths of the fingers. At the same time, fingerprint-based automatic personal authentication systems were widely used in law enforcement by the FBI and by US government departments. Subsequently, advances in hardware such as faster processing power and greater memory capacity made biometrics more feasible and effective. Since the 1990s, iris, retina, face, voice, palm print, signature and DNA technologies have joined the biometric family (Jain et al., 1999a; Zhang, 2000).

With the increasing demand for reliable and automatic solutions to security systems, biometric recognition is becoming ever more widely deployed in many commercial, government, and forensic applications. After the 911 terrorist attacks, the interest in biometrics-based security solutions and applications increased dramatically, especially in the need to identify individuals in crowds. Some airlines have implemented iris recognition technology in airplane control rooms to prevent any entry by unauthorized persons. In 2004, all Australian international airports implemented passports using face recognition technology for airline crews and this will eventually became available to all Australian passport holders (Jain et al., 1999a). Several governments are now using or will soon be using biometric recognition technology. The U.S. INSPASS immigration card and the Hong Kong

ID card, for example, both store biometric features for reliable and convenient personal authentication.

Generally speaking, any situation that allows an interaction between human and machine is capable of incorporating biometrics. Such situations may fall into a range of application areas. Biometrics is currently being used in areas such as computer desktops, networks, banking, immigration, law enforcement, telecommunication networks and monitoring the time and attendance of staff. Governments across the globe are tremendously involved in using and developing biometrics. National identity schemes, voting registration and benefit entitlement programs involve the management of millions of people and are rapidly incorporating biometric solutions. Fraud is an ever-increasing problem and security is becoming a necessity in many walks of life. Biometric applications can be simply categorized as follows (Zhang, 2000):

Law Enforcement: The law enforcement community is perhaps the largest user of biometrics. Police forces throughout the world use Automated Fingerprint Identification System (AFIS) technology to process suspects, match finger images and to process accused individuals. A number of biometric vendors are earning significant revenues in this area, primarily using AFIS and palm-based technologies.

Banking: Banks have been evaluating a range of biometric technologies for many years. Automated Teller Machines (ATMs) and transactions at the point of sale are particularly vulnerable to fraud and can be secured by biometrics. Other emerging markets such as telephone banking and Internet banking must also be totally secure for bank customers and bankers alike. A variety of biometric technologies are now striving to prove themselves throughout this range of diverse market opportunities.

Computer Systems (also known as Logical Access Control): Biometric technologies are proving to be more than capable of securing computer networks. This market area has phenomenal potential, especially if the biometric industry can migrate to large-scale Internet applications. As banking data, business intelligence, credit card number, medical information and other personal data become the target of attack, the opportunities for biometric vendors are rapidly escalating.

Physical Access: Schools, nuclear power stations, military facilities, theme parks, hospitals, offices and supermarkets, across the globe employ biometrics to minimize security threats. As security becomes more and more important for parents, employers, governments and other groups - biometrics will be seen as a more acceptable and therefore essential tool. The potential applications are infinite. Cars and houses, for example, the sanctuary of the ordinary citizen, are under constant threat of theft. Biometrics - if appropriately priced and marketed - could offer the perfect security solution.

Benefit Systems: Benefit systems like welfare especially need biometrics to struggle with fraud. Biometrics is well placed to capitalize on this phenomenal market opportunity and vendors are building on the strong relationship currently enjoyed with the benefits community.

Immigration: Terrorism, drug-running, illegal immigration and an increasing throughput of legitimate travellers is putting a strain on immigration authorities throughout the world. It is essential that these authorities can quickly and automatically process law-abiding travellers and identify law-breakers. Biometric technologies are being employed in a number of diverse applications to make this possible. The US Immigration and Naturalization Service is a major user and evaluator of a number of state-of-the-art biometric systems. Systems are currently in place throughout the US to automate the flow of legitimate travellers and deter illegal immigrants. Elsewhere biometrics is capturing the imagination of countries such as Australia, Bermuda, Germany, Malaysia and Taiwan.

National Identity: Biometric technologies are beginning to assist governments as they record population growth, identify citizens and prevent fraud from occurring during local and national elections. Often this involves storing a biometric template on a card that in turn acts as a national identity document. Finger scanning is particularly strong in this area and schemes are already under way in Jamaica, Lebanon, The Philippines and South Africa.

Telephone Systems: Global communication has truly opened up over the past decade, while telephone companies are under attack from fraud. Once again, biometrics is being called upon to defend against this onslaught. Speaker ID is obviously well suited to the telephone environment and is making in-roads into these markets.

Time, Attendance and Monitoring: Recording and monitoring the movement of employees as they arrive at work, have breaks and leave for the day were traditionally performed by time-card machines. Replacing the manual process with biometrics prevents any abuses of the system and can be incorporated with time management software to produce management accounting and personnel reports.

1.2 BIOMETRIC RECOGNITION TECHNOLOGIES

A biometric system can be regarded as a pattern recognition system, where a feature set is first extracted from the acquired data, and then is compared with the stored template set to make a decision on the identity of an individual. A biometric system can be operated in two modes, biometric verification and biometric identification. In biometric verification mode, the decision is whether a person is *"who he/she claims to be?"* In biometric identification mode, the decision is *"whose biometric data is this?"* Thus a biometric system can be formalized into a two-class or multi-class pattern recognition system.

A biometric system usually includes four major modules: data acquisition, feature extraction, matching, and system database (Jain, Ross, & Prabhakar, 2004). In the data acquisition module, the biometric data of an individual is acquired using a capture sensor. In the feature extraction module, the acquired data is processed to extract a set of discriminative features. In the matching module, the features are compared with the stored template set to make a decision on the identity of an individual. In the system database module, a database is built and maintained to store the biometric templates of the enrolled users. Feature extraction and matching are two of the most challenging problems in biometric recognition research, and have attracted researchers from different backgrounds: biometrics, computer vision, pattern recognition, signal processing, and neural networks.

Advances in sensor technology and increasing diverse demand of biometric systems cause the persistent progress on developing novel acquisition sensors and novel biometric technologies. Before 1980s, the *offline* "ink-technique" is the dominant approach to acquire fingerprint images. Nowadays, a number of *online* live-scan fingerprint sensors, e.g., optical, solid-state, and ultrasound, have been designed for fingerprint acquisition.

Although research on the issues of common biometric technologies have drawn considerable attention, and have been studied extensively over the last 25 years, there are still some limitations to varieties of existing applications. For example, some people have their fingerprints worn-away due to the hard work they do with their hands and some people are born with unclear fingerprints. Face-based and voice-based identification systems are less accurate and easier to be attacked using a mimic. Efforts geared towards improving the current personal identification methods will continue, and meanwhile new biometric technologies are under investigation. Currently, the major biometric technologies involve face, fingerprint, iris, palm print, signature, and voice recognition, as well as multi-biometric recognition technologies (Zhang, 2002). The following provides a brief introduction of these biometric traits:

Fingerprint: Because the patterns of ridges and valleys on an individual's fingertips are unique to that individual, fingerprints can be used for authenticating personal identity. For decades, law enforcement has been classifying and determining identity by matching key points of ridge endings and bifurcations. Fingerprints are so unique that even identical twins usually do not have the same fingerprint.

Iris: The patterns of the iris, the colored area that surrounds the pupil, are thought to be unique. Iris patterns can be obtained through a video-based image acquisition system. Iris scanning devices have been used in personal authentication applications. It has been demonstrated that iris-based biometric system can work with individuals without regard to ethnicity or nationality.

Palm Print: Palm print, the inner surface of the palm, carries several kinds of distinctive identification features for accurate and reliable personal recognition. Like fingerprints, palm print have permanent discriminative features including patterns of ridges and valleys, minutiae, and even pores in high resolution (>1000dpi) images. Except these quasi fingerprint features, palm print also carries other particular distinctive features including principal lines and wrinkles. Using a high resolution capture device, it is possible to extract all kinds of palm print features to construct a high accurate biometric system. In the early stage, palm print recognition techniques have been investigated to extract and match the singular points and minutia points from high resolution palm print images. High resolution palm print scanner, however, is expensive, and is time consuming to capture a palm print image, which restricts the potential applications of online palm print recognition systems. Subsequently, online capture device has been developed to collect real time low resolution palm print image, and low resolution palm print recognition has gradually received considerable recent interest in biometric community (Zhang, Kong, You, & Wong, 2003; Jain et al., 2004; Zhang, 2004).

Face: Images of a human face are highly suitable for use as a biometric trait for personal authentication because they can be acquired non-intrusively, hands-free, continuously, and usually in a way that is acceptable to most users (Zhao et al., 2003). The authentication of a person by their facial image can be done in a number of different ways, such as by capturing an image of the face in the visible spectrum using an inexpensive camera or by using the infrared patterns of facial heat emission. Facial recognition in visible light typically models key features from the central portion of a facial image.

Signature: Signature authentication involves the dynamic analysis of a signature to authenticate a person's identity. A signature-based system will measure the speed, pressure, and angle used by the person when producing a signature. This technology has potential applications in e-business, where signatures can be an accepted method of personal authentication.

Speech: Speech-based personal authentication, which has a history of about four decades, is regarded as a non-invasive biometric technology. Speech authentication uses the acoustic features of speech, which have been found to be different between individuals. These acoustic patterns reflect both anatomic (e.g., size and shape of the throat and mouth) and behavioral patterns (e.g., voice pitch, speaking style) of an individual. The incorporation of learned patterns into the voice templates (the latter called "voiceprints") has allowed speaker recognition to be recognized as a "behavioral biometric". Speech-based personal authentication systems employ three styles of spoken input: text-dependent, text-prompted and text-independent. Most speech authentication applications use text-dependent input, which involves selection and enrollment of one or more voice passwords. Text-prompted input is used whenever there is concern about imposters.

Retina: The vascular configuration of the retina is supposed to be a characteristic unique to each individual. The retina is regarded as one of the most secure biometric traits. Usually the acquisition of a retinal image requires the cooperation of the subject.

Gait: Gait, the peculiar way one walks, is a complex spatio-temporal biometric trait. Note that gait is a behavioral trait and may not remain the same over a long period of time, due to some factors such as changes in body weight. It is commonly considered that a gait-based biometric system can be used in some low-security applications. Gait authentication is also not intrusive and the acquisition of gait is similar to acquiring a facial image. Usually a gait-based biometric system analyzes a video-sequence to obtain the gait trait and it is generally computationally expensive.

Hand and Finger Geometry: A system may measure geometrical characteristics of either the hands or the fingers to perform personal authentication. These characteristics include length, width, thickness and surface area of the hand. Requiring only a small biometric sample of a few bytes is one interesting characteristic of this kind of biometric technology. The biometric system based on hand and finger geometry has been used in physical access control in commercial and residential applications, in time and attendance systems.

DNA: Deoxyribonucleic acid (DNA), which can be denoted by a one-dimensional code unique for every individual, is probably the most reliable biometric although personal authentication using DNA will fail in distinguishing the identities of identical twins. A biometric system using DNA also suffers from other problems such as privacy issues, possible contamination, and low-efficiency in DNA matching.

Ear: There is evidence to show that the shape of the ear and the structure of the cartilaginous tissue of the pinna are distinctive. As a result, the ear-based biometric system can be used for authenticating personal identity.

Odor: Each object, including people, spreads an odor that is characteristic of its chemical composition. This could be used for distinguishing various objects. This would be done with an array of chemical sensors, each sensitive to a certain group of compounds. However, deodorants and perfumes could compromise distinctiveness.

Multi-Biometrics: From an application standpoint, widespread deployment of a user authentication solution requires support for an enterprise's heterogeneous environment. Often, this requires a multi-faceted approach to security, deploying security solutions in combination. An authentication solution should seamlessly extend the organization's existing security technologies. We are now interested in understanding both how to build multi-biometric recognition systems and what possible improvements these combinations can produce. Currently there are several true multi-modal databases available for testing multi-biometric recognition algorithms. The most important resource available may be the extended M2VTS database, which is associated with the specific Lausanne protocol for measuring the performance of verification tasks. This database contains audio-visual material from 295 subjects (Poh & Bengio, 2006). To facilitate multi-biometric research, NIST presents an open resource of Biometric Scores Set - Release 1 (BSSR1), which includes true multimodel matching scores generated by face and fingerprint recognition algorithms (Grother & Tabassi, 2004).

1.3 MAIN PROBLEMS IN BIOMETRIC RECOGNITION

To enhance the recognition performance of the biometric system, this section suggests two advanced biometric recognition technologies, biometric data discrimination and multi-biometric technologies. In biometric data discrimination, we first introduce the fundamental of biometric data discrimination, and then suggest using a family of tensor discriminant analysis to deal with the diversity in forms of biometric data. In multi-biometrics, we introduce three categories of fusion strategies to enhance the performance and reliability of the biometric system.

Besides recognition performance, security and privacy issues should also be taken in account. In terms of security, there are many attacks, such as overplay, database and brute-force attacks, on biometric applications. In terms of privacy, biometric traits may carry additional sensitive personal information. For example, genetic disorders might be inferred from the DNA data used for personal identification.

1.3.1 Biometric Data Discrimination

Generally, biometric data mainly exists in the following three forms: 1D waveform (e.g. voice, signature data), 2D images (e.g. face images, fingerprints, palm prints, or image sequences, i.e., video), and 3D geometric data (such as 3-D facial or hand geometric shapes). Since the diversity in biometric data and feature forms, it is hardly difficult to develop a universal recognition technology which is capable to process all kinds of biometric data. Fortunately, recent progress in discriminant analysis sheds some light on the possibility on this problem.

Discriminant analysis, with the goal of dimensionality reduction and of retaining the statistical separation property between distinct classes, is a natural choice for biometric recognition. With the development of biometrics and its applications, many classical discriminant analysis technologies have been borrowed and applied to deal with biometric data. Among them, principal component analysis (PCA, or K-L transform) and Fisher linear discriminant analysis (LDA) have been very successful, in particular for face image recognition. These methods have themselves been greatly improved with respect to specific biometric data analyses and applications. Recently, non-linear projection analysis technology represented by kernel principal component analysis (KPCA) and kernel Fisher discriminant (KFD) has also shown great potential for dealing with biometric recognition problems. In summary, discrimination technologies play an important role in the implementation of biometric systems. They provide methodologies for automated personal identification or verification. In turn, the applications in biometrics also facilitate the development of discrimination methodologies and technologies, making discrimination algorithms more suitable for image feature extraction and recognition. Currently discriminant analysis has been widely applied to face, ear, fingerprint, gait recognition, and even multi-modal biometrics. Further, the increasing demand for reliable and convenient biometric system is also contributing to the development and improvement of linear/nonlinear discriminant analysis techniques.

A tensor is a higher order generalization of a vector or a matrix. In fact, a vector is a first-order tensor and a matrix is a tensor of order two. Furthermore speaking, tensors are multilinear mapping over a set of vector spaces. If we have data in three or more dimensions, then we mean to deal with a higher-order tensor. Tensor presents a generalized representation of biometric data. To deal with the diversity in biometric data forms, a family of tensor discriminant analysis technologies have been investigated. Nowadays, tensor principal compoenent analysis, tensor discriminant analysis, tensor independent component analysis, and other tensor analysis approaches have been successfully applied to face, palm print, and gait recognition.

Biometric data discrimination technologies can be briefly defined as automated methods of feature extraction and recognition based on given biometric data. It should be stressed that the biometric data discrimination technologies are not the simple application of classical discrimination techniques to biometrics, but are in fact improved or reformed discrimination techniques that are more suitable for biometric applications, for example by having a more powerful recognition performance or by being computationally more efficient for feature extraction or classification. In other words, the biometric data discrimination technologies are designed for extracting features from biometrics data, which are characteristically high-dimensional, large scale, and offer only a small sample size. The following explains these characteristics more fully.

High Dimensionality: In biometric recognition, high dimensional data usually are expected to be more powerful. The high-dimensionality of biometric data, however, would make direct classification (e.g. the so-called correlation method that uses a nearest neighbour classifier) in original data space almost impossible, firstly because the similarity (distance) calculation is very computationally expensive, secondly because it demands large amounts of storage. High dimensionality makes it necessary to use a dimension reduction technique prior to recognition.

Large Scale: Real-world biometric applications are often large-scale, which means biometric systems should be operated in large population databases. Typical examples of this would include welfare-disbursement, national ID cards, border control, voter ID cards, driver's licenses, criminal investigation, corpse identification, parenthood determination, and the identification of missing children. Given an input biometric sample, a large-scale biometric identification system determines whether the pattern is associated with any of a large number (e.g., millions) of enrolled identities. These large-scale biometric applications require high-quality and very generalizable biometric data discrimination technologies.

Sample Quality: Biometric systems automatically capture, detect and recognizing biometric image, making it inevitable that biometric data will sometimes be noisy or partially corrupted. The capture and communication of biometric data itself may introduce noise; some accessories will cause the partial corruption of biometric data, for example a scarf may occlude a facial image. Because all these factors are inevitable, the development of biometric system should always address the robust feature extraction and recognition of noisy or partially corrupted biometric data.

Small Sample Size: Unlike, for example, optical character recognition (OCR) problems, the training samples per class that are available in real-world biometric recognition problems are always very limited. Indeed, there may be only one sample available for each individual. Combined with high-dimensionality, small sample size creates the so-called small sample size (or under-sampled) problems. In these problems, the within-class scatter matrix is always singular because the training sample size is generally less than the space dimension. As a result, the classical LDA algorithm becomes infeasible in image vector space.

1.3.2 Multi-Biometrics

Verification or identification accuracy is always the first-of-all objective for biometric systems. Unibiometric system, the biometric system using a single biometric characteristic, usually suffers from some limitations and can not provide satisfactory recognition performance. For example, manual workers with damaged or dirty hands may not be able to provide high-quality fingerprint images, and thus failure to enrol would happen for single fingerprint recognition system.

Multi-biometric systems, which integrate information from multiple biometric traits, provide some effective means to enhance the performance and reliability of the biometric system. To combine information from individual biometric traits, there are three categories of fusion strategies, feature level fusion, matching score level fusion, and decision level fusion. In feature level fusion, the data obtained from each sensor is used to compute a feature vector. As the feature extracted from one biometric trait is independent of that extracted from the other, it is reasonable to concatenate the two vectors into a single new vector for performing multi-biometric based personal authentication. Note that the new feature vector now has a higher dimensionality than the original feature vector generated from each sensor. Feature reduction techniques may be employed to extract useful features from the set of the new feature vector. In matching score level fusion, each subsystem using one biometric trait of the multi-biometric system provides a matching score indicating the proximity of the feature vector with the template vector. These scores can be combined to assert the veracity of the claimed identity. In decision level fusion each sensor first acquire one of multiple biometric traits and the resulting feature vectors are individually classified into the two decisions---accept or reject the claimed identity. Then a scheme that exploits the known decisions to make the final decision is used. In the field of multi-biometrics, a great number of studies of feature level fusion, matching score level fusion and decision level fusion have been made. Though fusion of multi-biometrics are generally recognized as three classes as described above, in real-world applications of multi-modal biometric it is possible that the "Fusion Process" may be simultaneously involved in different levels such as in both the matching score level and the decision level.

1.4 BOOK PERSPECTIVE

In this book we will systematically introduce readers to two categories of advanced biometric recognition technologies, biometric data discrimination and multi-biometrics. This book addresses fundamental concerns of relevance to both researchers and practitioners using biometric data discrimination and multi-biometric technologies. The materials in the book are the product of many years of research on the part of the authors' and present the authors' recent academic achievements made in the field. For the sake of completeness, and readers may rest assured that wherever necessary this book also addresses the relevant work of other authors.

Recent decades have witnessed the development and prosperity of biometric data discrimination technologies. Various unsupervised/supervised, linear/nonlinear, vector/tensor discrimination technologies have been investigated and successfully applied to biometric recognition. At the beginning, linear unsupervised method, principal component analysis (PCA), was used to extract the holistic feature vectors for facial image representation and recognition (Sirovich & Kirby, 1987; Kirby & Sirovich, 1990; Turk & Pentland, 1991a & 1991b). Since then, PCA has been widely investigated and has become one of the most successful approaches to face recognition (Pentland, Moghaddam, & Starner, 1994; Pentland, 2000; Zhao & Yang, 1999; Moghaddam, 2002; Zhang, 2002; Kim, H. C., Kim, D., Bang, & Lee, 2004) and palm print recognition (Lu, Plataniotis, & Venetsanopoulos, 2003b). Other popular unsupervised methods, such as independent component analysis (ICA) and non-negative matrix factorization (NMF), have been applied to biometric recognition (Bartlett et al., 2002; Yuen & Lai, 2002; Liu & Wechsler, 2003; Draper, Baek, Bartlett, & Beveridge, 2003; Petridis & Perantonis, 2004).

Since the unsupervised methods do not utilize the class label information in the training stage, it is generally believed that the supervised methods are more effective in dealing with recognition problems. Fisher linear discriminant analysis (LDA), which aims to find a set of the optimal discriminant projection vectors that map the original data into a low-dimensional feature space, is then gaining popularity in biometric recognition research. In 1986, Fisher linear discriminant analysis was first applied to image classification (Tian, Barbero, Gu, & Lee, 1986). Further, LDA was applied to face recognition, and subsequently was developed into one of the most famous face recognition approaches, Fisherfaces (Liu, K. Cheng, Yang, & Liu, X. 1992; Swets & Weng, 1996; Belhumeur, Hespanha, & Kriengman, 1997). In biometric recognition, the data dimensionality is much higher than the size of the training set, leading to the well-known small sample size (SSS) problem. Currently there are two popular strategies to solve the SSS problem, the transform-based and the algorithm-based (Yang & Yang, 2003; Jian, Yang, Hu, & Lou, 2001; Chen, Liao, Lin, Kao, & Yu, 2000; Yu & Yang, 2001; Lu et al., 2003a; Liu & Wechsler, 2000 & 2001; Zhao et al., 1998; Loog, Duin, & Haeb-Umbach, 2001; Duin & Loog, 2004; Ye, 2004; Howland & Park, 2004). The transform-based strategy first reduces the dimensions of the original image data and then uses LDA for feature extraction. Typical transform-based methods include PCA+LDA and uncorrected LDA. The algorithm-based strategy finds an algorithm for LDA that can circumvent the SSS problem. Some representative algorithm-based methods can avoid the SSS problem, but most algorithm-based methods are computationally expensive or lose parts of important discriminatory information.

Biometric recognition usually is highly complex and can not be regarded as a linear problem. In the last few years, a class of nonlinear discriminant analysis techniques named as kernel-based discriminant analysis has been widely investigated for biometric data discrimination. Kernel principal component analysis (KPCA) and kernel Fisher discriminant (KFD) are two of the most representative nonlinear methods and have received considerable interests in the fields of biometrics, pattern recognition, and machine learning. By far, a number of kernel-methods, such as KPCA, KFD, complete kernel Fisher discriminant (CKFD), and kernel direct discriminant analysis (KDDA), have been developed from biometric recognition (Schölkopf et al., 1998; Mika Rätsch, Schölkopf, Smola, Weston, & Müller,1999a & 1999b; Baudat & Anouar, 2000; Roth & Steinhage, 2000; Mika, Rätsch, & Müller, 2001a & 2001b; Mika et al., 2003; Yang, 2002; Lu et al., 2003b; Xu, Zhang, & Li, 2001; Billings & Lee, 2002; Gestel, Suykens, Lanckriet, Lambrechts, De Moor, & Vanderwalle, 2002; Cawley & Talbot, 2003; Lawrence & Schölkopf, 2001; Liu, 2004; Yang, Zhang, & Lu, 2004a & 2004b; Xu, Yang, J. Y, & Yang, J., 2004; Yang, Zhang, Yang, Zhong, & Frangi, 2005). Most recently, manifold learning methods, such as isometric feature mapping (ISOMAP), locally linear embedding (LLE), and Laplacian eigenmaps, have also shown great potential in biometric recognition (Tenenbaum, 2000; Roweis & Saul, 2000; Belkin & Niyogi, 2002).

As a generalization of vector-based methods, a number of tensor discrimination technologies have been proposed. The beginning of tensor discrimination technology can be traced back to 1993, where a 2D image matrix based algebraic feature extraction method is proposed for image recognition (Liu, Cheng, & Yang, 1993). As a new development of the 2D image matrix based straightforward projection technique, a two-dimensional PCA (2DPCA) and uncorrelated image projection analysis were suggested for face representation and recognition (Yang, Zhang, Frangi, & Yang, 2004c; Yang. J, Yang, J. Y., Frangi, A. F., & Zhang, 2003b). To reduce the computational cost of 2DPCA, researchers have developed several BDPCA and generalized low rank approximation of matrices (GLRAM) approaches (Zuo, Wang, & Zhang, 2005; Ye, 2004; Liang & Shi 2005; Liang, Zhang, & Shi, 2007). Motivated by multilinear generalization of singular vector decomposition, a number of alterative supervised and unsupervised tensor analysis methods have been proposed for image or image sequence feature extraction (Lathauwer, Moor, & Vndewalle, 2000; Vasilescu, & Terzopoulos 2003; Tao, Li, Hu, Maybank, & Wu, 2005; Yan, Xu, Yang, Zhang, Tang, & Zhang, 2007).

Over the last several years, we have been devoted to biometric data discrimination research both in theory and in practice. A series of novel and effective technologies has been developed in the context of supervised and unsupervised statistical learning concepts. The class of new methods includes:

- **Extensions of Fisher's Discriminant Criterion:** We present three classification-oriented extensions of Fisher's discriminant criterion: large margin linear projection (LMLP), minimum norm minimum squared-error, and maximum scatter difference (MSD). All these three criteria are designed to deal with the small sample size problem;
- **Orthogonal Discriminant Analysis:** We investigate two novel orthogonal discriminant analysis methods: orthogonalized Fisher discriminant (OFD) and Fisher discriminant with Schur decomposition (FDS). Theoretical analysis and experimental studies showed that OFD and FDS are all optimal solutions to multiple Fisher discriminant Criterion;
- **Parameterized Discriminant Analysis:** We introduce three parameterized linear discriminant analysis methods, parameterized direct linear discriminant analysis, weighted nullspace linear discriminant analysis, and weighted linear discriminant analysis in the range of within-class scatter matrix;
- **New facial feature extraction methods:** We present two novel facial feature extraction methods, multiple maximum scatter difference (MMSD) and dDiscriminant based on coefficients of variances (DCV);
- **Tensor PCA:** We introduce the algorithms and discuss the properties of a group of tensor PCA methods;
- **Tensor LDA:** We investigate the algorithms and discuss the properties of a group of tensor LDA methods.

Multi-biometric system is designed to overcome the limitations of any single biometric systems by fusing information from multiple biometric traits. The fusion can be implemented in either of three levels, feature level, matching score level, and decision level. In feature level fusion, a new feature vector is constructed using the concatenation rule (Ross & Govindarajan, 2005), the parallel rule (Yang et al., 2003a; Yang, J., & Yang, J. Y., 2002), or the competitive rule (Kong, Zhang, & Kamel, 2006). In matching score level fusion, a number of transformation-based (Jain, Nandakumar, & Ross, 2005; Zuo, Wang, Zhang, D., & Zhang, H., 2007), classifier-based (Brunelli & Falavigna, 1995; Jain, Prabhakar, & Chen, 1999b; Fierrez-Aguilar, Ortega-Garcia, Gonzalez-Rodriguez, & Bigun, 2005), and density-based (Ulery, Hicklin, Watson, Fellner, & Hallinan, 2006; Nandakumar, Chen, Jain, & Dass, 2006) score fusion methods have been used to combine scores of multiple scores. In decision level fusion, boolean conjunctions, weighted decision methods, classical inference, Bayesian inference, Dempster–Shafer method, and voting have been proposed to make the final recognition decision (Gokberk, Salah, & Akarun, 2003; Jing, Zhang, D., & Yang, 2003).

In the last part of this book, we summarize our recent research on multi-biometrics. Our investigation covers all the three categories of multi-biometric technologies. The class of new methods includes:

- **Feature level fusion:** We investigate two novel feature level fusion methods, a pixel level fusion method to combine face and palm print traits, and a feature level fusion method to combine phase and orientation information of palm print images;
- **Matching score level fusion:** We present an example to illustrate the effectiveness of matching score level fusion in face and palm print recognition;
- **Decision level fusion:** We introduce a group decision-making combination approach to combine decisions of multiple face recognition algorithms.

This book is organized into three main parts. Chapter I first describes the basic concepts necessary for a premier understanding of biometric data discrimination and multi-biometrics. Section I explores some advanced biometric data discrimination technologies for the small sample size problem (SSS). Chapter II provides a brief introduction of LDA and SSS. Chapter III describes our researches on the pattern classification aspect of LDA for SSS problems. Chapter IV-VI present our studies on the feature extraction aspect of LDA for SSS problems. Specially, Chapter IV focuses on orthogonal discriminant analysis methods. Chapter V discusses parameterized discriminant analysis methods. Chapter VI describes two novel facial feature extraction methods.

Section II focuses on tensor-based biometric data discrimination technologies. Chapter VII describes the background materials for developing tensor-based discrimination technologies. In Chapter VIII, we develop some variants of classical PCA and discuss the properties of tensor PCA as a generalization of PCA. Chapter IX proposes two novel tensor discrimination technologies, two-dimensional LDA and two dimensional locality preserving projection. Chapter X describes tensor independent component analysis and tensor non-negative factorization, and Chapter XI introduces some other tensor discrimination technologies, such as tensor canonical correlation analysis and tensor partial least squares.

Section III states several multi-biometric technologies. Chapter XII introduces the fundamental conception and categories of multi-biometric technologies. In Chapter XIII, we develop two novel feature level fusion methods, a pixel level fusion method and a phase and orientation information fusion method. Chapter XIV dedicates to matching score level fusion. Chapter XV introduces decision level fusion and proposes a group decision-making combination approach.

REFERENCES

Bartlett, M. S., Movellan, J. R., & Sejnowski, T. J. (2002). Face recognition by independent component analysis. *IEEE Transactions on Neural Networks, 13*(6), 1450-1464.

Baudat, G., & Anouar, F. (2000). Generalized discriminant analysis using a kernel approach. *Neural Computation, 12*(10), 2385-2404.

Belhumeur, P. N., Hespanha, J. P., & Kriengman, D. J. (1997). Eigenfaces vs. Fisherfaces: Recognition using class specific linear projection. *IEEE Transactions on Pattern Analysis and Machine Intelligence, 19*(7), 711-720.

Belkin, M., & Niyogi, P. (2002). Laplacian eigenmaps and spectral techniques for embedding and clustering. *Advances in Neural Information Processing Systems, 14*, 585-591.

Billings, S. A., & Lee, K. L. (2002). Nonlinear Fisher discriminant analysis using a minimum squared error cost function and the orthogonal least squares algorithm. *Neural Networks, 15*(2), 263-270.

Bolle, R. M., Connell, J. H., Pankanti, S., Ratha, N. K., & Senior, A. W. (2004). *Guide to biometrics*. New York: Springer-Verlag.

Brunelli, R., & Falavigna, D. (1995). Person identification using multiple cues. *IEEE Transactions on Pattern Analysis and Machine Intelligence, 12*(10), 955–966.

Cawley, G. C., & Talbot, N. L. C. (2003). Efficient leave-one-out cross-validation of kernel fisher discriminant classifiers. *Pattern Recognition, 36***(11), 2585-2592.**

Chen, L. F., Liao, H. Y., Lin, J. C., Kao, M. D., & Yu, G. J. (2000). A new LDA-based face recognition system which can solve the small sample size problem. *Pattern Recognition, 33*(10), 1713-1726.

Draper, B. A., Baek, K., Bartlett, M. S., & Beveridge, J. R. (2003). Recognizing faces with PCA and ICA. *Computer Vision and Image Understandin,, 91*(1/2), 115-137.

Duin, R. P. W., & Loog, M. (2004). Linear dimensionality reduction via a heteroscedastic extension of LDA: the Chernoff criterion. *IEEE Transactions on Pattern Analysis and Machine Intelligence, 26*(6), 732-739.

Fierrez-Aguilar, J., Ortega-Garcia, J., Gonzalez-Rodriguez, J., & Bigun, J. (2005). Discriminative multimodal biometric authentication based on quality measure. *Pattern Recognition, 38*(5), 777-779.

Gestel, T. V., Suykens, J. A. K., Lanckriet, G., Lambrechts, A., De Moor, B., & Vanderwalle, J. (2002). Bayesian framework for least squares support vector machine classifiers, gaussian processs and kernel fisher discriminant analysis. *Neural Computation, 15*(5), 1115-1148.

Gokberk, B., Salah, A. A., & Akarun, L. (2003). Rank-based decision fusion for 3D shape-based face recognition. *Lecture Notes in Computer Science, 3546*, 1019-1028.

Grother, P., & Tabassi, E. (2004). NIST Biometric Scores Set - Release 1 (BSSR1). Available at http://www.itl.nist.gov/iad/894.03/biometricscores.

Howland, P., & Park, H. (2004). Generalizing discriminant analysis using the generalized singular va Lu e decomposition. *IEEE Transactions on Pattern Analysis and Machine Intelligence, 26*(8), 995-1006.

Jain, A., Bolle, R., & Pankanti, S. (1999a). Biometrics: Personal Identification in Networked Society. *Boston Hardbound: Kluwer Academic.*

Jain, A. K., Prabhakar, S., & Chen, S. (1999b). Combining multiple matchers for a high security fingerprint verification system. *Pattern Recognition Letters, 20*, 1371-1379.

Jain, A. K., Ross, A., & Prabhakar, S. (2004). An introduction to biometric recognition. *IEEE Trans. Circuits and Systems for Video Technology, 14*(1), 4-20.

Jain, A. K., Nandakumar, K., & Ross, A. (2005). Score normalization in multimodel biometric systems. *Pattern Recognition, 38*(5), 2270-2285.

Jin, Z., Yang, J. Y., Hu, Z. S., & Lou, Z. (2001). Face Recognition based on uncorrelated discriminant transformation. *Pattern Recognition, 34*(7), 1405-1416.

Jing, X.Y., Zhang, D., & Yang, J. Y. (2003). Face recognition based on a group decision-making combination approach. *Pattern Recognition, 36*(7), 1675-1678.

Kim, H. C., Kim, D., Bang, S. Y., & Lee, S. Y. (2004). Face recognition using the second-order mixture-of-eigenfaces method. *Pattern Recognition, 37*(2), 337-349.

Kirby, M., & Sirovich, L. (1990). Application of the KL procedure for the characterization of human faces, *IEEE Transactions on Pattern Analysis Machine Intelligence, 12*(1), 103-108.

Kong, A., Zhang, D., & Kamel, M. (2006). Palmprint identification using feature-level fusion, *Pattern Recognition, 39*, 478-487.

Lathauwer, L., Moor, B., & Vndewalle, J. (2000). A multilinear singular value decomposition. *SIAM Journal on Matrix Analysis and Application, 21*(4), 1233-1278.

Lawrence, N. D., & Schölkopf, B. (2001). Estimating a kernel Fisher discriminant in the presence of label noise. *Proceedings of 18th International Conference on Machine Learning. San Francisco, CA,* 306-313.

Liang, Z., & Shi, P. (2005). An analytical method for generalized low rank approximation matrices. *Pattern Recognition, 38*(11), 2213-2216.

Liang, Z., Zhang, D., & Shi, P. (2007). The theoretical analysis of GRLDA and its applications. *Pattern Recognition, 40*(3), 1032-1041.

Liu, K., Cheng, Y. Q., Yang, J. Y., & Liu, X. (1992). An efficient algorithm for Foley-Sammon optimal set of discriminant vectors by algebraic method. *International Journal of Pattern Recognition and Artificial Intelligence, 6*(5), 817-829.

Liu, K., Cheng, Y. Q., & Yang, J. Y. (1993). Algebraic feature extraction for image recognition based on an optimal discriminant criterion. *Pattern Recognition, 26*(6), 903-911.

Liu, C., & Wechsler, H. (2000). Robust coding schemes for indexing and retrieval from large face databases. *IEEE Transactions on Image Processing, 9*(1), 132-137.

Liu, C., & Wechsler, H. (2001). A shape- and texture-based enhanced Fisher classifier for face recognition. *IEEE Transactions on Image Processing, 10*(4), 598-608.

Liu, C., & Wechsler, H. (2003). Independent component analysis of Gabor features for face recognition. *IEEE Transactions on Neural Networks, 14*(4), 919-928.

Liu, C. (2004). Gabor-based kernel PCA with fractional power polynomial models for face recognition. *IEEE Transactions on Pattern Analysis and Machine Intelligence, 26*(5), 572-581.

Loog, M., Duin, R. P. W., & Haeb-Umbach, R. (2001). Multiclass linear dimension reduction by weighted pairwise Fisher criteria. *IEEE Transactions on Pattern Analysis and Machine Intelligence, 23*(7), 762-766.

Lu, J. W., Plataniotis, K. N., & Venetsanopoulos, A. N. (2003a). Face recognition using LDA-based algorithms. *IEEE Transactions on Neural Networks, 14*(1), 195-200.

Lu, J., Plataniotis, K. N., & Venetsanopoulos, A. N. (2003b). Face recognition using kernel direct discriminant analysis algorithms. *IEEE Transactions on Neural Networks, 14*(1), 117-126.

Lu, G., Zhang, D., & Wang, K. (2003). Palmprint Recognition using Eigenpalms Features, *Pattern Recognition Letters, 24*(9-10), 1463-1467.

Miller, B. (1994). Vital signs of identity. *IEEE Spectrum, 31*(2), 22-30.

Mika, S., Rätsch, G., Weston, J., Schölkopf, B., & Müller, K. R. (1999a). Fisher discriminant analysis with kernels. *IEEE International Workshop on Neural Networks for Signal Processing, Madison, Wisconsin, August 23-25* (pp. 41-48).

Mika, S., Rätsch, G., Schölkopf, B., Smola, A., Weston, J., & Müller, K. R. (1999b). Invariant feature extraction and classification in kernel spaces. *Advances in Neural Information Processing Systems, 12*, 526-532.

Mika, S., Rätsch, G., & Müller, K. R. (2001a). A mathematical programming approach to the Kernel Fisher algorithm. *Advances in Neural Information Processing Systems, 13*, 591-597.

Mika, S., Smola, A. J., & Schölkopf, B. (2001b). An improved training algorithm for kernel fisher discriminants. *International Workshop on Artificial Intelligence and Statistics, San Francisco, CA, January 4-7*, 98-104.

Mika, S., Rätsch, G., Weston, J., Schölkopf, B., Smola, A., & Müller, K. R. (2003). Constructing descriptive and discriminative non-linear features: Rayleigh coefficients in kernel feature spaces. *IEEE Transactions on Pattern Analysis and Machine Intelligence, 25*(5), 623-628.

Moghaddam, B. (2002). Principal manifolds and probabilistic subspaces for visual recognition. *IEEE Transactions on Pattern Analysis Machine Intelligence, 24*(6), 780-788.

Nandakumar, K., Chen, Y., Jain, A. K., & Dass, S. (2006). Quality-based score level fusion in multibiometric systems. *Proceedings of International Conference on Pattern Recognition, Hong Kong, August 20-24* (pp. 473-476).

Pentland, A., Moghaddam, B., & Starner, T. (1994). View-based and mododular eigenspaces for face recognition. *IEEE Conference on Computer Vision and Pattern Recognition, Seattle, June 21-23* (pp. 84-91).

Pentland, A. (2000). Looking at people: sensing for ubiquitous and wearable computing. *IEEE Transactions on Pattern Analysis Machine Intelligence, 22*(1), 107-119.

Petridis, S., & Perantonis, S. T. (2004). On the relation between discriminant analysis and mutual information for supervised linear feature extraction. *Pattern Recognition, 37*(5), 857-874.

Poh, N., & Bengio, S. (2006). Database, protocol and tools for evaluating score-level fusion algorithms in biometric authentication. *Pattern Recognition, 39*(2), 223-233.

Ross, A., & Govindarajan, R. (2005). Feature level fusion using hand and face biometrics. *Proceedings of SPIE Conference on Biometric Technology for Human Identification, Orlando, USA, March 28* (pp. 196-204).

Roth, V., & Steinhage, V. (2000). Nonlinear discriminant analysis using kernel functions. *Advances in Neural Information Processing Systems, 12*, 568-574.

Roweis, S. T., & Saul, L. K. (2000). Nonlinear dimensionality reduction by locally linear embedding. *Science, 290*, 2323-2326.

Schölkopf, B., Smola, A., & Muller, K. R. (1998). Nonlinear component analysis as a kernel eigenvalue problem. *Neural Computation, 10*(5), 1299-1319.

Sirovich, L., & Kirby, M. (1987). Low-dimensional procedure for characterization of human faces. *Journal of Optical Society of America A, 4,* 519-524.

Swets, D. L., & Weng, J. (1996). Using discriminant eigenfeatures for image retrieval. *IEEE Transactions on Pattern Analysis and Machine Intelligence, 18*(8), 831-836.

Tao, D., Li, X., Hu, W., Maybank, S. J., & Wu, X. (2005). Supervised tensor learning. *IEEE International Conference on Data Mining*, Houston, Texas, November 27-30 (pp. 450-457).

Tenenbaum, J. B., de Silva, V., & Langford, J. C. (2000). A global geometric framework for nonlinear dimensionality reduction. *Science, 290*, 2319-2323.

Tian, Q., Barbero, M., Gu, Z. H., & Lee, S. H. (1986). Image classification by the Foley-Sammon transform. *Optical Engineering, 25*(7) 834-839.

Turk, M., & Pentland, A. (1991a). Eigenfaces for recognition. *Journal of Cognitive Neuroscience, 3*(1), 71-86.

Turk, M., & Pentland, A. (1991b). Face recognition using Eigenfaces. *IEEE Conference on Computer Vision and Pattern Recognition*, Maui, Hawaii, June 3-6 (pp. 586-591).

Ulery, B., Hicklin, A. R., Watson, C., Fellner, W., & Hallinan, P. (2006). Studies of biometric fusion. *NIST Technical Report IR7346*.

Vasilescu, M. A. O., & Terzopoulos, D. (2003). Multilinear subspace analysis of image ensembles. *IEEE Conference on Computer Vision and Pattern Recognition*, Madison, Wisconsin, June 16-22 (pp. 93-99).

Wayman, J. (2005). *Biometric systems: Technology, design and performance evaluation*. London: Springer.

Wu, X., Zhang, D., & Wang, K. (2003). Fisherpalms based Palmprint recognition. *Pattern Recognition Letters, 24*(15), 2829-2838.

Xu, J., Zhang, X., & Li, Y. (2001). Kernel MSE algorithm: a unified framework for KFD, LS-SVM, and KRR. *Proceedings of the International Joint Conference on Neural Networks*, Washington, D.C., July 15-19 (pp. 1486-1491).

Xu, Y., Yang, J. Y., & Yang, J. (2004). A reformative kernel Fisher discriminant analysis. *Pattern Recognition, 37*(6), 1299-1302.

Yan, S., Xu, D., Yang, Q., Zhang, L., Tang, X., & Zhang, H. J. (2007). Multilinear discriminant analysis for face recognition. *IEEE Transactions on Image Processing, 16*(1), 212-220.

Yang, M. H. (2002). Kernel Eigenfaces vs. kernel Fisherfaces: Face recognition using kernel methods. *Proceedings of the Fifth IEEE International Conference on Automatic Face and Gesture Recognition (RGR'02)*, Washington D. C., May 21 (pp. 215-220).

Yang, J., & Yang, J. Y. (2002). Generalized K-L transform based combined feature extraction. *Pattern Recognition, 35*(1), 295-297.

Yang, J., & Yang, J. Y. (2003). Why can LDA be performed in PCA transformed space? *Pattern Recognition, 36*(2), 563-566.

Yang, J., Yang, J. Y., Zhang, D., & Lu, J. F. (2003a). Feature fusion: parallel strategy vs. serial strategy. *Pattern Recognition, 36*(6), 1369-1381.

Yang, J., Yang, J. Y., Frangi, A. F., & Zhang, D. (2003b). Uncorrelated projection discriminant analysis and its application to face image feature extraction. *International Journal of Pattern Recognition and Artificial Intelligence, 17*(8), 1325-1347.

Yang, J., Jin, Z., Yang, J. Y., Zhang, D., & Frangi, A. F. (2004a). Essence of Kernel Fisher Discriminant: KPCA plus LDA. *Pattern Recognition, 37*(10), 2097-2100.

Yang, J., Frangi, A. F., & Yang, J. Y. (2004b). A new kernel Fisher discriminant algorithm with application to face recognition, *Neurocomputing, 56,* 415-421.

Yang, J., Zhang, D., Frangi, A. F., & Yang, J. Y. (2004c). Two-dimensional PCA: A new approach to face representation and recognition. *IEEE Transactions on Pattern Analysis and Machine Intelligence, 26*(1), 131-137.

Yang, J., Zhang, D., Yang, J. Y., Zhong, J., & Frangi, A. F. (2005). KPCA plus LDA: A complete kernel Fisher discriminant framework for feature extraction and recognition. *IEEE Transactions on Pattern Analysis and Machine Intelligence, 27*(2), 230-244.

Ye, J. (2004). Generalized low rank approximations of matrices. *The Twenty-First International Conference on Machine Learning,* Bonn, Germany, August 7-11.

Ye, J., Janardan, R., Park, C. H., & Park, H. (2004). An optimization criterion for generalized discriminant analysis on undersampled problems. *IEEE Transactions on Pattern Analysis and Machine Intelligence, 26*(8), 982-994.

Yu, H., & Yang, J. (2001). A direct LDA algorithm for high-dimensional data—with application to face recognition. *Pattern Recognition,* 34(10), 2067-2070.

Yuen, P. C., & Lai, J. H. (2002). Face representation using independent component analysis. *Pattern Recognition,* 35(6), 1247-1257.

Zhang, D. (2000). *Automated biometrics: tecnologies and systems.* Boston Hardbound: Kluwer Academic.

Zhang, D. (2002). *Biometrics solutions for authentication in an e-world.* Boston Hardbound: Kluwer Academic.

Zhang, D. (2004). *Palmprint authentication.* Boston Hardbound: Kluwer Academic Publishers.

Zhang, D., Peng, H., Zhou, J., & Pal, S. K. (2002). A novel face recognition system using hybrid neural and dual eigenfaces methods. *IEEE Transactions on System, Man, and Cybernetics, Part A, 32*(6), 787-793.

Zhang, D., Kong, W. K., You, J., & Wong, M. (2003). On-line palmprint identification. *IEEE Transactions on Pattern Analysis Machine Intelligence,* 25(9), 1041-1050.

Zhao, L., & Yang, Y. (1999). Theoretical analysis of illumination in PCA-based vision systems. *Pattern Recognition, 32*(4), 547-564.

Zhao, W., Krishnaswamy, A., Chellappa, R., Swets, D., & Weng, J. (1998). Discriminant analysis of principal components for face recognition. In H. Wechsler, P.J. Phillips, V. Bruce, F.F. Soulie , & T.S. Huang (Eds.), *Face Recognition: From Theory to Applications* 73-85, Berlin: *Springer-Verlag.*

Zhao, W., Chellappa, R., & Rosenfeld, A. (2003). Face recognition: a literature survey. *ACM Computing Survey, 36*(4), 399-458.

Zuo, W., Wang, K., & Zhang, D. (2005). Bi-directional PCA with assembled matrix distance metric. *International Conference on Image Processing* Genova, Italy, September 11-14 (pp. 958-961).

Zuo, W., Wang, K., Zhang, D., & Zhang, H. (2007). Combination of two novel LDA-based methods for face recognition. *Neurocomputing,* 70(4-6), 735-742.

Section I
Biometric Discriminant Analysis

Chapter II
Discriminant Analysis for Biometric Recognition

ABSTRACT

This chapter is a brief introduction to biometric discriminant analysis technologies — Section I of the book. Section 2.1 describes two kinds of linear discriminant analysis (LDA) approaches: classification-oriented LDA and feature extraction-oriented LDA. Section 2.2 discusses LDA for solving the small sample size (SSS) pattern recognition problems. Section 2.3 shows the organization of Section I.

2.1 LINEAR DISCRIMINANT ANALYSIS

Linear discriminant analysis (LDA) method has been widely studied in and successfully applied to biometric recognition such as face, fingerprint, and palm print identification or verification.

The essence of LDA is to construct a linear discriminant criterion which can be used to build a binary classifier or a feature extractor. To differentiate LDA for binary classification from LDA for feature extraction, hereafter we name the former as classification-oriented LDA, and the later feature extraction-oriented LDA.

2.1.1 Classification-Oriented Linear Discriminant Analysis

Linear discriminant analysis was initially developed for binary classification in the seminal work of LDA (Fisher, 1936). Among various discriminant criteria, one of the most famous is Fisher discriminant criterion (FDC) for binary linear discriminant analysis. FDC tries to seek an optimal projection direction such that the between-class variance is maximized while the within-class variance is minimized if samples from two distinct classes are projected along this projection direction. Besides FDC, there exist other linear discriminant criteria for binary classification. Among them, perceptron and minimum squared-error (MSE) (Duda, Hart, & Stork, 2001) criteria are two well-known examples.

The mathematical form of each linear discriminant criterion can be characterized as an optimization model which is used to calculate the weight and sometimes the bias of a binary classifier. Similarly, the mathematical form of linear support vector machine (LSVM) (Burges, 1998) is also an optimization model to calculate the weight and bias for a binary classifier. Thus, LSVM can be viewed as a kind of classification-oriented LDA method.

Classification-oriented LDA methods are in fact binary linear classifiers and can not directly be applied to multiple pattern classification tasks. They should be used in combination with one of the implementation strategies described in Section 3.1.3 if they are applied to these tasks.

2.1.2 Feature Extraction-Oriented Linear Discriminant Analysis

Based on Fisher's work, Wilks (1962) extended the concept of optimal projection direction to a set of discriminant vectors by extending Fisher discriminant criterion to multiple Fisher discriminant criterion. While the former is used to calculate the weight of the Fisher classifier, the latter is used to compute a set of Fisher discriminant vectors. By using these discriminant vectors as a transformation matrix, Wilks successfully reduced a complicated classification problem in a high-dimensional input space into a simple one in a low-dimensional feature space. The procedure which compresses the data from the input space into a feature space by utilizing a transformation matrix is called linear feature extraction. The feature extraction method using Fisher discriminant vectors is called Fisher linear discriminant (FLD).

In general, Fisher discriminant vectors are unnecessarily orthogonal to each other. Many researchers believed that the discriminant capability of FLD could be enhanced by removal of linear dependence among Fisher discriminant vectors. Based on this intuition, Foley-Sammon discriminant (FSD) — a feature extraction method which used a set of orthogonal discriminant vectors was subsequently developed (Sammon, 1970; Foley & Sammon, 1975; Duchene & Leclercq, 1988).

2.2 LDA FOR SOLVING THE SMALL SAMPLE SIZE PROBLEMS

2.2.1 The Small Sample Size Pattern Recognition Problems

Since FDC, MSE, FLD, and FSD all involve the computation of the inverse of one or several scatter matrices of sample data, it is a precondition that these matrices should be nonsingular. In the small sample size (SSS) pattern recognition problems such as appearance-based face recognition, the ratio of dimensionality of input space to the number of samples is so large that the matrices involved are all singular. As a result, standard LDA methods cannot directly be applied to these SSS problems. Due to the prospective applications to biometric identification and computer vision, LDA for solving the SSS problems becomes one of the hottest research topics in pattern recognition.

2.2.2 Studies on Classification-Oriented LDA for SSS Problems

In comparison with rich literature in feature extraction-oriented LDA for SSS problems, studies on pattern classification aspect of LDA for SSS problems are quite few. To the best of our knowledge, except for large margin linear projection (LMLP) (Song, Yang, & Liu, 2004a), minimum norm minimum squared-error (MNMSE) (Song, Yang & Liu, 2004b), and maximum scatter difference (MSD) (Song, Cheng, Yang & Liu, 2004; Song, Zhang, Chen & Wang, 2007) there is almost no endeavor in this direction.

2.2.3 Studies on Feature Extraction-Oriented LDA for SSS Problems

Linear discriminant feature extraction methods for solving the SSS problems generally fall into two categories. One is computation-oriented; the other is sub-space-based. Some researchers think that the trouble that standard LDA methods encounter in the SSS problems is only computational and can be avoided by using approximated calculation. Typical computation-oriented methods include the pseudo-inverse method (Tian, Barbero, Gu & Lee, 1986), the singular value disturbance method (Hong & Yang, 1991), and the regularization method (Zhao, Chellappa, & Phillip, 1999).

By treating the standard LDA method as an ill-posed optimization model with respect to SSS problems, many researchers focus their attentions on the modification of the optimization model corresponding to the LDA method, especially on the feasible region of the optimization model. Representative subspace-based methods include Fisherface (Belhumeur, Hespanha & Kriengman, 1997), nullspace LDA (N-LDA) (Chen, Liao, Ko, Lin & Yu, 2000), direct LDA (D-LDA) (Yu & Yang, 2001), and complete LDA (C-LDA) (Yang & Yang, 2003). Belhumeur Hespanha and Kriengman (1997) tried to seek discriminant vectors in a subspace of the range of the total scatter matrix. Chen, Liao, Ko, Lin and Yu (2000) tried to seek discriminant vectors in the null space of the within-class scatter matrix. Yu and Yang (2001) tried to seek discriminant vectors in the range of the between-class scatter matrix. Yang and Yang (2003) tried to seek discriminant vectors both in the range of the between-class scatter matrix and in the null space of the within-class scatter matrix.

2.3 ORGANIZATION OF SECTION I

The first section of the book presents some of our recent studies on LDA for solving the SSS problems and its applications for biometric recognitions. It consists of five chapters. Chapter II provides a brief introduction. Chapter III describes our researches on the pattern classification aspect of LDA for SSS problems. Chapter IV-VI present our studies on the feature extraction aspect of LDA for SSS problems. More specifically, Chapter IV focuses on orthogonal discriminant analysis methods. Chapter V discusses parameterized discriminant analysis methods, and Chapter VI describes two novel facial feature extraction methods, multiple maximum scatter difference and discriminant based on coefficients of variances.

REFERENCES

Belhumeur, P. N., Hespanha, J. P., & Kriengman, D. J. (1997). Eigenfaces vs. fisherfaces: recognition using class specific linear projection. *IEEE Trans. Pattern Anal. Machine Intell., 19*(7), 711-720.

Burges, C. J. C. (1998). A tutorial on support vector machines for pattern recognition. *Data Mining and Knowledge Discovery, 2*(2), 121–167.

Chen, L., Liao, H., Ko, M., Lin, J., & Yu, G. (2000). A new lda-based face recognition system which can solve the small sample size problem. *Pattern Recognition, 33*(10), 1713-1726.

Duchene, J., & Leclercq, S. (1988). An optimal transformation for discriminant and principal component analysis. *IEEE Trans. Pattern Anal. Machine Intell., 10*(6), 978-983.

Duda, R. O., Hart, P. E., & Stork, D. G. (2001). *Pattern Classification*. New York: John Wiley & Sons.

Fisher, R. (1936). The use of multiple measurements in taxonomic problems. *Annals of Eugenics*, 7(2), 178-188.

Foley, D. H., & Sammon, J. W. (1975). An optimal set of discriminant vectors. *IEEE Trans. Computer*, 24(3), 281-289.

Hong, Z. Q., & Yang, J. Y. (1991). Optimal discriminant plane for a small number of samples and design method of classifier on the plane. *Pattern Recognition*, 24(4), 317-324.

Sammon, J. W. (1970). An Optimal discriminant plane. *IEEE Trans. Computer*, C-19(9), 826-829.

Song, F. X., Cheng, K., Yang, J. Y., & Liu, S. H. (2004). Maximum scatter difference, large margin linear projection and support vector machines. *Acta Automatica Sinica (in Chinese)*, 30(6), 890-896.

Song, F. X., Yang, J. Y., & Liu, S. H. (2004a). Large margin linear projection and face recognition. *Pattern Recognition*, 37(9), 1953-1955.

Song, F. X., Yang, J. Y., & Liu, S. H. (2004b). Pattern recognition based on the minimum norm minimum squared-error classifier. *Proceedings of the Eighth International Conference on Control, Automation, Robotics and Vision (ICARCV 2004)*, (pp. 1114-1117).

Song, F. X., Zhang, D., Chen, Q. L., & Wang, J. Z. (2007). Face recognition based on a novel linear discriminant criterion. *Pattern Analysis & Applications*, 10(3), 165-174.

Tian, Q., Barbero, M., Gu, Z. H., & Lee, S. H. (1986). Image classification by the Foley-Sammon transform. *Optical Engineering*, 25(7), 834-840.

Wilks, S. S. (1962). *Mathematical Statistics*, New York: Wiley.

Yang, J., & Yang, J. Y. (2003). Why can lda be performed in pca transformed space? *Pattern Recognition*, 36(2), 563-566.

Yu, H., & Yang, J. (2001). A direct LDA algorithm for high-dimensional data—with application to face recognition. *Pattern Recognition*, 34(10), 2067-2070.

Zhao, W., Chellappa, R., & Phillip, P. J. (1999). *Subspace linear discriminant analysis for face recognition (CAR-TR-914)*. University of Maryland, Center for Automatic Research.

Chapter III
Discriminant Criteria for Pattern Classification

ABSTRACT

As mentioned in Chapter II, there are two kinds of LDA approaches: classification-oriented LDA and feature extraction-oriented LDA. In most chapters of this session of the book, we focus our attention on the feature extraction aspect of LDA for SSS problems. On the other hand,, with this chapter we present our studies on the pattern classification aspect of LDA for SSS problems. In this chapter, we present three novel classification-oriented linear discriminant criteria. The first one is large margin linear projection (LMLP) which makes full use of the characteristic of the SSS problems. The second one is the minimum norm minimum squared-error criterion which is a modification of the minimum squared-error discriminant criterion. The third one is the maximum scatter difference which is a modification of the Fisher discriminant criterion.

3.1 INTRODUCTION

3.1.1 Linear Discriminant Function and Linear Classifier

Let $\mathbf{x}_1,...,\mathbf{x}_N \in R^d$ be a set of training samples from two classes ω_1 and ω_2 with N_i samples from ω_i, and let $y_1,...,y_N \in \{1,-1\}$ be their corresponding class labels. Here $y_j = 1$ means that $\mathbf{x}_j$ belongs to ω_1 whereas $y_j = -1$ means that $\mathbf{x}_j$ belongs to ω_2. A linear discriminant function is a linear combination of the components of a feature vector $\mathbf{x} \in R^d$ which can be written as:

$$g(\mathbf{x}) = \mathbf{w}^T \mathbf{x} + w_0 \qquad (3.1)$$

where the vector $\mathbf{w} \in R^d$ and the scalar w_0 are called weight and bias respectively. The hyperplane $\mathbf{w}^T \mathbf{x} + w_0 = 0$ is a decision surface which is used to separate samples with positive class labels from samples with negative ones.

A linear discriminant criterion is an optimization model which is used to seek the weight for a linear discriminant function. The chief goal of classification-oriented LDA is to set up an appropriated linear discriminant criterion and to calculate the optimal projection direction, i.e. the weight. Here "optimal" means that after samples are projected onto the weight, the resultant projections of samples from two distinct classes ω_1 and ω_2 are fully separated.

Once the weight $\mathbf{w}^*$ has been derived from a certain linear discriminant criterion, the corresponding bias w_0 can be computed using:

$$w_0 = -\mathbf{w}^{*T} \mathbf{m} \qquad (3.2)$$

or

$$w_0 = -\mathbf{w}^{*T} \left(\frac{\mathbf{m}_1 + \mathbf{m}_2}{2} \right) \qquad (3.3)$$

where $\mathbf{m}$ and $\mathbf{m}_i$ are respectively the mean training sample and the mean of training samples from the class ω_i. They are defined as

$$\mathbf{m} = \frac{1}{N} \sum_{\mathbf{x} \in \omega_1 \cup \omega_2} \mathbf{x}, \qquad (3.4)$$

and

$$\mathbf{m}_i = \frac{1}{N_i} \sum_{\mathbf{x} \in \omega_i} \mathbf{x}. \qquad (3.5)$$

For simplicity, we calculate the bias using the Eq. (3.2) throughout this chapter.

Let $m_1 = \dfrac{1}{N_1} \sum_{\mathbf{x} \in \omega_1} \mathbf{w}^{*T} \mathbf{x} = \mathbf{w}^{*T} \mathbf{m}_1$

denote the mean of the projected training samples from the class ω_1. Thus, the binary linear classifier based on the weight $\mathbf{w}^*$ and the bias w_0 is defined as follow:

$$f(\mathbf{x}) = sign(\mathbf{w}^{*T}\mathbf{x} + w_0) \cdot sign(m_1 + w_0), \tag{3.6}$$

which assigns a class label $sign(\mathbf{w}^{*T}\mathbf{x} + w_0) \cdot sign(m_1 + w_0)$ to an unknown sample $\mathbf{x}$. Here, *sign* is the sign function. That is, once the weight in a linear discriminant function has been worked out the corresponding binary linear classifier is fixed.

3.1.2 Linear Support Vector Machine

Linear support vector machine (LSVM) (Burges, 1998) is one of the top performing classifiers in the field of pattern recognition. It has been successfully applied to text mining, machine learning, and computer vision. LSVM is one of the most important statistical learning methods which are based on the structural risk minimization principle (Vapnik, 1995). It is a binary classifier in nature and tries to seek an optimal hyperplane which maximizes the margin between samples from two distinct classes.

When training samples are linearly separable, the weight $\mathbf{w}$ and the bias b of the optimal decision superplane $\mathbf{w}^T\mathbf{x} - b = 0$ are calculated by the following model:

$$\min \frac{1}{2}\|\mathbf{w}\|^2$$
$$y_i(\mathbf{w}^T\mathbf{x}_i - b) \geq 1. \tag{3.7}$$

If training samples are linearly inseparable, the weight $\mathbf{w}$ and the bias b of the optimal separated superplane can be derived from the following model:

$$\min \frac{1}{2}\|\mathbf{w}\|^2 + C \cdot \sum_{i=1}^{N} \xi_i$$
$$y_i(\mathbf{w}^T\mathbf{x}_i - b) \geq 1 - \xi_i$$
$$\xi_i \geq 0, i = 1, ..., N \tag{3.8}$$

Here $\xi_i, i = 1, ..., N$ are slack variables and the parameter C controls the tradeoff between large margin and small training error. C has only positive values.

3.1.3 Using Binary Classifiers for Multiclass Classification

It is well known that binary classifiers cannot be directly applied to multiclass classification problems. To use binary classifiers for multiclass classification we have to divide a multiclass problem into a series of binary classification problems using one of the three implementation strategies: one-vs-rest, one-vs-one, and directed-acyclic-graph (Hsu & Lin, 2002).

In the one-vs-rest strategy, an l-class problem is divided into l binary problems. In the ith problem a binary classifier is trained with all samples from the ith class with positive class labels, and all other samples with negative class labels. Thus we obtain l linear discriminant functions $g_i(\mathbf{x}) = \mathbf{w}_i^T \mathbf{x} + w_0^i, i = 1,...,l$. An unknown sample $\mathbf{x}$ is assigned to the jth class if $g_j(\mathbf{x}) = \max_{1 \le i \le l} g_i(\mathbf{x})$.

In the one-vs-one strategy, an l-class problem is divided into $l(l-1)/2$ binary problems: $\mathbf{P}(1, 2), ..., \mathbf{P}(i, j), ..., \mathbf{P}(l-1, l)$. In the problem $\mathbf{P}(i, j)$, a binary classifier is trained with all samples from the ith class with positive class labels, and all samples from the jth class with negative class labels. This classifier assigns each unknown sample $\mathbf{x}$ to the ith class or the jth class according to the output value of the learned linear discriminant function. Thus, each unknown sample $\mathbf{x}$ holds a set of $l(l-1)/2$ class labels. The final class label of the sample $\mathbf{x}$ is j if j appears most frequently in the set of class label of $\mathbf{x}$.

The training phase of the directed-acyclic-graph strategy is the same as the one-vs-one strategy by training $l(l-1)/2$ binary classifiers. However, in the testing phase, it uses a rooted binary directed acyclic graph (see Figure 3.1) which has $l(l-1)/2$ internal nodes and l leaves. Each node is a binary classifier of the ith and

Figure 3.1. Rooted binary directed acyclic graph

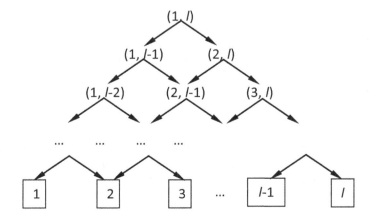

the jth classes. Given an unknown sample $\mathbf{x}$, starting at the root node, the binary linear discriminant function is evaluated. Then it moves to either left or right depending on the output value. Therefore, we go through a path before reaching a leaf node which indicates the predicted class. Since numerous studies have shown that the one-vs-one implementation strategy is most effective, this implementation strategy is used in this book.

3.2 LARGE MARGIN LINEAR PROJECTION CLASSIFIER

3.2.1 Fisher Discriminant Criterion

The Fisher discriminant criterion (FDC) (Duda, Hart, & Stork, 2001) tries to seek an optimal projection direction such that along that direction the within-class variance of projected training samples is minimized while the between-class variance of projected samples is maximized. The weight derived from FDC is called Fisher weight, and is denoted as $\mathbf{w}_F$.

Specifically, the FDC maximizes the generalized Rayleigh quotient (Duda, Hart and Stork, 2001):

$$J_f(\mathbf{w}) = \frac{\mathbf{w}^T S_b \mathbf{w}}{\mathbf{w}^T S_w \mathbf{w}}, \tag{3.9}$$

where S_b and S_w are respectively the between- and within-class scatter matrices for binary classification problems, which are defined as:

$$S_b = (\mathbf{m}_1 - \mathbf{m}_2)(\mathbf{m}_1 - \mathbf{m}_2)^T, \tag{3.10}$$

$$S_w = \sum_{i=1}^{2} \sum_{\mathbf{x} \in \omega_i} (\mathbf{x} - \mathbf{m}_i)(\mathbf{x} - \mathbf{m}_i)^T, \tag{3.11}$$

The Fisher weight can be computed in closed-form using the formula:

$$\mathbf{w}_F = S_w^{-1}(\mathbf{m}_1 - \mathbf{m}_2), \tag{3.12}$$

if the within-class scatter matrix S_w is nonsingular.

In the SSS problems such as appearance-based face recognition, the matrix S_w is always singular. Thus, how to deal with the singularity of the within-class scatter matrix is one of the important problems in the field of LDA (Belhumeur, Hespanha, & Kriengman, 1997).

3.2.2 Model and Algorithm

If the within-class scatter matrix S_w is singular, there is at least one nonzero vector $\mathbf{w}$ such that $\mathbf{w}^T S_w \mathbf{w} = 0$. In this case, $\max J_f(\mathbf{w})$ becomes an ill-posed optimization problem. It is natural to transform the optimization model of FDC into the following one:

$$\max_{\mathbf{w}^T S_w \mathbf{w}=0} \frac{\mathbf{w}^T S_b \mathbf{w}}{\mathbf{w}^T \mathbf{w}}. \tag{3.13}$$

The discriminant criterion corresponding to this optimization model is called large margin linear projection (LMLP) (Song, Yang, & Liu, 2004). The weight derived from LMLP is called LMLP weight, and is denoted as $\mathbf{w}_L$.

The LMLP weight $\mathbf{w}_L$ can be computed in two distinct ways. We first present the first approach.

Let $\mathbf{v}_1,...,\mathbf{v}_n$ be an orthonormal basis for the nullspace of the within-class scatter matrix S_w, $N(S_w)$. According to Theorem 3 in Liu, Cheng and Yang (1992), the constraint $\mathbf{w}^T S_w \mathbf{w} = 0$ is equivalent to $\mathbf{w} \in N(S_w)$. As a result, the optimization model (3.13) can be rewritten as

$$\max \frac{\mathbf{u}^T V^T S_b V \mathbf{u}}{\mathbf{u}^T \mathbf{u}}. \tag{3.14}$$

Here $V = [\mathbf{v}_1,...,\mathbf{v}_n]$. Using the Lagrangian multiplier method (Bian & Zhang, 2000), the LMLP weight can be calculated using the formula

$$\mathbf{w}_L = V\mathbf{u}_1. \tag{3.15}$$

Here $\mathbf{u}_1$ is the eigenvector of the matrix $V^T S_b V$ corresponding to the largest eigenvalue.

Since solving an orthonormal basis for the nullspace of a large scale matrix is extremely time-expensive, the LMLP weight is seldom calculated using the formula (3.15).

Now we discuss the second approach for computing the LMLP weight.

From the constraint $\mathbf{w}^T S_w \mathbf{w} = 0$ in the optimization model (3.13) and the definition of S_w in (3.11), it is easy to conclude that there are at most two distinct projected points m_1 and m_2, and each of which corresponds to one class of samples, after all the samples are projected onto $\mathbf{w}$. Since

$$\frac{\mathbf{w}^T S_b \mathbf{w}}{\mathbf{w}^T \mathbf{w}} = \frac{(m_1 - m_2)^2}{\|\mathbf{w}\|^2},$$

thus maximizing $\dfrac{\mathbf{w}^T S_b \mathbf{w}}{\mathbf{w}^T \mathbf{w}}$

is maximizing the margin or the distance between the projected samples from the two classes.

Let $Q_1 \in R^{N_1 \times d}$ and $Q_2 \in R^{N_2 \times d}$ denote sample matrices for classes ω_1 and ω_2 respectively. The model (3.13) can be reformulated as:

$$\max(m_1 - m_2)^2, \text{ subject to,} \begin{cases} Q_1 \mathbf{w} = m_1 \mathbf{1}_{N_1} \\ Q_2 \mathbf{w} = m_2 \mathbf{1}_{N_2} \\ \|\mathbf{w}\| = 1 \end{cases} \tag{3.16}$$

where $\mathbf{1}_n$ is a n-dimensional column vector whose elements are all constant 1.

Without losing generality, let $m_1 = -m_2 = m$, and substitute $\mathbf{w}$ with $\mathbf{w}/m$, then the optimal model described by (3.16) can be further converted to:

$$\min \frac{1}{2}\|\mathbf{w}\|^2, \text{ subject to } \begin{cases} Q_1 \mathbf{w} = \mathbf{1}_{N_1} \\ Q_2 \mathbf{w} = -\mathbf{1}_{N_2} \end{cases}. \tag{3.17}$$

Thus, we can rewrite the optimization model again as:

$$\min_{y_i \mathbf{w}^T \mathbf{x}_i = 1} \frac{1}{2}\|\mathbf{w}\|^2. \tag{3.18}$$

It is a quadratic programming problem which can be solved using various ready algorithms efficiently.

In fact, LMLP is a special type of LSVM which assumes that training samples are linearly separable. Thus LMLP inherits the excellent properties of LSVM.

The feasible region of the quadratic programming model (3.18) is nonempty if and only if training samples satisfy the following two conditions:

Consistent condition If $\mathbf{x}_i = \mathbf{x}_j$, then $y_i = y_j$;
Separable condition If Q denotes the feature by sample matrix, then $rank(Q) \leq d$.

The consistent condition is a precondition for any pattern recognition problem. If there do exist two samples which have the same feature vector but different class labels, they should be removed from the sample data. In SSS problems the separable condition is always true.

3.2.3 Experimental Evaluation

The performance of LMLP is tested on the ORL face image database. ORL database is provided by Olivetti research lab (ORL, http://www.cam-or.co.uk/Facedatabase. html). This set of data consists of 40 distinct persons, with each containing 10 different images with variation in pose, illumination, facial expression (open/closed eyes, smiling/not smiling) and facial details (glasses / no glasses). All the images are taken against a dark homogeneous background with the subjects in an upright, frontal position with a tolerance for some tilting and rotation of the face of up to 20 degrees. Moreover, there is also some variation in the scale of up to about 10 percent. All images were taken in grayscale with a 256-level and normalized to a resolution of 112×92 pixels. Five sample images of one individual from the ORL database are shown in Figure 3.2. In this experiment, the first five images of each individual are used for training and the remaining five for testing. Thus the total amount of the training samples and the testing samples are both 200. Table 3.1 shows the best recognition rates obtained by using the nearest neighbor classifier in combination with each of the three important facial feature extraction methods: Fisherface (Belhumeur, Hespanha, & Kriengman, 1997), Eigenfaces (Turk & Pentland, 1991), and uncorrelated linear discriminant analysis (U-LDA) (Jin, Yang, Hu, & Lou, 2001) as well as the recognition rate obtained by using LMLP classifier.

To further compare the performance of LMLP with that of LSVM, the best recognition rates, the worst recognition rates, the mean recognition rates, and the

Figure 3.2. Sample images from the ORL face image database

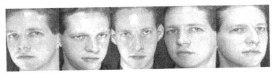

Table 3.1 Comparison of the best recognition rates (%) of the three classical LDA techniques with that of LMLP

Fisherface	Eigenface	Uncorrelated discriminant	LMLP
88.5	93.5	88.0	94.5

Table 3.2. Comparison of the performance of LMLP with that of LSVM

		resolution	112×92	56×46	28×23	14×12	7×6
Classifier	LSVM	max	99.0	99.0	99.0	99.0	99.0
		min	90.5	90.5	91.0	90.5	89.5
		mean	95.9	96.0	96.2	95.9	95.8
		std	1.64	1.58	1.55	1.57	1.82
	LMLP	max	99.5	99.0	99.5	99.0	99.0
		min	91.5	91.5	91.5	91.0	89.5
		mean	95.6	95.8	96.2	96.1	95.7
		std	1.54	1.47	1.41	1.41	1.68

standard deviation of the two binary linear classifiers based on 252 runs are shown in Table 3.2. The five different resolutions considered in the experiment are 112×92, 56×46, 28×23, 14×12 and 7×6 obtained as in Jin, Yang, Hu and Lou (2001). The results listed in Table 3.2 are derived from 252 $(= C_{10}^5)$ distinct runs for each resolution. In each of the tests the ith, jth, kth, lth, and mth images of each individual are used for training and the remaining five for testing $(1 \le i < j < k < l < m \le 10)$. The total time for training and testing consuming by LMLP and LSVM for various resolutions is shown in Table 3.3. From these experimental results we can conclude that LMLP is a promising binary classifier for face recognition.

3.3 MINIMUM NORM MINIMUM SQUARED-ERROR CLASSIFIER

3.3.1 Minimum Squared-Error Criterion

Let $\mathbf{x}_1,...,\mathbf{x}_N \in R^d$ be a set of d-dimensional training samples from two classes ω_1 and ω_2 with N_i samples from ω_i, and $y_1,...,y_N \in \{1,-1\}$ to be their class labels. Let $\mathbf{y}_i = [\mathbf{x}_i^T \ \ 1]^T \cdot y_i$ be the normalized augmented vector of $\mathbf{x}_i$, Y be the N-by-d matrix (

Table 3.3. The total time (sec) for training and classification consuming by LMLP and LSVM

	112×92	56×46	28×23	14×12	7×6
LMLP	85.9	25.5	10.1	7.0	6.0
LSVM	89.5	28.2	12.9	10.1	10.3

$\hat{d} = d + 1$) whose ith row is the transpose of the vector $\mathbf{y}_i$, and $\mathbf{b}$ be a vector composed of positive numbers $\mathbf{b} = (b_1, ..., b_N)^T$. The minimum squared-error (MSE) criterion tries to calculate the weight and the bias of a linear discriminant function by seeking a solution to a set of linear equations

$$Y\mathbf{a} = \mathbf{b}. \tag{3.19}$$

If Y is nonsingular, there is a unique solution $\mathbf{a} = Y^{-1}\mathbf{b}$. When Y is singular or rectangular, the inverse matrix of Y does not exist. As an alternative choice, MSE tries to seek a vector which minimizes the following discriminant criterion function

$$J_s(\mathbf{a}) = \|Y\mathbf{a} - \mathbf{b}\|^2 = \sum_{i=1}^{N}(\mathbf{a}^T\mathbf{y}_i - b_i)^2. \tag{3.20}$$

Once the optimal vector $\mathbf{a}$ has been worked out, the weight $\mathbf{w}$ and the bias w_0 are fixed by

$$[\mathbf{w}^T \ w_0]^T = \mathbf{a}. \tag{3.21}$$

If the $\hat{d}$-by-$\hat{d}$ matrix Y^TY is nonsingular, we can solve for $\mathbf{a}$ uniquely as

$$\mathbf{a} = (Y^TY)^{-1}Y^T\mathbf{b}. \tag{3.22}$$

But if the matrix Y^TY is singular, as is often the case in the SSS problems, there are infinitely many solutions $\mathbf{a}$ such that $J_s(\mathbf{a}) = 0$. In these cases conventional MSE solutions can not assure the optimal decision surface.

3.3.2 Minimum Norm Minimum Squared-Error Weight

In terms of matrix algebra, a vector $\mathbf{a}$ which minimizes the discriminant criterion function $J_s(\mathbf{a})$ is a MSE solution for the matrix equation (3.19). No matter whether the vector $\mathbf{a}$ is over-determined or underdetermined by Eq. (3.19), a MSE solution for it always exists.

While there might be infinite MSE solutions, the minimum norm minimum squared-error solution is unique

$$\mathbf{a} = Y^+\mathbf{b}, \tag{3.23}$$

where Y^+ is the Moore-Penrose inverse of the matrix Y.

Y^+ can be computed in two ways (Cheng, 1989):

1. $Y^+ = VS^{-1}U^T$, if the singular value decomposition of Y is USV^T;
2. $Y^+ = V(U^TYV)^{-1}U^T$, if the rank decomposition of Y is UV^T.

Let $\mathbf{1}_N$ be the column vector whose elements are all ones. The minimum norm minimum squared-error (MNMSE) weight is fixed by

$$[\mathbf{w}^T \quad w_0]^T = Y^+\mathbf{1}_N. \tag{3.24}$$

The physical explanation of the MNMSE weight is presented as following.

When there are fewer equality constraints than unknown variables and constraints are consistent in Eq. (3.19), a MSE solution degenerates into a solution of the underdetermined linear system.

Let $\mathbf{w}$ be the weight corresponding to a solution $\mathbf{a}$ for $Y\mathbf{a} = \mathbf{1}_N$. Thus, along the direction $\mathbf{w}$ all samples from the class ω_1 are projected to the point 1 and all samples from the class ω_2 are projected to the point -1, i.e.

$$\begin{cases} \mathbf{w}^T\mathbf{x}^+ = 1 \\ \mathbf{w}^T\mathbf{x}^- = -1, \end{cases} \tag{3.25}$$

where $\mathbf{x}^+$ and $\mathbf{x}^-$ stand for a sample from ω_1 and ω_2 respectively.

It is easy to understand that the margin between the two projected points is $2/\|\mathbf{w}\|$. Therefore while all MSE solutions separate the positive samples from the negative ones correctly, the MNMSE weight separates them with the largest margin.

3.3.3 Experimental Evaluation

To properly evaluate the performance of MNMSE a series of experiments are carried out in this subsection. The first experiment is conducted on the Yale face image database. The Yale face image database contains 165 images of 15 individuals (each person has 11 different images) under various facial expressions and lighting conditions. All images are grayscale and normalized to a resolution of 100×80 pixels. Sample images of one person from the Yale database are shown in Figure 3.3.

Besides LSVM and LMLP, four facial feature extractor: Eigenface, independent component analysis (ICA) (Bartlett, Movellan, & Sejnowski, 2002), two-dimensional principal component analysis (2DPCA) (Yang, Zhang, Frangi, & Yang, 2004), and kernel Eigenface (Yang, 2002) are also evaluated in the experiment. The leave-one-out evaluation strategy is adopted, that is, each sample is used as a testing sample while the others are used as training samples. Again, the nearest neighbor classifier is used in combination with feature extraction methods. Experimental results are

Figure 3.3. Sample images of one person from Yale face database

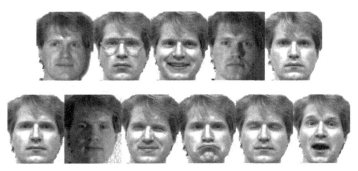

Table 3.4. Comparison of the recognition rates of MNMSE with those of other face recognition techniques using Yale database

Method	PCA	ICA	KPCA	2DPCA	LSVM	LMLP	MNMSE
Accuracy	71.52%*	71.52%*	72.73%*	84.24%†	90.91%	92.73%	92.73%

listed in Table 3.4. Here PCA stands for Eigenface and KPCA stands for Kernel Eigenface. The results with symbol "*" are from (Yang et al., 2004). The result with symbol "†" is from (Bartlett, Movellan, & Sejnowski, 2002). It is showed that MNMSE is superior to all of face recognition techniques except for LMLP in terms of recognition rate on this dataset.

The second experiment is performed on Concordia University CENPARMI handwritten numeral database. In this database, there are 600 samples for each of ten digits (from 0 to 9), in which the first 400 ones are used for training and the rest for testing. Sample images of the digit zero from the CENPARMI database are shown in Figure 3.4. In the experiment two kinds of original features: 256-dimensional Gabor transformation feature and 121-dimensional Legendre moment feature extracted by Hu, Lou, Yang, Liu and Sun, (1999) are used respectively. The best recognition rates using Foley-Sammon discriminant (FSD) (Foley and Sammon, 1975), uncorrelated linear discriminant analysis (U-LDA), and LSVM, as well as the accuracy using MNMSE are shown in Table 3.5. Note that the results with asterisk are from (Yang, 2002). The accuracy of MNMSE is superior to all of face recognition techniques except for LSVM.

The third experiment is performed on seven datasets available from the UCI machine learning repository (Murphy & Aha, 1992). The recognition rates and consumed time using LSVM and MNMSE are listed in Table 3.6. Statistical tests (*t*-test and rank-sum test) both show that there is no significant difference between

Figure 3.4 Sample images of the digit zero from the CENPARMI database

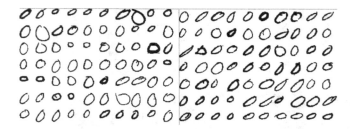

Table 3.5. Comparison of the accuracies of MNMSE with those of FSD, U-LDA, and LSVM using CENPARMI database

	FSD	U-LDA	LSVM	MNMSE
Gabor feature	54.3%*	84.7%*	86.9%	85.8%
Legendre feature	51.7%*	90.3%*	93.35%	92.1%

Table 3.6. Comparison of the recognition rates (%) and the consumed time (sec) of MNMSE with those of LSVM on seven machine learning datasets

Dataset		LSVM		MNMSE	
name	dimension	Rate	time	Rate	time
Heart	270×13	83.70	8940	83.70	1.42
Ionosphere	351×34	87.46	21.3	86.61	4.30
Iris	150×4	98.00	1.06	98.00	4.55
Liver disorder	345×6	70.14	772	62.90	1.52
Sonar	208×60	76.44	5.06	73.08	3.97
Tic Tac Toe	958×9	65.34	107	61.27	10.0
Wine	178×13	94.38	2300	97.19	1.08

the recognition rates of the two methods at a significance level of 0.05. But there does exit a significant difference between the times consuming by the two methods. Considering the fact that the MNMSE is realized by the plain Matlab language whereas the LSVM was realized by a special SVM tool (Ma, Zhao, & Ahalt, 2001) the difference is amazing.

3.4 MAXIMUM SCATTER DIFFERENCE CLASSIFIER

By viewing Fisher discriminant criterion as a special realization of a multi- objective programming problem, another realization of the same multi-objective programming problem leads to a novel classification-oriented linear discriminant criterion called maximum scatter difference (MSD) (Song, Cheng, Yang, & Liu, 2004; Song, Zhang, Chen, & Wang, 2007).

3.4.1 Model and Algorithm

Between-class scatter $\dfrac{\mathbf{w}^T S_b \mathbf{w}}{\mathbf{w}^T \mathbf{w}}$

and within-class scatter $\dfrac{\mathbf{w}^T S_w \mathbf{w}}{\mathbf{w}^T \mathbf{w}}$

are two useful measures of the separability of projected samples. The larger the score of between-class scatter is, the more separable the projected samples are; the smaller the score of within-class scatter is, the more separable the projected samples are.

Thus, the problem of finding the optimal projection direction can be formulated as a multi-objective programming problem:

$$\text{Maximize: } \frac{\mathbf{w}^T S_b \mathbf{w}}{\mathbf{w}^T \mathbf{w}}, \qquad\qquad (3.26)$$

$$\text{Minimize: } \frac{\mathbf{w}^T S_w \mathbf{w}}{\mathbf{w}^T \mathbf{w}}. \qquad\qquad (3.27)$$

There are mainly two ways to translate a multi-objective programming problem into a single-objective programming problem. The first is the goal programming approach in which one of the objectives is optimized while the remaining objectives are converted into constraints. The second is the combining objective approach in which all objectives are combined into one scalar objective (Eschenauer, Koski, & Osyczka, 1990).

Though the goal programming approach may also lead to a new linear discriminant criterion, we will concern ourselves with the combining objective one here. There exist two different principles to combine objectives. The first is multiplicative and the second is additive. By applying the multiplicative principle to the multi-objective programming problem one can obtain the Fisher discriminant criterion. If the additive principle is used the maximum scatter difference (MSD) discriminant criterion is followed.

Let $J_M(\mathbf{w})$ denote $\dfrac{\mathbf{w}^T(S_b - C \cdot S_w)\mathbf{w}}{\mathbf{w}^T\mathbf{w}}$.

The optimization model corresponding to MSD discriminant criterion is as follow:

$$\max J_M(\mathbf{w}), \tag{3.28}$$

where the parameter C is a nonnegative constant which balances the relative merits of the first objective (3.26) to the second objective (3.27). The physical meaning of the parameter will be discussed in detail in Subsection 3.4.3.

The Lagrangian function of the quadratic programming problem (3.28) is:

$$L(\mathbf{w},\lambda) = J_M(\mathbf{w}) - \lambda \cdot (\|\mathbf{w}\| - 1) = \mathbf{w}^T(S_b - C \cdot S_w)\mathbf{w} - \lambda(\mathbf{w}^T\mathbf{w} - 1). \tag{3.29}$$

Let $\dfrac{\partial L(\mathbf{w},\lambda)}{\partial \mathbf{w}} = 0$, then we have:

$$(S_b - C \cdot S_w)\mathbf{w} = \lambda \cdot \mathbf{w}. \tag{3.30}$$

By substituting Eq. (3.30) into $J_M(\mathbf{w})$ we obtain $J_M(\mathbf{w}) = \lambda$.

Thus, the optimal projection direction determined by MSD is the eigenvector of the matrix $(S_b - C \cdot S_w)$ corresponding to the largest eigenvalue. The optimal weight calculated by MSD discriminant criterion is called MSD weight and is denoted by $\mathbf{w}^*$. It is obvious that $\mathbf{w}^*$ is a function of the parameter C.

Unlike Fisher discriminant criterion which is inapplicable to the case where S_W is singular and LMLP discriminant criterion which is applicable only to these special cases, the optimal projection direction of MSD discriminant criterion always exists no matter whether the matrix S_W is singular or not.

3.4.2 Relations between MSD Classifier and Other Classifiers

Relations between the MSD weight $\mathbf{w}^*$ and weights calculated by certain well known classifiers are revealed in this subsection.

3.4.2.1 On Nonsingular Within-Class Scatter Matrix

Let $\mathbf{w}^*(c)$ be the optimal projection direction determined by MSD when the parameter C assumes the value c, and

$$F(c) = \frac{\mathbf{w}^*(c)^T (S_b - c \cdot S_w) \mathbf{w}^*(c)}{\mathbf{w}^*(c)^T \mathbf{w}^*(c)} = J_M(\mathbf{w}^*(c)) \qquad (3.31)$$

be the separability measure of projected samples along the direction $\mathbf{w}^*(c)$.

Since $F(c) = \max\limits_{\mathbf{w} \neq 0} \dfrac{\mathbf{w}^T (S_b - c \cdot S_w) \mathbf{w}}{\mathbf{w}^T \mathbf{w}}$,

$F(c)$ is equal to the largest eigenvalue of the matrix $(S_b - c \cdot S_w)$ according to the extremum property of generalized Rayleigh quotient.

Theorem 3.1 $F(c)$ is a monotone decreasing function. Especially, $F(c)$ will be a strictly monotone decreasing function if the within-class scatter matrix S_w is non-singular and the limit of $F(c)$ is negative infinity when c is approaching infinity.

Proof: Let $c_1 < c_2$, and $\mathbf{w}_i$ be the unit eigenvector of the matrix $(S_b - c \cdot S_w)$ corresponding to the largest eigenvalue, $i = 1, 2$. It is obvious that

$$F(c_1) = \mathbf{w}_1^T (S_b - c_1 \cdot S_w) \mathbf{w}_1 \geq \mathbf{w}_2^T (S_b - c_1 \cdot S_w) \mathbf{w}_2$$

$$= \mathbf{w}_2^T (S_b - c_2 \cdot S_w) \mathbf{w}_2 + (c_2 - c_1) \mathbf{w}_2^T S_w \mathbf{w}_2$$

$$= F(c_2) + (c_2 - c_1) \mathbf{w}_2^T S_w \mathbf{w}_2.$$

Since S_w is semi-positive definite, we have $\mathbf{w}_2^T S_w \mathbf{w}_2 \geq 0$. Thus, $F(c_1) \geq F(c_2)$, i.e., $F(c)$ is a monotone decreasing function.

Especially, when S_w is non-singular, S_w is positive definite. Thus, for any unit vector $\mathbf{w}$, we always have

$$\mathbf{w}^T S_w \mathbf{w} \geq \lambda_w > 0, \qquad (3.32)$$

where λ_w is the smallest eigenvalue of S_w.

In this case, $F(c_1) > F(c_2)$, i.e., $F(c)$ is a strictly monotone decreasing function.

Figure 3.5 The curve of the function F(c): (a) Sw is nonsingular; (b) Sw is singular

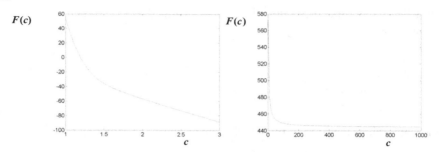

Let λ_b denote the largest eigenvalue of the matrix S_b. Then, for any unit vector **w**, the following inequality always holds

$$\mathbf{w}^T S_b \mathbf{w} \leq \lambda_b. \tag{3.33}$$

Combining Eq. (3.32) and Eq. (3.33), we have

$$F(c) = \mathbf{w}^*(c)^T S_b \mathbf{w}^*(c) - c \cdot \mathbf{w}^*(c)^T S_w \mathbf{w}^*(c) \leq \lambda_b - c \cdot \lambda_w.$$

It is obvious that $\lim_{c \to \infty} F(c) = -\infty$.
Thus we complete the proof of Theorem 3.1.
The curve of the function $F(c)$ is illustrated in Figure 3.5.

Lemma 3.1 $F(c)$ is a continuous real-value function of variable c (Cao, 1980).

Theorem 3.2 If S_w is nonsingular, there exists a unique positive root c_0 of the equation $F(c) = 0$ such that the unit eigenvector of the matrix $(S_b - c_0 \cdot S_w)$ corresponding to the largest eigenvalue is the Fisher weight.

Proof: It is obvious that $F(0) = \max_{\mathbf{w} \neq 0} \dfrac{\mathbf{w}^T S_b \mathbf{w}}{\mathbf{w}^T \mathbf{w}} = \lambda_b > 0$.

From the proof of Theorem 3.1, we know that $F(c^*) < 0$ when $c^* > \dfrac{\lambda_b}{\lambda_w}$.

Since $F(c)$ is a continuous function, there must exist a point c_0 in the interval $(0, c^*)$ such that $F(c_0) = 0$.

Considering that $F(c)$ is a strictly monotone function, we know that the point c_0 is unique.

From $F(c_0) = 0$, i.e., $(S_b - c_0 \cdot S_w)\mathbf{w}^*(c_0) = 0$, one can easily conclude that $S_b\mathbf{w}^*(c_0) = c_0 \cdot S_w\mathbf{w}^*(c_0)$.

Since the matrix S_b has only one positive eigenvalue, $\mathbf{w}^*(c_0)$ is just the Fisher weight $\mathbf{w}_F$.

Theorem 3.2 implies that Fisher classifier is a special MSD classifier when the within-class scatter matrix is nonsingular.

3.4.2.2 Asymptotic Property of MSD

Theorem 3.3. If S_W is singular, the weight $\mathbf{w}^*(C)$ determined by MSD is approaching the LMLP weight $\mathbf{w}_L$ when the parameter C is approaching infinity.

Proof: Let $\mathbf{w}_b$, $\mathbf{w}_c$ denote the unit eigenvectors of matrices S_b, $(S_b - C \cdot S_W)$ corresponding to the largest eigenvalues λ_b, λ_c respectively.

Since S_W is a singular matrix there exists a nonzero unit vector $\mathbf{w}_0$ such that $S_W \mathbf{w}_0 = 0$. Considering the fact that S_b is a semi-positive matrix we have:

$$\lambda_c = \max_{\|\mathbf{w}\|=1} \mathbf{w}^T(S_b - C \cdot S_w)\mathbf{w} \geq \mathbf{w}_0^T S_b \mathbf{w}_0 - C \cdot \mathbf{w}_0^T S_w \mathbf{w}_0 = \mathbf{w}_0^T S_b \mathbf{w}_0 \geq 0.$$

(3.34)

From the meanings of λ_c and $\mathbf{w}_c$ the following equation is always true for any positive real number C:

$$(S_b - C \cdot S_w)\mathbf{w}_c = \lambda_c \mathbf{w}_c.$$

(3.35)

Using equality (3.35), inequality (3.34) and the meaning of λ_b we obtain:

$$\mathbf{w}_c^T S_w \mathbf{w}_c = \frac{1}{C}(\mathbf{w}_c^T S_b \mathbf{w}_c - \lambda_c) \leq \frac{1}{C}\mathbf{w}_c^T S_b \mathbf{w}_c \leq \frac{1}{C}\lambda_b.$$

(3.36)

Noticing that the matrix S_W is also semi-positive we find:

$$\mathbf{w}_c^T S_w \mathbf{w}_c \geq 0.$$

(3.37)

By combining facts (3.36) and (3.37) we can simply conclude that

$$\lim_{C \to \infty} \mathbf{w}_c^T S_w \mathbf{w}_c = 0.$$

(3.38)

Thus we complete the proof of Theorem 3.3.

Theorem 3.3 implies that LMLP classifier is in fact an asymptotic form of the MSD classifier when the within-class scatter matrix is singular.

Theorem 3.4. If S_w is nonsingular, the weight $\mathbf{w}^*(C)$ determined by MSD is approaching the unit eigenvector of the within-class scatter matrix corresponding to the smallest eigenvalue when the parameter C is approaching positive infinity.

Proof: Let $\mathbf{w}_0$ denote the unit eigenvector of matrix S_w corresponding to the smallest eigenvalue λ_0, and $\mathbf{w}_c$ be the unit eigenvector of matrix $(S_b - C \cdot S_w)$ corresponding to the largest eigenvalue. Then, for any unit vector $\mathbf{w}$, we have:

$$\mathbf{w}_c^T (S_b - C \cdot S_w)\mathbf{w}_c \geq \mathbf{w}^T (S_b - C \cdot S_w)\mathbf{w}. \tag{3.39}$$

Let $\mathbf{v}_c = \mathbf{w}_0 \, \mathbf{w}_c$. Thus, the following inequality holds:

$$(\mathbf{v}_c + \mathbf{w}_0)^T (S_b - C \cdot S_w)(\mathbf{v}_c + \mathbf{w}_0) \geq \mathbf{w}_0^T (S_b - C \cdot S_w)\mathbf{w}_0. \tag{3.40}$$

It can be simplified as:

$$C \cdot (\mathbf{v}_c^T S_w \mathbf{v}_c + 2\mathbf{v}_c^T S_w \mathbf{w}_0) \leq \mathbf{w}_c^T S_b \mathbf{w}_c - \mathbf{w}_0^T S_b \mathbf{w}_0 \leq \mathbf{w}_c^T S_b \mathbf{w}_c + \mathbf{w}_0^T S_b \mathbf{w}_0 \leq 2\lambda_b. \tag{3.41}$$

Here λ_b is the largest eigenvalue of the matrix S_b.

Since $S_w \mathbf{w}_0 = \lambda_0 \mathbf{w}_0$, the inequality (3.41) can be rewritten as:

$$\mathbf{v}_c^T S_w \mathbf{v}_c + 2\lambda_0 \mathbf{v}_c^T \mathbf{w}_0 \leq 2\lambda_b / C. \tag{3.42}$$

Considering the fact $\mathbf{w}_c = \mathbf{v}_c + \mathbf{w}_0$ and $\mathbf{w}_c^T \mathbf{w}_c = \mathbf{w}_0^T \mathbf{w}_0 = 1$ we have:

$$\mathbf{v}_c^T \mathbf{v}_c = -2\mathbf{v}_c^T \mathbf{w}_0. \tag{3.43}$$

Thus, by substituting the equation (3.43) into the inequality (3.41) the following inequality holds for any positive number C:

$$\mathbf{v}_c^T S_w \mathbf{v}_c - \lambda_0 \mathbf{v}_c^T \mathbf{v}_c \leq 2\lambda_b / C. \tag{3.44}$$

Since λ_0 is the smallest eigenvalue of the matrix S_w, it means that:

$$\lim_{C \to \infty} \mathbf{v}_c^T S_w \mathbf{v}_c = \lambda_0 \mathbf{v}_c^T \mathbf{v}_c. \tag{3.45}$$

From the definition of $\mathbf{v}_c$ we know that $\lim\limits_{C\to\infty}\mathbf{v}_c = 0$, i.e.,

$$\lim_{C\to\infty}\mathbf{w}_c = \mathbf{w}_0. \tag{3.46}$$

Thus we complete the proof of Theorem 3.4.

The binary linear classifier based on the weight $\mathbf{w}_0$ is called the smallest within-class scatter classifier in this book.

3.4.2.3 Maximum Scatter Difference with C = 0

If the parameter C assumes zero value the MSD weight will degenerate into the eigenvector of the matrix S_b corresponding to the largest eigenvalue. By the definition of S_b in (3.10) we know that it has an unique positive eigenvalue $(\mathbf{m}_1 - \mathbf{m}_2)^T (\mathbf{m}_1 - \mathbf{m}_2)$. The corresponding unit eigenvector is

$$\mathbf{w}_b = \frac{\mathbf{m}_1 - \mathbf{m}_2}{\|\mathbf{m}_1 - \mathbf{m}_2\|}. \tag{3.47}$$

In this case MSD classifier assigns a unknown sample $\mathbf{x}$ with the same label as the nearest mean sample (or centroid) $\mathbf{m}_i, i = 1,2$. This is a binary minimum distance algorithm with Euclidean distance. We call this classifier as Centroid classifier.

Figure 3.6. A sample curve of r(c) when the within-class scatter matrix is nonsingular

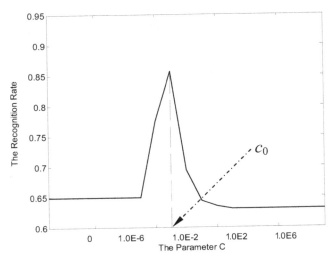

3.4.3 Discussion on the Parameter C

Now we discuss the physical meaning of the parameter C in some detail. Let $r(c)$ be the recognition rate obtained by MSD classifier for a certain recognition problem when the parameter C assumes value c.

If the within-class scatter matrix is nonsingular one sample curve of the function $r(c)$ is illustrated in Figure 3.6 (The plot is based on experiments performed on Australian dataset available from the UCI machine learning repository (Murphy & Aha, 1992).)

From Figure 3.6 we find that there is a pulse in the sample curve. When the parameter C is small enough the recognition rate obtained by MSD classifier is the same as the one of the Centroid classifier; when the parameter C is large enough the recognition rate obtained by MSD classifier is equal to the recognition rate of the smallest within-class scatter classifier. When the parameter C is approaching c_0 the recognition rate obtained by MSD classifier is approaching the maximum value— the recognition rate of Fisher classifier. It implies that the recognition rate obtained by MSD classifier is not robust on the parameter C when the within-class scatter matrix is nonsingular.

If the within-class scatter matrix is singular one sample curve of the function $r(c)$ is illustrated in Figure 3.7 (The plot is based on experiments performed on ORL face image dataset with the first five images of each person used for training and the rest images used for test.)

Figure 3.7. A sample curve of r(c) when the within-class scatter matrix is singular

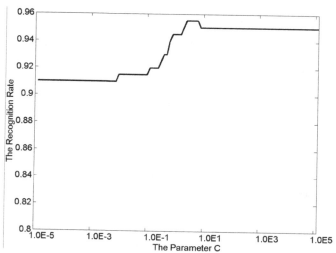

Figure 3.8. The parameter controls the tradeoff between the weights $\mathbf{w}_b$ *and* $\mathbf{w}_e$

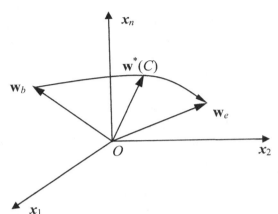

From Fig 3.7 we find that $r(c)$ is nearly a nondecreasing function. When the parameter C is small enough the recognition rate obtained by MSD classifier is the same as the one of the Centroid classifier; when the parameter C is large enough the recognition rate obtained by MSD classifier is equal to the recognition rate of LMLP classifier. It implies that the MSD classifier can be applied to small size problem such as face recognition without the need of parameter tuning.

Let $\mathbf{w}_b$ denote the unit eigenvector of matrix S_b corresponding to the largest eigenvalue, $\mathbf{w}_e$ be the unit eigenvector of matrix S_w corresponding to the smallest eigenvalue if S_w is nonsingular, or the LMLP weight $\mathbf{w}_L$ if S_w is singular. Thus, when the parameter C increases from zero to positive infinity MSD weight $\mathbf{w}^*(C)$ will swerve from $\mathbf{w}_b$ to $\mathbf{w}_e$ gradually as illustrated in Figure 3.8. Moreover, the end point of Fisher weight $\mathbf{w}_F$ is always in the arc if it exists, i.e., the within-class scatter matrix S_w is nonsingular. We can conclude that when S_w is nonsingular the parameter C should be close to c_0 (see Theorem 3.2) such that $\mathbf{w}^*(C)$ is close to Fisher weight $\mathbf{w}_F$. When S_w is singular the parameter C can be any large number.

3.4.4 Experimental Evaluation

The performance of MSD classifier is evaluated on ORL, Yale, a subset of FE-RET (Phillips, Moon, Rizvi, & Rauss, 2000; Yang, Yang, & Frangi, 2003), and a subset of AR (Yang, Zhang, Frangi, & Yang, 2004; Martinez & Benavente, 1998) face image databases. In comparison with MSD, experimental results of certain linear classifiers such as LSVM, LMLP, and Centroid are also included. In addition, experimental results of well known facial feature extraction methods such as Eigenface, Fisherface, orthogonal complementary space (OCS) (Liu, Cheng, & Yang, 1992), nullspace LDA (N-LDA) (Chen, Liao, Ko, Lin and Yu, 2000), and direct LDA (D-LDA) (Yu & Yang, 2001) in combination with the nearest neighbor classifier are also reported here.

The experiment conducted on the ORL dataset contains ten runs. In each of the ten runs, five images of each person are used for training and the remaining five for testing. The images of each person numbered 1 to 5, 2 to 6, ..., 10 to 4 are used as training samples for the first, second,..., and the tenth run respectively. The average recognition rates of various face recognition methods are reported. In the experiment performed on the Yale face image database, the leave-one-out evaluation strategy was adopted.

The subset of FERET face image database used in this experiment includes 1400 images of 200 individuals (each individual has seven images). This subset involves variations in facial expression, illumination, and pose. In the experiment, the facial portion of each original image was automatically cropped based on the location of eyes and the cropped image was resized to 80×80 pixels and preprocessed by histogram equalization. In each of the seven runs, four images of each person are used for training and the remaining three images for testing. The images of each

Figure 3.9 Sample images from FERET database

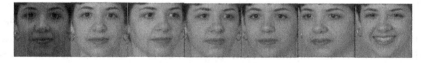

Figure 3.10. All images of one individual from the AR database

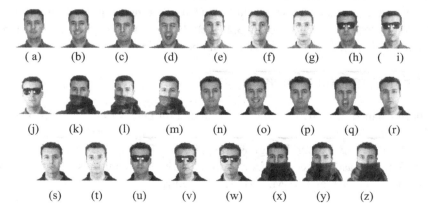

person numbered 1 to 4, 2 to 5, …, 7 to 3 are used as training samples for the first, second, …, and seventh run respectively. Sample images of one individual from the subset of FERET database are illustrated in Figure 3.9.

The AR face database contains over 4,000 color face images of 126 people (70 men and 56 women), including frontal views of faces with different facial expressions, lighting conditions and occlusions. The pictures of most persons were taken in two sessions (separated by two weeks). Each section contains 13 color images and 119 individuals (65 men and 54 women) participated in both sessions. The images of these 119 individuals were selected and used in the experiment. All color images have been transformed into gray images. Each original image was denoted by a 768×576 matrix and had 256 gray levels. Figure 3.10 shows all samples of one individual from the AR database, where (a)–(m) are from Session 1 and (n)–(z) are from Session 2. The details of the images are: (a) and (n), neutral expression; (b) and (o), smile; (c) and (p), anger; (d) and (q), scream; (e) and (r), left light on; (f) and (s), right light on; (g) and (t), all sides light on; (h) and (u), wearing sun glasses; (i) and (v), wearing sun glasses and left light on; (j) and (w), wearing sun glasses and right light on; (k) and (x), wearing scarf; (l) and (y) wearing scarf and left light on; and (m) and (z), wearing scarf and right light on.

Only the full facial images were considered here (no attempt was made to handle occluded face recognition in each session). All images are normalized with a resolution of 50×40 and pre-processed by histogram equalization. The normalized images of one person are shown in Figure 3.11, where Figs. 3.11a, 3.11b, 3.11c, 3.11d, 3.11e, 3.11e, 3.11f, and 3.11g are from Session 1, and Figs. 3.11n, 3.11o, 3.11p, 3.11q, 3.11r, 3.11s, and 3.11t are from Session 2.

Figure 3.11. Normalized images of one individual from the AR database

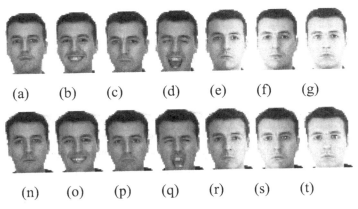

<table>
<tr><td>(a)</td><td>(b)</td><td>(c)</td><td>(d)</td><td>(e)</td><td>(f)</td><td>(g)</td></tr>
<tr><td>(n)</td><td>(o)</td><td>(p)</td><td>(q)</td><td>(r)</td><td>(s)</td><td>(t)</td></tr>
</table>

Table 3.7. Comparison of the accuracies of MSD classifier with those of other face recognition techniques

		Datasets			
		ORL	Yale	FERET	AR
Methods	Centroid	90.25%	91.52%	55.90%	63.33%
	LSVM	95.25%	90.91%	62.95%	66.19%
	LMLP	94.95%	94.55%	62.19%	65.95%
	MSD	95.15%	92.73%	62.98%	66.07%
	Eigenface	93.25%	81.82%	55.71%	65.12%
	Fisherface	91.00%	97.58%	27.55%	59.88%
	OCS	95.90%	98.18%	*	59.88%
	N-LDA	96.25%	98.18%	52.10%	60.12%
	Direct LDA	94.95%	98.79%	47.62%	63.45%

Figure 3.12. Sample recognition rate curves of MSD and LSVM classifiers

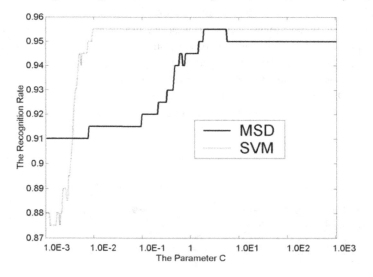

In the experiment, seven images of each person in the first session are used for training and the seven images in the second session for testing. The symbol "*" means that orthogonal complementary space method is not applicable to large face image databases such as FERET in our experiments. It is too time consuming. Since the dimensions of input space in all datasets are very high, in order to save computing time, input spaces are compressed by PCA transform before feature extraction or classifier training. The recognition rates of various face recognition methods on datasets ORL, Yale, FERET, and OR are reported in Table 3.7. From the experimental results we find that in comparison with state-of-the-art face recognition methods MSD is very promising.

To check the robustness of MSD classifier for SSS problems we compare the recognition rate curve of MSD with that of LSVM on the ORL face image dataset when the parameter C varies from 0.001 to 1000. Here, the training sample set consists of the first five images of each individual, and test sample set consists of the rest of the images. The experimental results are illustrated in Figure 3.12. As a result, we can conclude that MSD classifier is rather robust and can achieve very high recognition rate.

3.5 SUMMARY

With this chapter, we first provide a brief introduction to linear classification and then present three novel classification-oriented linear discriminant criteria. The first one is the large margin linear projection which makes full use of the characteristic of the SSS problems. Theoretical analysis demonstrates that LMLP is a special linear support vector machine. Therefore it inherits the advantages of LSVM. As LMLP is especially developed for the SSS problems, it is not applicable to other type of pattern recognition problems. The second one is the minimum norm minimum squared-error criterion which is a modification of the minimum squared-error discriminant criterion. MNMSE has a unique closed-form solution which avoids suboptimal points of traditional gradient descent approaches for MSE. The third one is the maximum scatter difference which is a modification of Fisher discriminant criterion. Neither like FDC which is only applicable to situations when the within-class scatter matrix is nonsingular, nor like LMLP which is only applicable to situations when the within-class scatter matrix is singular, MSD can be used in both cases. Theory analysis shows that MSD is an extension of Fisher discriminant criterion when the within-class scatter matrix is nonsingular, and its asymptotic form is LMLP when the parameter approaches infinity and the within-class scatter matrix is singular.

REFERENCES

Bartlett, M. S., Movellan, J. R., & Sejnowski, T. J. (2002). Face recognition by independent component analysis. *IEEE Trans. Neural Networks*, *13*(6), 1450-1464.

Belhumeur, P. N., Hespanha, J. P., & Kriengman, D. J. (1997). Eigenfaces vs. fisherfaces: recognition using class specific linear projection. *IEEE Trans. Pattern Anal. Machine Intell.*, *19*(7), 711-720.

Bian, Z. Q., & Zhang, X. G. (2000). *Pattern Recognition (in Chinese)*. Beijing: Qinghua University Press.

Burges, C. J. C. (1998). A tutorial on support vector machines for pattern recognition. *Data Mining and Knowledge Discovery*, *2*(2), 121-167.

Cao, Z. H. (1980). *Eigenvalue problems (in Chinese)*. Shanghai: Shanghai Science and Technology Press.

Chen, L., Liao, H., Ko, M., Lin, J., & Yu, G. (2000). A new lda-based face recognition system which can solve the small sample size problem. *Pattern Recognition*, *33*(10), 1713-1726.

Cheng, Y. P. (1989). *Matrix Theory (in Chinese)*. Xi'an: North-west Industry University Press.

Duda, R. O., Hart, P. E., & Stork, D. G. (2001). *Pattern Classification*. New York: John Wiley & Sons.

Eschenauer, H., Koski, J., & Osyczka, A. (1990). *Multicriteria Design Optimization*. Berlin: Springer-Verlag.

Foley, D. H., & Sammon, J. W. (1975). An optimal set of discriminant vectors. *IEEE Trans. Computer*, *24*(3), 281-289.

Hsu, C., & Lin, C. (2002). A comparison of methods for multiclass support vector machines. *IEEE Transaction on Neural Networks*, *13*(2), 415-425.

Hu, Z. S., Lou, Z., Yang, J.Y., Liu, K., & Sun, C. Y. (1999). Handwritten digit recognition based on multi-classifier combination. *Chinese J. Comput. (in Chinese)*, *22* (4), 369-374.

Jin, Z., Yang, J. Y., Hu, Z. S., & Lou, Z. (2001). Face recognition based on the uncorrelated discriminant transformation. *Pattern Recognition*, *34*(7), 1405-1416.

Liu, K., Cheng, Y. Q., & Yang, J. Y. (1992). An efficient algorithm for Foley-Sammon optimal set of discriminant vectors by algebraic method. *International Journal of Pattern Recognition and Artificial Intelligence*, *6*(5), 817-829.

Ma, J., Zhao, Y., & Ahalt., S. (2001). OSU SVM Classifier Matlab Toolbox (ver 3.00). From http: //www.eleceng.ohio-state.edu/~maj/osu_svm.

Martinez, A. M., & Benavente, R. (1998). The AR Face Database. *CVC Technical Report*, no. 24.

Murphy, P. M., & Aha, D. W. (1992). *UCI repository of machine learning databases.* http://www.ics.uci.edu/~mlearn/MLRepository.html.

Phillips, P. J., Moon, H., Rizvi, S. A., & Rauss, P. J. (2000). The FERET evaluation methodology for face recognition algorithms. *IEEE Trans. Pattern Analysis and Machine Intelligence, 20*(10), 1090-1104.

Song, F. X., Cheng, K., Yang, J. Y., & Liu, S. H. (2004). Maximum scatter difference, large margin linear projection and support vector machines. *Acta Automatica Sinica (in Chinese), 30*(6), 890-896.

Song, F. X., Yang, J. Y., & Liu, S. H. (2004). Large margin linear projection and face recognition. *Pattern Recognition, 37*(9), 1953-1955.

Song, F. X., Zhang, D., Chen, Q. L., & Wang, J. Z. (2007). Face recognition based on a novel linear discriminant criterion. *Pattern Analysis & Applications, 10*(3), 165-174.

Turk, M., & Pentland, A. (1991). Face recognition using eigenfaces. *Proc. IEEE Conf. Computer Vision and Pattern Recognition*, (pp. 586-591).

Vapnik, V. (1995). *The Nature of Statistical Learning Theory.* New York: Springer-Verlag.

Yang, J. (2002). *Linear projection analysis: theory, algorithms, and application in Feature Extraction (in Chinese).* Unpublished doctoral dissertation, Nanjing University of Science & Technology, Nanjing, China.

Yang, J., Yang, J. Y., & Frangi, A. F. (2003). Combined fisherfaces framework. *Image and Vision Computing, 21*(12), 1037-1044.

Yang, J., Zhang, D., Frangi, A. F., & Yang, J. Y. (2004). Two-dimensional pca: a new approach to appearance-based face representation and recognition. *IEEE Trans. Pattern Analysis and Machine Intelligence, 26*(1), 131-137.

Yang, M. H. (2002). Kernel Eigenfaces vs. kernel Fisherfaces: face recognition using kernel methods. *Proc. Fifth IEEE Int'l Conf. Automatic Face and Gesture Recognition*, (pp. 215-220).

Yu, H., & Yang, J. (2001). A direct lda algorithm for high-dimensional data—with application to face recognition. *Pattern Recognition, 34*(10), 2067-2070.

Chapter IV
Orthogonal Discriminant Analysis Methods

ABSTRACT

In this chapter, we first give a brief introduction to Fisher linear discriminant, Foley-Sammon discriminant, orthogonal component discriminant, and application strategies for solving the SSS problems. We then present two novel orthogonal discriminant analysis methods, orthogonalized Fisher discriminant and Fisher discriminant with Schur decomposition. At last, we compare the performance of several main orthogonal discriminant analysis methods under various SSS strategies.

4.1 INTRODUCTION

4.1.1 Fisher Linear Discriminant

Fisher linear discriminant (FLD) (Duda, Hart, & Stork, 2001) operates by learning a discriminant matrix which maps a d-dimensional input space into an r-dimensional feature space by maximizing the multiple Fisher discriminant criterion.

Specifically, a Fisher discriminant matrix is an optimal solution of the following optimization model:

$$\max_{W \in R^{d \times r}} J_F(W) = \frac{\left| W^T S_B W \right|}{\left| W^T S_W W \right|}. \tag{4.1}$$

Here $W \in R^{d \times r}$ is an arbitrary matrix, and S_B and S_W are the between- and within-class scatter matrices, and $|A|$ is the determinant of a square matrix A.

The between-class scatter matrix S_B and the within-class scatter matrix S_W are defined as follows,

$$S_B = \sum_{i=1}^{l} N_i (\mathbf{m}_i - \mathbf{m})(\mathbf{m}_i - \mathbf{m})^T, \tag{4.2}$$

and $$S_W = \sum_{i=1}^{l} S_i = \sum_{i=1}^{l} \sum_{\mathbf{x} \in \omega_i} (\mathbf{x} - \mathbf{m}_i)(\mathbf{x} - \mathbf{m}_i)^T. \tag{4.3}$$

Here N_i and $\mathbf{m}_i$ are respectively the number and the mean of samples from the ith class ω_i, $\mathbf{m}$ the mean of samples from all classes, and l the number of classes.

It has been proved that if S_W is nonsingular, the matrix composed of unit eigenvectors of the matrix $S_W^{-1} S_B$ corresponding to the first r largest eigenvalues is an optimal solution of the optimization model defined in Eq. (4.1) (Wilks, 1962). The matrix $S_W^{-1} S_B$ is the Fisher discriminant matrix commonly used in Fisher linear discriminant.

Since the matrix $S_W^{-1} S_B$ is usually asymmetric, Fisher discriminant vectors, i.e. column vectors of the Fisher discriminant matrix are unnecessary orthogonal to each other.

4.1.2 Foley-Sammon Discriminant

Many researchers think that it is helpful to eliminate linear dependencies among discriminant vectors by making them orthogonal to each other. Foley-Sammon discriminant (FSD) is a feature extraction method that does this using the optimal discriminant vectors. Optimal discriminant vectors are derived from the multiple Fisher discriminant criterion which is subject to orthogonality constraints initially for binary classification tasks (Sammon, 1970; Foley & Sammon, 1975). In detail, the first discriminant vector of FSD is the first Fisher discriminant vector, i.e. a unit eigenvector of the matrix $S_W^{-1} S_B$ corresponding to the largest eigenvalue. After the first k $(1 \le k < r)$ discriminant vectors $\mathbf{w}_1, ..., \mathbf{w}_k$ have been calculated, the $(k+1)$th discriminant vector $\mathbf{w}_{k+1}$ of FSD is then one of the optimal solutions to the following optimization model

$$\max_{\mathbf{w}_i^T \mathbf{w} = 0, \, i=1,...,k} J_0(\mathbf{w}) = \frac{\mathbf{w}^T S_B \mathbf{w}}{\mathbf{w}^T S_W \mathbf{w}}. \tag{4.4}$$

Here, $J_0(\mathbf{w})$ is a special form of the multiple Fisher discriminant criterion function, $J_F(W)$ in the model (4.1) in the case of $r = 1$.

Duchene and Leclercq (1998) extended FSD to multiclass classification problems and presented an algorithm for calculating FSD discriminant vectors. Subsequently, Jin, Yang, Hu, and Lou (2001) further simplified the calculation procedure. They showed that a unit eigenvector of the matrix $S_W^{-1} P S_B$ corresponding to the largest eigenvalue could be the $(k+1)$th discriminant vector of FSD. The matrix P is calculated by the formula

$$P = I - D^T (D S_W^{-1} D^T)^{-1} D S_W^{-1}. \tag{4.5}$$

Here I is an identity matrix, and $D = [\mathbf{w}_1, ..., \mathbf{w}_k]^T$.

4.1.3 Orthogonal Component Discriminant

Previously studies demonstrated that FSD was quite effective in pattern recognition. Unfortunately, the calculation procedure for FSD discriminant vectors is too complex and time- consuming. To overcome the drawbacks of FSD, many orthogonal discriminant analysis methods have been proposed in succession. Orthogonal component discriminant (OCD) (Sun and Wu, 2003) is one example of them.

Sun and Wu (2003) proposed OCD based on intuition. They used the following discriminant criterion instead of the multiple Fisher discriminant criterion,

$$\max_{W \in R^{d \times r}} J_S(W) = \frac{|W^T S_B S_W^{-1} W|}{|W^T S_W W|}. \tag{4.6}$$

It can be proved that the matrix composed of unit eigenvectors of the matrix $S_W^{-1} S_B S_W^{-1}$ corresponding to the first r largest eigenvalues is an optimal solution of the optimization model (4.6). The column vectors of this eigenvector matrix are discriminant vectors of OCD. Since the matrix $S_W^{-1} S_B S_W^{-1}$ is symmetrical, there is a set of orthogonal eigenvectors of the matrix. These orthogonal eigenvectors are the discriminant vectors of OCD.

4.1.4 Application Strategies for Small Sample Size Problems

A SSS problem arises when the dimensionality of an input space is larger than the number of training samples. In such cases, since the within-class scatter matrix S_W is singular, it is not possible to properly calculate the discriminant vectors for FLD,

FSD, OCD, or other standard LDA methods. As a result, these discriminant feature extraction methods cannot be applied directly to SSS problems.

In order to make standard discriminant feature extraction methods applicable to SSS problems with either no or only minor modification, it is necessary to adopt one of application strategies for SSS problems. For convenience, we call these application strategies for SSS problems as SSS strategies. A SSS strategy is a procedure in which a high-dimensional input space is compressed into a low-dimensional intermediate space such that in which standard or extended feature extraction methods are applicable. In the following we present three such SSS strategies.

4.1.4.1 Strategy One

SSS Strategy One is primarily used in combination with FLD in the famous facial feature extraction method—Fisherface (Belhumeur, Hespanha, & Kriengman, 1997; Swets & Weng, 1996). This strategy first uses principal component analysis (PCA) transformation to compress a high-dimensional input space into the range of the total scatter matrix (the sum of the between-class scatter matrix and the within-class scatter matrix) of training samples. It then selects the largest n ($n \leq N - l$) principal components of the samples. Here, N is the number of training samples, and l is the number of classes. Finally, standard feature extraction methods such as FLD, FSD, and OCD are performed on this n-dimensional subspace. Actually, Fisherface is SSS Strategy One + FLD.

Strategy One has widely been criticized for two drawbacks. First, it might lose some useful discriminant information by abandoning some minor components in the PCA stage. Second, theoretically it can not guarantee the non-singularity of the within-class scatter matrix. A similar SSS strategy has been proposed by Liu and Wechsler (2000). It is also believed to only partially solve the SSS problem and fails to obviate the risk of losing useful discriminant information.

4.1.4.2 Strategy Two

Strategy Two first compresses a high-dimensional input space into the range of the total scatter matrix of training samples by PCA transformation. Then, extended versions of standard feature extraction methods are applied on this reduced space.

Extended Fisher linear discriminant (EFLD) is proposed as a substitute for FLD (Fukunaga, 1990). The key idea is to replace the within-class scatter matrix S_w in FLD with the total scatter matrix S_T. Liu, Cheng, Yang and Liu (1992) had showed that EFLD was equivalent to FLD if the matrix S_w was nonsingular. The idea of EFLD has been extensively investigated in pattern recognition literature

(Fukunaga, 1990; Liu, Cheng, Yang, & Liu, 1992; Guo, Li, Yang, Shu, & Wu, 2003; Jing, Zhang, & Tang, 2004).

The extended multiple Fisher discriminant criterion is defined as,

$$\max_{W \in R^{d \times r}} J_E(W) = \frac{\left| W^T S_B W \right|}{\left| W^T S_T W \right|}. \tag{4.7}$$

Here $S_T = S_B + S_W$ is the total scatter matrix. The first r discriminant vectors of EFLD are unit eigenvectors of the matrix $S_T^{-1} S_B$ corresponding to the first r largest eigenvalues. Similarly, we can extend FSD and OCD to extended FSD (EFSD) and extended OCD (EOCD), by replacing S_W with S_T in calculation procedures for FSD and OCD discriminant vectors.

Discriminant vectors of EFSD should meet the following requirements. The first discriminant vector of EFSD is a unit eigenvector corresponding to the largest eigenvalue of the matrix $S_T^{-1} S_B$. After the first k ($1 \le k < r$) discriminant vectors, $\mathbf{w}_1, ..., \mathbf{w}_k$ have been calculated, the $(k+1)$th discriminant vector $\mathbf{w}_{k+1}$ of EFSD is a unit eigenvector of the matrix $S_T^{-1} P S_B$ corresponding to the largest eigenvalue. The matrix P is calculated by the formula

$$P = I - D^T (D S_T^{-1} D^T)^{-1} D S_T^{-1}. \tag{4.8}$$

Here I is again an identity matrix, and $D = [\mathbf{w}_1, \mathbf{w}_2, ..., \mathbf{w}_k]^T$. The first r discriminant vectors of EOCD are unit eigenvectors of $S_T^{-1} S_B S_T^{-1}$ corresponding to the first r largest eigenvalues.

Although EFLD, EFSD, and EOCD cannot be directly applied to SSS problems, they can safely be performed in the range of S_T. That is, SSS problems can be completely solved in theory if these extended feature extraction methods are used in combination with a PCA transformation. It follows the SSS Strategy Two.

4.1.4.3 Strategy Three

Whereas the first two SSS strategies both involve a Karhunen-Loeve expansion based on the total scatter matrix, Strategy Three uses another kind of Karhunen-Loeve expansion. SSS Strategy Three first compresses a high-dimensional input space into the range of the within-class scatter matrix of training samples by a Karhunen-Loeve expansion based on the within-class scatter matrix. Then, the standard feature extraction methods such as FLD, FSD, and OCD are safely performed on this reduced space.

The procedure for calculating discriminant vectors of FLD, FSD, and OCD under Strategy Three is as follows.

Step 1. Perform eigenanalysis on the matrix S_W through singular value decomposition theorem (Golub & Loan, 1996). Let $P = [\mathbf{p}_1, \mathbf{p}_2, ..., \mathbf{p}_n]$ be the matrix composed of unit eigenvectors of S_W corresponding to nonzero eigenvalues. Here $n = rank(S_W)$ is the rank of S_W.

Step 2. Compress the input space into the range of S_W by projecting an input vector $\mathbf{x}$ to $P^T\mathbf{x}$.

Step 3. Calculate the between- and within-class scatter matrices of projected samples by using formulae $\tilde{S}_B = P^T S_B P$ and $\tilde{S}_W = P^T S_W P$.

Step 4. Calculate the discriminant matrix V based on $\tilde{S}_B$ and $\tilde{S}_W$ using FLD, FSD, or OCD.

Step 5. Let $W = PV$. The column vectors of W are discriminant vectors what we seek.

4.2 ORTHOGONALIZED FISHER DISCRIMINANT

Although orthogonal component discriminant successfully decreases the computational complexity of Foley-Sammon discriminant, the theoretical background of OCD is poor. There is no convincing explanation for its high accuracy. In this section, a more convincing orthogonal discriminant feature extraction method — orthogonalized Fisher discriminant (OFD) is presented.

4.2.1 Model and Algorithm

Suppose $\mathbf{w}_1, ..., \mathbf{w}_r$ are r Fisher discriminant vectors and $\mathbf{v}_1$ is $\mathbf{w}_1$. Assume k vectors $\mathbf{v}_1, ..., \mathbf{v}_k$ $(1 \leq k \leq r-1)$ have been obtained. The $(k+1)$th OFD vectors $\mathbf{v}_{k+1}$ is calculated as follows:

$$\mathbf{v}_{k+1} = \mathbf{w}_{k+1} - \sum_{i=1}^{k} \frac{\mathbf{v}_i^T \mathbf{w}_{k+1}}{\mathbf{v}_i^T \mathbf{v}_i} \mathbf{v}_i. \tag{4.9}$$

It is easy to verify that discriminant vectors $\mathbf{v}_1, ..., \mathbf{v}_k, \mathbf{v}_{k+1}$ are orthogonal to each other.

We can rewrite Eq. (4.9) as $\mathbf{v}_k = \mathbf{w}_k + \sum_{i=1}^{k-1} \alpha_{ik} \mathbf{w}_i$, here $\alpha_{ik}, i = 1,...,k-1, k = 2,...,r$ are real numbers. Let $V = [\mathbf{v}_1,...,\mathbf{v}_r]$, then we have $V = W\Lambda$, where Λ is an upper triangular matrix with main diagonal elements being all one. Thus,

$$J_F(V) = J_F(W\Lambda) = \frac{\left| \Lambda^T (W^T S_B W)\Lambda \right|}{\left| \Lambda^T (W^T S_W W)\Lambda \right|} = \frac{\left| \Lambda^T \right| \left| W^T S_B W \right| \left| \Lambda^T \right|}{\left| \Lambda^T \right| \left| W^T S_W W \right| \left| \Lambda^T \right|} = \frac{\left| W^T S_B W \right|}{\left| W^T S_W W \right|} = J_F(W)$$

$$(4.10)$$

It means that the matrix which consists of OFD discriminant vectors is also an optimal solution to the optimization model (4.1).

4.2.2 Experimental Evaluation

To evaluate the performance of OFD eight datasets are used in this subsection. The first is a subset of the FERET face database (please refer to Section 3.4.4). The used subset contains 700 images from 100 individuals (each person has 7 different images). Each image was preprocessed using the same approach shown in Section 3.4.4. For each person three images are randomly selected as training samples and the remaining four are used for testing. Thus the total amount of training and testing samples are 300 and 400 respectively. The accuracy is estimated by using a ten-run average.

The second dataset is the CENPARMI handwritten numeral database (please refer to Section 3.3.3). This experiment uses the same training set and the same testing test as the second experiment in Section 3.3.3. The 256-dimensional Gabor transformation feature and the 121-dimensional Legendre moment feature are also used in the experiment. The third dataset is the NUST603 handwritten Chinese character database built in Nanjing University of Science and Technology. The database contains 19 groups of Chinese characters, which are collected from bank checks. There are 400 samples for each character (7600 in total), in which the first 200 ones are used for training and the others for testing. Sample images from the NUST603 handwritten Chinese character database are showed in Figure 4.1. Two kinds of features: 128-dimensionl cross feature and 128-dimensional peripheral feature are used in the experiment. The other five datasets are from the UCI Machine Learning Repository (Murphy & Aha, 1992). Accuracies are estimated by using the leave-one-out strategy.

Figure 4.1. Sample images from the NUST603 handwritten Chinese character database

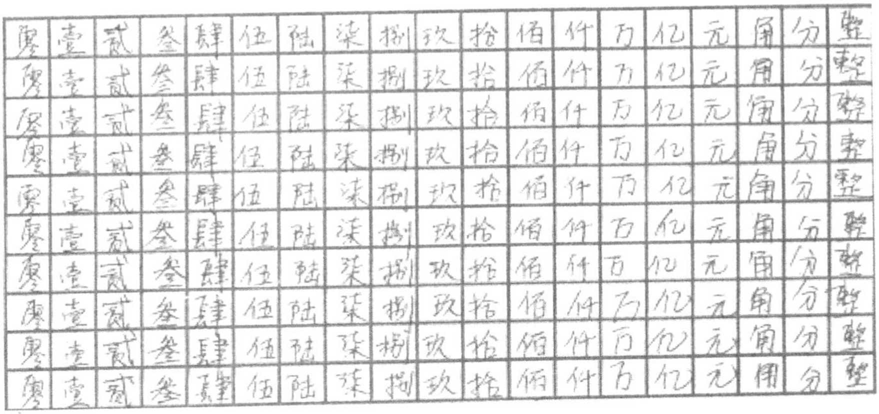

In the experiment on the FERET face image database SSS Strategy One was used. In experiments performed on all datasets except for CENPARMI and NUST603, the nearest neighbor classifier is used. In experiments on the CENPARMI handwritten digit database and the NUST603 handwritten Chinese character database, the quadratic Bayesian classifier is used. The performance of FSD and OFD on the FERET database is shown in Table 4.1. The accuracies of the FSD and OFD on the CENPARMI handwritten numeral database are shown in Table 4.2. The experimental results of the FSD and OFD on the NUST603 handwritten Chinese character database and the five UCI Machine Learning datasets are shown in Table 4.3 and Table 4.4, respectively. These experimental results demonstrate that OFD is more accurate and much more efficient than FSD.

4.3 FISHER DISCRIMINANT WITH SCHUR DECOMPOSITION

In this section, another promising orthogonal discriminant feature extraction method—Fisher discriminant with Schur decomposition (FDS) is provided.

Table 4.1. Comparison of performance of FSD and OFD on the FERET database

Average time for feature extraction and pattern classification (sec)		Average accuracy (%)	
FSD	OFD	FSD	OFD
55.88	12.84	66.43	67.11

Table 4.2. Accuracies and total times for feature extraction on the CENPARMI database

Number of extracted features	Gabor feature		Legendre feature	
	FSD (%)	OFD (%)	FSD (%)	OFD (%)
1	28.05	28.05	30.40	30.40
3	39.25	45.50	35.05	64.65
6	43.05	73.95	39.35	84.45
9	49.35	80.75	43.90	89.35
Time (sec)	9.5940	1.7970	1.0470	0.4530

Table 4.3. Accuracies and total times for feature extraction on the NUST603 database

Number of extracted features	Cross feature		Peripheral feature	
	FSD (%)	OFD (%)	FSD (%)	OFD (%)
1	30.24	30.24	23.63	23.63
6	46.34	85.92	81.53	90.16
12	76.18	93.03	90.61	95.21
18	81.92	93.13	91.03	96.05
Time (sec)	12.938	12.359	14.078	12.796

Table 4.4. Performance comparison of OFD and FSD on five UCI datasets

Dataset	Dimension	No. of classes	No. of features	FSD		OFD	
				Accuracy (%)	Time (sec)	Accuracy (%)	Time (sec)
Glass	214×9	6	5	54.67	2.500	68.69	1.860
Iris	150×4	3	2	97.33	0.907	96.00	0.844
Vehicle	846×18	4	3	70.33	28.187	74.82	28.422
Wine	178×13	3	2	92.13	1.344	98.88	1.328
Zoo	101×16	7	6	96.04	2.843	96.04	2.563

It is well-known that Schur decomposition is a natural extension of and good substitution for eigenanalysis when the matrix indented to be analyzed is asymmetric (Golub and Loan, 1996). Let A be a real square matrix, its Schur decomposition is $A = UTU^T$. Here U is an orthogonal matrix, and T is a pseudo upper diagonal matrix with the real eigenvalues of the matrix A on the diagonal and the complex eigenvalues in 2-by-2 blocks on the diagonal.

Instead of performing eigenanalysis on the matrix $S_W^{-1}S_B$ in FLD, Schur decomposition is carried out on $S_W^{-1}S_B$ in FDS. Let the Schur decomposition of $S_W^{-1}S_B$ be denoted by UTU^T, and $\mathbf{u}_1,...,\mathbf{u}_d$ be all column vectors of the matrix U, i.e. Schur vectors of $S_W^{-1}S_B$. It is obvious that $\mathbf{u}_1,...,\mathbf{u}_d$ are orthogonal to each other. Assume $\mathbf{u}_1,...,\mathbf{u}_r$ to be Schur vectors of $S_W^{-1}S_B$ corresponding to the first r largest eigenvalues, i.e. the first r largest diagonal elements of the matrix T. Thus, we can compress a high-dimensional input space R^d into a low-dimensional feature space R^r by a mapping, $\mathbf{x} \mapsto V^T \mathbf{x}$. Here $V = [\mathbf{u}_1,...,\mathbf{u}_r]$ is the discriminant matrix of FDS, and $\mathbf{u}_1,...,\mathbf{u}_r$ are FDS discriminant vectors.

Similar to FLD and OFD, the discriminant matrix of FDS is also an optimal solution to the optimization model (4.1). The following theorem reveals the fact.

Theorem 4.1 Let $\mathbf{u}_1,\mathbf{u}_2,...,\mathbf{u}_r$ be discriminant vectors of FDS. Thus, we have

$$J_F([\mathbf{u}_1,...,\mathbf{u}_r]) = \frac{\left|[\mathbf{u}_1,\mathbf{u}_2,...,\mathbf{u}_r]^T S_B [\mathbf{u}_1,\mathbf{u}_2,...,\mathbf{u}_r]\right|}{\left|[\mathbf{u}_1,\mathbf{u}_2,...,\mathbf{u}_r]^T S_W [\mathbf{u}_1,\mathbf{u}_2,...,\mathbf{u}_r]\right|} = \max_{W \in R^{d \times r}} J_F(W). \quad (4.11)$$

Proof. Since $\mathbf{u}_1,\mathbf{u}_2,...,\mathbf{u}_r$ are Schur vectors of the matrix $S_W^{-1}S_B$ corresponding to the first r largest eigenvalues, we have

$$S_W^{-1}S_B \mathbf{u}_j = \lambda_j \mathbf{u}_j, \, j = 1,...,r. \quad (4.12)$$

Here λ_j is the jth largest eigenvalue of the matrix $S_W^{-1}S_B$.

From the formula (4.12) it follows that

$$[\mathbf{u}_1,...,\mathbf{u}_r]^T S_B [\mathbf{u}_1,...,\mathbf{u}_r] = diag(\lambda_1,..., \lambda_r)[\mathbf{u}_1,...,\mathbf{u}_r]^T S_W [\mathbf{u}_1,...,\mathbf{u}_r].$$

$$(4.13)$$

Thus, we have

$$J_F([\mathbf{u}_1,...,\mathbf{u}_r]) = \frac{\left|[\mathbf{u}_1,...,\mathbf{u}_r]^T S_B [\mathbf{u}_1,...,\mathbf{u}_r]\right|}{\left|[\mathbf{u}_1,...,\mathbf{u}_r]^T S_W [\mathbf{u}_1,...,\mathbf{u}_r]\right|} = \prod_{j=1}^{r} \lambda_j = \max_{W \in R^{d \times r}} J_F(W).$$

$$(4.14)$$

4.3.2 Experimental Evaluation

The performance of FDS is evaluated using two benchmark datasets: the ORL (please refer to Section 3.2.3) and AR (please refer to Section 3.4.4) face image databases. For the ORL database, ten tests are conducted on this database for each dimensionality reduction method. In each test five images of each individual are used for training and the remaining five for testing. Thus the total amount of training samples and testing samples are both 200. The training samples are taken in turn. That is, the images of each person numbered 1 to 5, 2 to 6, ..., 10 to 4 are used as training samples respectively. For the AR database, 1666 images from 119 individuals are used for experiments (each has fourteen different images with seven taken in the first session and seven taken in the second session). All images are also normalized and preprocessed using histogram equalization as shown in Section 3.4.4. In the experiment, seven images of each person in the first session are used for training and the seven images in the second session for testing.

In all experiments in this subsection, SSS Strategy One is used for FLD, FSD, and FDS. As usual, the nearest neighbor classifier with Euclidean distance is used. In order to evaluate the performance of FDS properly, experimental results of N-LDA proposed by Chen, Liao, Ko, Lin and Yu (2000) are also included. It is interesting that discriminant vectors of N-LDA are also orthogonal to each other.

Figure 4.2. Average recognition rates of FLD, FSD, N-LDA, and FDS vs. the number of extracted features on the ORL face image database

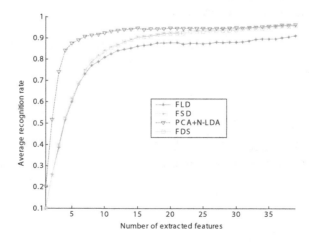

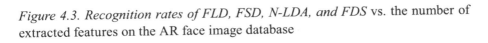

Figure 4.3. Recognition rates of FLD, FSD, N-LDA, and FDS vs. the number of extracted features on the AR face image database

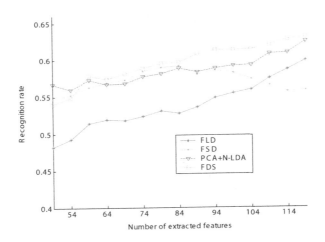

Although N-LDA can directly compress a high-dimensional input space in theory, its memory- and time-cost are extremely high. As a rule N-LDA is usually used in combination with a PCA transformation in face recognition, i.e. PCA + N-LDA.

Figure 4.2 displays trends of average recognition rates of various dimensionality reduction methods on the ORL face image database when the number of extracted features increases. We find that FDS is as accurate as FSD, better than FLD, and competes with N-LDA when the number of extracted features is large enough. Figure 4.3 shows trends of recognition rate of various dimensionality reduction methods on the AR face image database when the number of extracted features is increasing. We find that FDS is the most accurate technique for feature dimensionality reduction.

Table 4.5 lists average times consumed by various dimensionality reduction methods and the corresponding standard deviations on the ORL database when 39 features are extracted. From Table 4.5 we find that FDS is near the most efficient dimensionality reduction method N-LDA, and much more efficient than FSD. Table 4.6 lists times consumed by various dimensionality reduction techniques on the AR database when 119 features are extracted. From Table 4.6 we find that FDS is the most efficient dimensionality reduction method and much more efficient than FSD. It should be pointed out that the poor efficiency of FSD is mainly due to its iterative calculation procedure for discriminant vectors.

Table 4.5. Average times and standard deviations of various methods on the ORL database when 39 features are extracted (sec.)

	Dimensionality Reduction Methods			
	FLD	FSD	N-LDA	FDS
mean	0.8124	7.2626	0.5502	0.7608
std	0. 0321	0. 0.0732	0. 0178	0. 0129

Table 4.6. Times spent for dimensionality reduction of various methods on the AR database when 119 features are extracted (sec.)

	Dimensionality Reduction Methods			
	FLD	FSD	N-LDA	FDS
Time	23.312	1916.2	58.828	16.765

4.4 COMPARISON OF ORTHOGONAL DISCRIMINANT ANALYSIS METHODS

The performance of several typical orthogonal discriminant analysis methods, i.e. FSD, OCD, OFD, and FDS is evaluated using the three SSS strategies on the ORL and FERET face image databases. For comparison, we also present the experimental results of FLD. In all experiments the nearest neighbor classifier with Euclidean distance is used.

4.4.1 Database and Experimental Settings

The ORL (please refer to Section 3.2.3) is a typical small-scale uniform face image database. We conducted ten runs on this dataset for each combination of a feature extraction method and an SSS strategy. In each runs five images of each person were used for training and the remaining five for testing. This made a total of 200 training and 200 testing samples. The training samples are taken in turn. That is, the images of each person numbered 1 to 5, 2 to 6, …, 10 to 4 are used as training samples.

The FERET (please refer to Section 3.4.4) is a typical large-scale noisy face image database. In this section the same subset of FERET including 1400 images of 200 individuals as shown in Section 3.4.4 was used Each image was also preprocessed

Figure 4.4. Average recognition rates of FLD, FSD, OCD, OFD, and FDS under SSS Strategy One vs. the number of extracted features on two face image databases

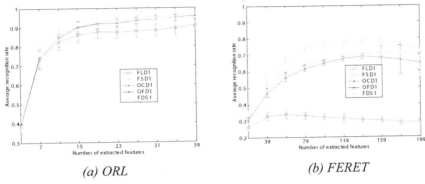

(a) ORL   (b) FERET

Strategy One vs. the number of extracted features on two face image databases

using the same approach shown in Section 3.4.4. Three images of each individual were randomly chosen for training and the remaining four images were used for testing. Thus, the training sample set size is 600 and the testing sample set size is 800. We ran the system ten times and obtained ten different training and testing sample sets.

Figure 4.5. Average recognition rates of FLD, FSD, OCD, OFD, and FDS under SSS Strategy Two vs. the number of extracted features on two face image databases

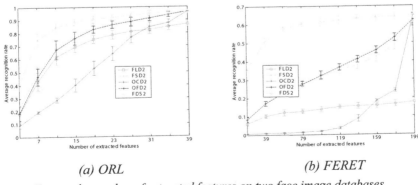

(a) ORL   (b) FERET

Strategy Two vs. the number of extracted features on two face image databases

4.4.2 Accuracy of Various Methods under the SSS Strategy One

Figure 4.4 shows error bars of recognition rates of various feature extraction methods under the SSS Strategy One on the ORL and FERET face image databases with varying number of extracted features. Here, FLD1, FSD1, OCD1, OFD1, and FDS1 stand for FLD, FSD, OCD, OFD, and FDS in combination with SSS Strategy One respectively. In fact, FLD1 is the well-known Fisherface.

4.4.3 Accuracy of Various Methods under the SSS Strategy Two

Figure 4.5 shows error bars of recognition rates of various feature extraction methods under the SSS Strategy Two on the ORL and FERET face image databases with varying number of extracted features. From Figure 4.5 we can conclude that FLD is significantly inferior to all orthogonal discriminant analysis methods except OCD.

4.4.4 Accuracy of Various Methods under the SSS Strategy Three

Figure 4.6 shows error bars of recognition rates of various feature extraction methods under the SSS Strategy Three on the ORL and FERET face image databases with varying number of extracted features. From Figure 4.6 we find that FLD is almost as effective as OCD, OFD, and FDS, and significantly more effective than FSD.

Figure 4.6. Average recognition rates of FLD, FSD, OCD, OFD, and FDS under SSS Strategy Three vs. the number of extracted features on two face image databases

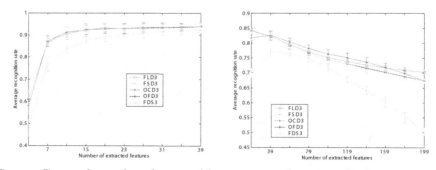

Strategy Two vs. the number of extracted features on two face image databases

Figure 4.7. Average times for feature extraction of various methods under the three SSS strategies on two databases when 39 or 199 features are extracted

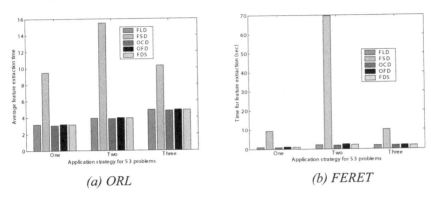

(a) ORL (b) FERET

4.4.5 Efficiency Comparison of Various Methods

Figure 4.7 shows the average times spent for feature extraction of various methods under the three SSS strategies on the ORL and FERET databases when 39 or 199 features are extracted. The time unit is second. From Figure 4.7, we see that FDS, FLD, OCD, and OFD are similar in efficiency, and they are much more efficient than FSD no matter what kind of SSS strategy is used.

Figure 4.8. Average recognition rates of FLD under SSS Strategy One, Two, and Three vs. the number of extracted features on two face image databases

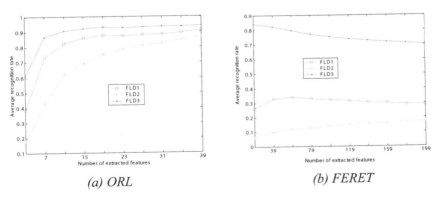

(a) ORL (b) FERET

Figure 4.9. Average recognition rates of FSD under SSS Strategy One, Two, and Three vs. the number of extracted features on two face image databases

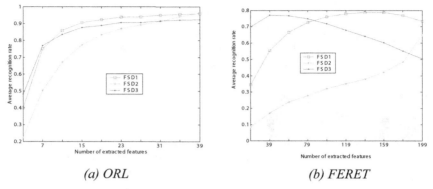

(a) ORL   (b) FERET

Figure 4.10. Average recognition rates of OCD under SSS Strategy One, Two, and Three vs. the number of extracted features on two face image databases

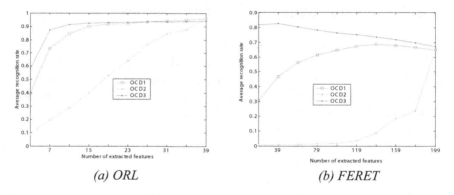

(a) ORL   (b) FERET

Figure 4.11. Average recognition rates of OFD under SSS Strategy One, Two, and Three vs. the number of extracted features on two face image databases

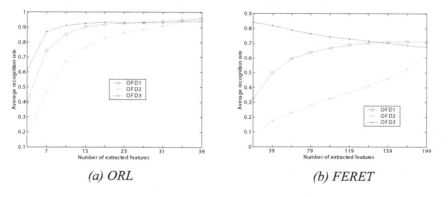

(a) ORL   (b) FERET

Figure 4.12. Average recognition rates of FDS under SSS Strategy One, Two, and Three vs. the number of extracted features on two face image databases

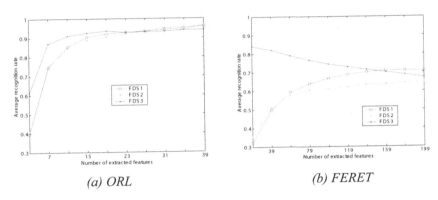

(a) ORL   (b) FERET

4.4.6 Discussions on SSS Strategies

It is generally believed that since SSS Strategy Two holds all discriminant information it is definitely superior to the other two SSS Strategies. But our experimental results demonstrate that it is not always true.

Figure 4.8-4.12 shows curves of average recognition rates of FLD, FSD, OCD, OFD, and FDS under the SSS Strategy One, Two, and Three on the ORL and FERET face image databases with the varying number of extracted features. From Figure 4.8-4.12 we find that SSS Strategy Three is the most effective and SSS Strategy Two is the least effective in general.

4.5 SUMMARY

In this chapter we first briefly review orthogonal discriminant analysis and its related application strategies to small sample size problems. Then we present two novel orthogonal discriminant analysis methods: one is orthogonalized Fisher discriminant; the other is Fisher discriminant with Schur decomposition. Theoretical analysis and experimental studies showed that OFD and FDS are all optimal solutions to multiple Fisher discriminant criterion, and they can compete with FSD in accuracy and more efficient than the latter. At last we thoroughly compare the performance of several main orthogonal discriminant analysis methods under various SSS strategies.

REFERENCES

Belhumeur, P. N., Hespanha, J. P., & Kriengman, D. J. (1997). Eigenfaces vs. fisher-faces: recognition using class specific linear projection. *IEEE Trans. Pattern Anal. Machine Intell., 19*(7), 711-720.

Chen, L., Liao, H., Ko, M., Lin, J., & Yu, G. (2000). A new lda-based face recognition system which can solve the small sample size problem. *Pattern Recognition, 33*(10), 1713-1726.

Duchene, J., & Leclercq, S. (1988). An optimal transformation for discriminant and principal component analysis. *IEEE Trans. Pattern Anal. Machine Intell., 10*(6), 978-983.

Duda, R. O., Hart, P. E., & Stork, D. G. (2001). *Pattern Classification*. New York: John Wiley & Sons.

Foley, D. H., & Sammon, J. W. (1975). An optimal set of discriminant vectors. *IEEE Trans. Comput., 24*(3), 281-289.

Fukunaga, K. (1990). *Introduction to Statistical Pattern Recognition*. New York: Academic.

Golub, G. H., & Loan, C. F. V. (1996). *Matrix Computations*. Baltimore and London: The Johns Hopkins University Press.

Guo, Y. F., Li, S. J., Yang, J. Y., Shu, T. T., & Wu, L. D. (2003). A generalized Foley-Sammon transform based on generalized Fisher discriminant criterion and its application to face recognition. *Pattern Recognition Letters, 24*(1-3), 147-158.

Jin, Z., Yang, J. Y., Hu, Z. S., & Lou, Z. (2001). Face recognition based on uncorrelated discriminant transformation. *Pattern Recognition, 34*(7), 1405-1416.

Jing, X. Y., Zhang, D., Tang, Y. Y. (2004). An improved LDA approach. *IEEE Transactions on Systems, Man, and Cybernetics, Part B: Cybernetics, 34*(5), 1942-1951.

Liu , C. J., & Wechsler, H. (2000). Robust coding schemes for indexing and retrieval from large face databases. *IEEE Trans. Image Processing, 9*(1), 132-137.

Liu, K., Cheng, Y. Q. Yang, J. Y., & Liu, X. (1992). An efficient algorithm for Foley-Sammon optimal set of discriminant vectors by algebraic method. *International Journal of Pattern Recognition and Artificial Intelligence, 6*(5), 817-829.

Murphy, P. M., & Aha, D. W. (1992). *UCI repository of machine learning databases*. http://www.ics.uci.edu/~mlearn/MLRepository.html.

Sammon, J.W. (1970). An optimal discriminant plane. *IEEE Trans. Comput., C-19,* 826-829.

Sun, D. R., & Wu, L. N. (2003). Face recognition using orthonormal discriminant subspace method. *Proceedings of the International Conference on Active Media Technology,* (pp.314-319).

Swets, D. L., & Weng, J. (1996). Using discriminant eigenfeatures for image retrieval. *IEEE Trans. Pattern Anal. Machine Intell., 18*(8), 831-836.

Wilks, S. S. (1962). *Mathematical Statistics.* New York: Wiley.

Chapter V
Parameterized Discriminant Analysis Methods

ABSTRACT

In this chapter, we mainly present three kinds of weighted LDA methods. In Sections 5.1, 5.2 and 5.3, we respectively present parameterized direct linear discriminant analysis, weighted nullspace linear discriminant analysis and weighted LDA in the range of within-class scatter matrix. We offer a brief summery of the chapter in Section 5.4.

5.1 PARAMETERIZED DIRECT LINEAR DISCRIMINANT ANALYSIS

5.1.1 Introduction

Direct LDA (D-LDA) (Yu & Yang, 2001) is an important feature extraction method for SSS problems. It first maps samples into the range of the between-class scatter matrix, and then transforms these projections using a series of regulating matrices. D-LDA can efficiently extract features directly from a high-dimensional input space without the need to first apply other dimensionality reduction techniques such as PCA transformations in Fisherfaces (Belhumeur, Hespanha, & Kriengman, 1997) or pixel grouping in nullspace LDA (N-LDA) (Chen, Liao, Ko, Lin, & Yu, 2000), and as a result has aroused the interest of many researchers in the field of pattern recognition and computer vision. Indeed, there are now many extensions of D-LDA, such as fractional D-LDA (Lu, Plataniotis, & Venetsanopoulos, 2003a), regularized D-LDA (Lu, Plataniotis, &Venetsanopoulos, 2003b; Lu, Plataniotis, & Venetsano-poulos, 2005), kernel D-LDA (Lu, Plataniotis, & Venetsanopoulos, 2003c), and boosting D-LDA (Lu, Plataniotis, Venetsanopoulos, & Li, 2006).

But there nonetheless remain some questions as to its usefulness as a facial feature extraction method. First, as been pointed out in Lu, Plataniotis and Venetsanopoulos (2003b; Lu, Plataniotis, & Venetsanopoulos, 2005), D-LDA performs badly when only two or three samples per individual are used. Second, regulating matrices in D-LDA are either redundant or probably harmful. The second drawback of D-LDA has not been seriously addressed in previous studies.

In this section, we present a new feature extraction method—parameterized direct linear discriminant analysis (PD-LDA) for SSS problems (Song, Zhang, Wang, Liu, & Tao, 2007). As an improvement of D-LDA, PD-LDA inherits advantages of D-LDA such as "direct" and "efficient". Meanwhile, it greatly enhances the accuracy and robustness of D-LDA.

5.1.2 Direct Linear Discriminant Analysis

5.1.2.1 The Algorithm of D-LDA

Let S_B and S_W denote the between- and the within-class scatter matrices respectively. The calculation procedure of D-LDA is as follows:

Step 1. Perform eigenvalue decomposition on the between-class scatter matrix S_B

Let $\Lambda = diag(\lambda_1, ..., \lambda_d)$ be the eigenvalue matrix of S_B in decreasing order and V $= [\mathbf{v}_1, ..., \mathbf{v}_d]$ be the corresponding eigenvector matrix. It follows that

$$V^T S_B V = \Lambda. \tag{5.1}$$

Let r be the rank of the matrix S_B. Let $Y = [\mathbf{v}_1, ..., \mathbf{v}_r]$ and $D_b = diag(\lambda_1, ..., \lambda_r)$, and we have

$$Y^T S_B Y = D_b. \tag{5.2}$$

Step 2. Map each sample vector $\mathbf{x}$ to get its intermediate representation $Z^T \mathbf{x}$ using the projection matrix $Z = YD_b^{-1/2}$

Step 3. Perform eigenvalue decomposition on the within-class scatter matrix of the projected samples, S_W which is given by

$$\tilde{S}_W = Z^T S_W Z. \tag{5.3}$$

Let $D_w = diag(\mu_1,...\mu_r)$ be the eigenvalue matrix of $\tilde{S}_W$ in ascending order and $U = [\mathbf{u}_1,...,\mathbf{u}_r]$ be the corresponding eigenvector matrix. It follows that

$$U^T \tilde{S}_W U = D_w. \tag{5.4}$$

Step 4. Calculate the discriminant matrix W and map each sample $\mathbf{x}$ to $W^T \mathbf{x}$
The discriminant matrix of D-LDA is given by

$$W = YD_b^{-1/2}UD_w^{-1/2}. \tag{5.5}$$

5.1.2.2 The Mechanism of D-LDA

From the calculation procedure for discriminant matrix of D-LDA, we find that D-LDA first maps samples into the range of the between-class scatter matrix using the matrix Y, and then transforms these projections using a series of regulating matrices $D_b^{-1/2}$, U, and $D_w^{-1/2}$.

The matrix Y itself can be used as a discriminant matrix for feature extraction. Since it is derived from the Karhunen-Loève decomposition of the between-class scatter matrix, the feature extraction method based on the matrix Y is abbreviated as KLB. The discriminant matrix of D-LDA W is the multiplication of Y and $D_b^{-1/2}UD_w^{-1/2}$. Thus, D-LDA is in fact a modified version of KLB.

Now, we study the impact of these regulating matrices on the feature representation capability of D-LDA.

By expanding the matrix $Z = YD_b^{-1/2}$ we have

$$Z = [\mathbf{v}_1,...,\mathbf{v}_r] \begin{bmatrix} 1/\sqrt{\lambda_1} & \cdots & 0 \\ \cdots & \cdots & \cdots \\ 0 & \cdots & 1/\sqrt{\lambda_r} \end{bmatrix} = [\frac{1}{\sqrt{\lambda_1}}\mathbf{v}_1,...,\frac{1}{\sqrt{\lambda}}\mathbf{v}_r]. \tag{5.6}$$

This implies that column vectors of Z are weighted column vectors of Y. The eigenvalue λ_i reflects the separability of training samples when they are projected onto the discriminant vector $\mathbf{v}_i$. The larger the eigenvalue λ_i, the better the discriminant vector $\mathbf{v}_i$. According to previous assumption, $\lambda_1 \geq ... \geq \lambda_r > 0$, the discriminant vector $\mathbf{v}_i$ is more important than the discriminant vector $\mathbf{v}_j$, if $i > j$. Since weight coefficients

$$\Big/ \sqrt{\lambda_i}, i=1,...,r,$$

are in inverse proportion to λ_i, they deemphasize important discriminant vectors of KLB. It results in a degraded version of KLB. Thus, the regulating matrix $D_w^{-1/2}$ cannot enhance the discriminant capability of the matrix Y and should be discarded.

In D-LDA, the matrix Z is regulated by matrices U and $D_w^{-1/2}$ such that its discriminant capability changes greatly.

The expansion of the matrix $D_w^{-1/2}$ is

$$[\mathbf{u}_1,...,\mathbf{u}_r] \begin{bmatrix} \dfrac{1}{\sqrt{\mu_1}} & \cdots & 0 \\ \cdots & \cdots & \cdots \\ 0 & \cdots & \dfrac{1}{\sqrt{\mu_r}} \end{bmatrix} = [\dfrac{1}{\sqrt{\mu_1}}\mathbf{u}_1,...,\dfrac{1}{\sqrt{\mu_r}}\mathbf{u}_r]. \qquad (5.7)$$

The role of the matrix $D_w^{-1/2}$ is in weighting column vectors of the matrix U. The eigenvalue μ_i also reflects the separability of training samples when they are projected onto the projection vector $\mathbf{u}_i$. The smaller the eigenvalue μ_i, the better the projection vector $\mathbf{u}_i$. The projection vector $\mathbf{u}_i$ is more important than the projection vector $\mathbf{u}_j$, if $\mu_i < \mu_j$. Thus, weight coefficients

$$\Big/ \sqrt{\mu_i}, i=1,...,r,$$

will emphasize important projection vectors and depress unimportant projection vectors in some ideal cases.

In other cases, however, when an eigenvalue μ is either very small or large, the corresponding weight coefficient

$$\Big/ \sqrt{\mu}$$

might be either too large or small, and thus over-emphasize projection vectors with tiny eigenvalues or over-depress projection vectors with huge eigenvalues. In sum, this is why D-LDA performed well in some cases and failed in others.

5.1.3 Model and Algorithm

5.1.3.1 The Algorithm of PD-LDA

The following describes in detail the calculation procedure of PD-LDA:

Step 1. Perform eigenvalue decomposition on the between-class scatter matrix S_B to obtain the discriminant matrix of KLB, Y

Step 2. Map each sample vector $\mathbf{x}$ to obtain its intermediate representation $Y^T\mathbf{x}$

Step 3. Perform eigenvalue decomposition on the within-class scatter matrix of projected samples, $\tilde{S}_W$ which is given by

$$\hat{S}_W = Y^T S_W Y. \tag{5.8}$$

Let $N = diag(\mu_1, \dots \mu_r)$ be the eigenvalue matrix of $\tilde{S}_W$ in ascending order and $U = [\mathbf{u}_1, \dots, \mathbf{u}_r]$ be the corresponding eigenvector matrix. It follows that

$$U^T \hat{S}_W U = N. \tag{5.9}$$

Step 4. Choose a parameter value β and calculate the regulating matrix $\Phi(\beta)$ using the following formula

$$\Phi(\beta) = diag((1+\mu_1)^\beta, \dots, (1+\mu_r)^\beta). \tag{5.10}$$

Here, the parameter β is used to emphasize projection vectors with small eigenvalues and to depress projection vectors with large ones.

It should be pointed out that the constant one in weight coefficients $(1+\mu_i)^\beta$, $i = 1, \dots, r$, plays a key role in preventing the over-emphasis of projection vectors with tiny eigenvalues.

Step 5. Calculate the discriminant matrix W and map each sample $\mathbf{x}$ to $W^T\mathbf{x}$

The discriminant matrix of PD-LDA is given by

$$W = YU\Phi(\beta). \tag{5.11}$$

To alleviate the computational burden in high-dimensional input space, the matrix Y can be calculated using the singular value decomposition theorem as shown in Yu and Yang (2001).

5.1.3.2 Discussions on the Parameter

Obviously, how to tune the parameter β is a crucial problem for PD-LDA. As discussed in Section 5.1.2.2, the weight coefficient $(1+\mu_1)^\beta$ for $\mathbf{u}_1$ should be larger than the weight coefficient $(1+\mu_r)^\beta$ for $\mathbf{u}_r$. It follows that $\beta \leq 0$.

When $\beta = 0$, the discriminant matrix of PD-LDA is $W = YU$. Since U is an orthogonal matrix, the discriminant matrix YU is equivalent to Y in terms of the recognition rate of a nearest neighbor classifier using Euclidean distance. Therefore, PD-LDA degenerates to KLB if $\beta = 0$.

As weighting coefficients, $(1+\mu_i)^\beta$, $i = 1,...,r$, what important is not their absolute but relative values. The ratio of the maximum weight coefficient $(1+\mu_i)^\beta$ to the minimum weight coefficient $(1+\mu_i)^\beta$ is crucial for the discriminant capability of PD-LDA. Let

$$\alpha = (1+\mu_1)^\beta / (1+\mu_r)^\beta. \tag{5.12}$$

Then, the parameter β is given by

$$\beta = \log(\alpha) / \log[(1+\mu_1)/(1+\mu_r)]. \tag{5.13}$$

It is obvious that $\alpha \geq 1$. If $\alpha = 1$, the regulating matrix $\Phi(\beta)$ is an identity matrix. In this case all eigenvectors of $\hat{S}_W$ are equally weighted. With the increase of α, the representation capability of PD-LDA is gradually enhanced due to properly emphasizing eigen-vectors of $\hat{S}_W$ corresponding to small eigenvalues. When α is large enough, with the increase of α, the representation capability of PD-LDA is gradually weakened due to over-emphasizing. As a result, the curve of recognition rate of PD-LDA is similar to a parabola.

Now we try to experientially estimate the optimal value of α.

In the following experiment, we use the ORL face image database (please refer to Section 3.2.3). Five randomly selected images of each person are used for training and the remaining five for testing. Thus the total amount of training samples and testing samples are both 200. There is no overlapping between the training set and the testing set. Figure 5.1 displays the curve of average recognition rate of PD- LDA with varying α over ten runs. Here, the nearest neighbor classifier with Euclidean distance is used in the experiment.

Figure 5.1. Average recognition rate of PD-LDA vs. the ratio of the maximum weight coefficient to the minimum weight coefficient

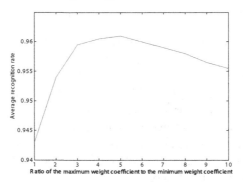

From Figure 5.1 we find that the curve of the average recognition rate is nearly a parabola as we expect, and it achieves the maximum around 5. Apparently, the optimal value of α (and the corresponding optimal value of β) might be database-dependent. It even depends on the partition of a dataset. The value 5 is only an rough approximation of the optimal value of α.

For simplicity, we let $\alpha = 5$ and the parameter be calculated using the formula (5.13) in all the experiments in this book. An astounding fact is that although the parameter β has not been finely tuned, the recognition rates of PD- LDA are significantly higher than those of D-LDA, KLB, Eigenface, and Fisherfaces.

5.1.4 Experimental Evaluation

The proposed PD-LDA feature extraction method is used for face recognition and tested on two benchmark datasets, i.e., the AR and FERET face image databases. To evaluate PD-LDA properly, we also include experimental results for D-LDA, KLB, and two benchmark facial feature extraction methods, Eigenface (Turk & Pentland, 1991) and Fisherface (Belhumeur, Hespanha, & Kriengman, 1997). In all experiments, we use the nearest neighbor classifier with Euclidean distance.

5.1.4.1 Experimental Results on the AR Database

The 120 individuals each having 26 face images taken in two sessions of the AR face database (please refer to Section 3.4.4) were selected and used in our experiment. Only the full facial images were considered here. The face portion of the image was manually cropped and normalized to 50×40 pixels as in Yang, Zhang, Frangi and Yang (2004).

In this experiment, images from the first session are used for training, and images from the second session are used for testing. Thus, the total number of training samples was 840. Since the two sessions were separated by an interval of two weeks, the aim of this experiment was to compare the performance of PD-LDA with other facial feature extraction methods under the conditions where there are changes over time.

Figure 5.2 demonstrates how recognition rates of D-LDA, KLB, Eigenface, Fisherface and PD-LDA vary with the number of extracted features on the AR face image database. Here, the Fisherface is the LDA performed on the subspace spanned by the first 120 prinicipal components.From Figure 5.2 we find that PD-LDA significantly outperforms D-LDA and Fisherface, as well as or a little better than KLB and Eigenface.

5.1.4.2 Experimental Results on the FERET Database

The same subset of the FERET database as shown in Section 3.4.4 are used. All images are also resized and pre-processed using the same approch as shown in Section 3.4.4. The experiment consists of five tests and each test consists of seven

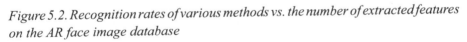

Figure 5.2. Recognition rates of various methods vs. the number of extracted features on the AR face image database

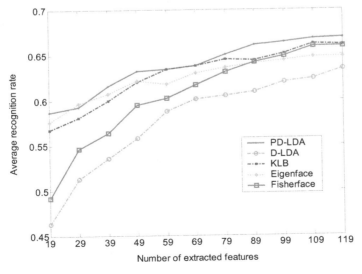

Table 5.1. Average recognition rates and standard deviations of different methods in the test on the FERET dataset

Method	D-LDA	KLB	Eigenface	Fisherface	PD-LDA
No. of features	199	199	799	199	199
Mean	0.4762	0.5910	0.5619	0.5219	0.6445
Std	0.1305	0.0640	0.0070	0.1160	0.0890

runs. In each run of the ith test, i images of each individual are used for training and the remaining $(6 - i)$ images for testing. Images of each person numbered 1 to $(i + 1)$, 2 to $(i + 2)$, …, 7 to i are used as training samples in the first, second,…, senventh run respectively.

Table 5.1 shows average recognition rates and standard deviations of D-LDA, KLB, Eigenface, Fisherface, and PD-LDA in the test on the FERET face image database. That is, in each of seven runs, four images of each individual are used for training and the remaining three images for testing. Here the number of extracted features for each method assumes its maximum value. From Table 5.1, we see that the PD-LDA is the most accurate method among the five tested facial feature extraction methods.

Figure 5.3. Average recognition rates of various methods vs. the number of training samples per individual on the FERET face image database

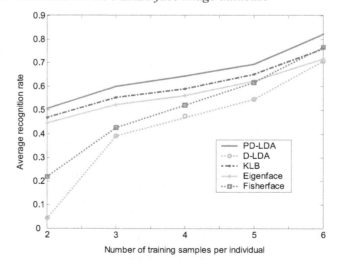

Figure 5.3 shows how average recognition rates of D-LDA, KLB, Eigenface, Fisherface and PD-LDA vary with the number of training samples per individual on the FERET face image database. In each test, the Fisherface is the LDA performed on the subspace spanned by the first 200 principal components. From Figure 5.3 we find that PD-LDA outperforms the other four facial feature extraction methods no matter how many training samples per individual are used.

5.2 Weighted Nullspace Linear Discriminant Analysis

5.2.1 Related Works

Nullspace LDA (N-LDA) (Chen, Liao, Ko, Lin, & Yu, 2000) is one of the most important variations on linear discriminant analysis (LDA) for SSS problems. Since standard LDA methods are not applicable to SSS problems due to the singular within-class scatter matrix S_W. N-LDA avoids this problem by first compressing the high-dimensional input space into the nullspace of S_W, i.e. $N(S_W)$ and then seeking a discriminant matrix which maximizes the between-class scatter in the subspace. Numerous studies have demonstrated that N-LDA is very accurate for facial feature extraction and outperforms two popular facial feature extraction methods: Eigenface and Fisherface. Nonetheless, N-LDA has two drawbacks. First, as it uses a singular value decomposition of a large scale matrix in its calculation procedure, N-LDA is computationally rather complex. Second, its separability criterion is not directly related with classification accuracy and as a consequence, as in other LDA methods, it is not guaranteed that N-LDA will find the optimal discriminant matrix.

Many researchers have addressed the issue of the computational complexity of N-LDA. Chen, Liao, Ko, Lin and Yu (2000) initially used a pixel grouping technique to alleviate the burden of computation. Huang, Liu, Lu and Ma (2002) proposed a two-stage N-LDA approach, PCA + N-LDA. This approach first uses principal component analysis (PCA) to compress a high-dimensional input space into the range of the total scatter matrix S_T, i.e. $R(S_T)$ and then performs N-LDA on this reduced subspace. The essence of this approach is performing the singular value decomposition to the between-class scatter matrix in a much smaller subspace $R(S_T) \cap N(S_W)$ rather than in the high-dimensional subspace $N(S_W)$. Zheng, Zhao and Zou (2004) later presented a similar strategy but replaced the orthogonality constraints with conjugate orthogonality constraints. Recently, Zhao, Yuen and Yang (2005) theoretically proved that the discriminant matrix of PCA + N-LDA is equivalent to that of N-LDA.

In the past several years, much work has been done to improve the relationship between a discriminant criterion and its classification accuracy. One of the most widely-applied approaches has been to introduce a weighting strategy to modify the between-class scatter matrix S_B. Weighting strategies have been used by Lotlikar and Kothari (2000), Lu, Plataniotis and Venetsanopoulos (2003a), Liang, Gong, Pan and Li (2005), and Qin, Suganthan and Loog (2006). All of these studies used the weighted between-class scatter matrix

$$\hat{S}_B = \sum_{i=1}^{c-1} \sum_{j=i+1}^{c} P_i P_j w_{ij}(d_{ij})(\mathbf{m}_i - \mathbf{m}_j)(\mathbf{m}_i - \mathbf{m}_j)^T, \qquad (5.14)$$

to substitute for the between-class scatter matrix

$$S_B = \sum_{i=1}^{c-1} \sum_{j=i+1}^{c} P_i P_j (\mathbf{m}_i - \mathbf{m}_j)(\mathbf{m}_i - \mathbf{m}_j)^T. \qquad (5.15)$$

Here, P_i is the class priori probability of the ith class, $w_{ij}(\cdot)$ the monotonically decreasing function, $d_{ij} = (\mathbf{m}_i - \mathbf{m}_j)^T S_W^{-1}(\mathbf{m}_i - \mathbf{m}_j)$ the Mahalanobis distance between two classes, and $\mathbf{m}_i$ the mean sample of the ith class. The principal reason for this substitution is that discriminant vectors based on S_B attempt to preserve the distances between already well-separated classes while neglecting the small distances of adjacent class pairs.

In this section, we present a novel facial feature extraction method, weighted nullspace LDA (WN-LDA) which successfully overcomes the two limitations of N-LDA. As in PCA + N-LDA (Huang, Liu, Lu, & Ma, 2002;   Zheng, Zhao, & Zou, 2004; Zhao, Yuen, & Yang, 2005), WN-LDA also incorporates a PCA stage into its computation procedure. However, instead of weighting the between-class scatter matrix, we enhance the discriminative capability of N-LDA by directly weighting its discriminant vectors. More specifically, unlike most LDA techniques which assume discriminant vectors to be isotropic, the presented method assumes that discriminant vectors are anisotropic and that important discriminant vectors should be endowed with larger weights. The proposed method is direct and simple yet very accurate and efficient. Extensive experimental studies conducted on the benchmark face image database, FERET demonstrate that WN-LDA is more accurate than most popular facial feature extraction methods such as Eigenface, Fisherface, N-LDA, and direct LDA (D-LDA).

Algorithm 5.1. A general WN-LDA algorithm

> **Input:** A group of labeled training samples $\mathbf{x}_1,...\mathbf{x}_N \in R^d$, the number of extracted features r, and the weight function $f(\cdot)$
> **Output:** WN-LDA discriminant matrix $V \in R^{d\times r}$

1. Compute the between-class scatter matrix S_B, the within-class scatter matrix S_W, and the total scatter matrix S_T.

2. Calculate the matrix $P \in R^{d\times t}$ of all eigenvectors of S_T corresponding to nonzero eigenvalues using the singular value decomposition theorem. Here t is the rank of S_T.

3. Work out the between- and within-class scatter matrices in the range of S_T using the formula

$$\tilde{S}_B \leftarrow P^T S_B P,$$
and
$$\tilde{S}_W \leftarrow P^T S_W P.$$

4. Seek the matrix $Q \in R^{t\times s}$ of all eigenvectors of $\tilde{S}_W$ corresponding to zero eigenvalues. Here s is the dimension of the subspace $N(\tilde{S}_W)$.

5. Figure out the between-class scatter matrix in the nullspace of $\tilde{S}_W$ using the formula

$$\tilde{\tilde{S}}_B \leftarrow Q^T \tilde{S}_B Q = (PQ)^T S_B (PQ).$$

6. Derive the eigenvector- and eigenvalue-matrices $U = [\mathbf{u}_1,...,\mathbf{u}_s]$ and $\Lambda = diag(\lambda_1,..., \lambda_s)$ of the matrix $\tilde{\tilde{S}}_B$.

7. Compute the WN-LDA discriminant matrix V using the formula

$$V \leftarrow PQ \cdot [\mathbf{u}_1,...,\mathbf{u}_r] \cdot diag(f(\lambda_1),...,f(\lambda_r)).$$

5.2.2 Model and Algorithm

5.2.2.1 The Idea behind WN-LDA

While the concept of feature weight has widely been investigated for feature selection, for example in text representation (Sebastiani, 2002; Gómez, 2003), it is a new idea in feature extraction.

The initial motivation of weighted nullspace linear discriminant analysis (WN-LDA) is demonstrated as follows. Let S_B and S_W be respectively the between- and the within-class scatter matrices, $\mathbf{q}_1,...,\mathbf{q}_s$ an orthonormal basis for the nullspace of S_W, $Q = [\mathbf{q}_1,...,\mathbf{q}_s]$, and $\tilde{S}_B = Q^T S_B Q$. Let $\mathbf{u}_1,...,\mathbf{u}_s$ be eigenvectors of the matrix $\tilde{S}_B$ corresponding to eigenvalues $\lambda_1,..., \lambda_s$ in descending order, the first r ($r \leq rank(S_B)$) discriminant vectors of N-LDA are $\mathbf{u}_1,...,\mathbf{u}_r$. The eigenvalue λ_i reflects the separability of training samples when they are projected onto the discriminant vector $\mathbf{u}_i$. The larger the eigenvalue λ_i, the better the discriminant vector $\mathbf{u}_i$. Maintaining the previous assumption, $\lambda_1 \geq ... \geq \lambda_r$, the discriminant vector $\mathbf{u}_i$ is more important than the discriminant vector $\mathbf{u}_j$, if $i < j$. It is easy to see that the discriminative capability of a discriminant matrix will be enhanced if important discriminant vectors are properly emphasized. Thus, WN-LDA tries to enhance the discriminative capability of N-LDA by multiplying its discriminant matrix $U = [\mathbf{u}_1, \mathbf{u}_2,...,\mathbf{u}_r]$ with a diagonal matrix $f(\Lambda) = diag(f(\lambda_1),...,f(\lambda_r))$. Here $f(\cdot) \geq 0$ is a monotonically increasing function. We call the matrix $f(\Lambda)$ the weight matrix, $f(\lambda_1),...,f(\lambda_r)$ the feature weight coefficients.

5.2.2.2 The WN-LDA Algorithm

The following is a general algorithm for WN-LDA which marries the ideas of PCA + N-LDA and feature weight.

5.2.2.3 Choosing the Weight Function

Now, the problem is how to properly choose the weight function $f(\cdot)$ so as to improve the discriminative capability of the N-LDA discriminant matrix. In this chapter, we are going to investigate a family of simple weight functions with one parameter, i.e. power functions $f(\lambda) = \lambda^\alpha$ with $\alpha > 0$. These functions are monotonically increasing such that important discriminant vectors are endowed with larger weight coefficients.

Apparently, absolute values of feature weight coefficients are not important and what is really important is their relative scores. Besides the form of a weigh function, the discriminative capability of WN-LDA crucially depends upon the ratio of the maximum feature weight coefficient $f(\lambda_1)$ to the minimum feature weight coefficient $f(\lambda_r)$,

$$\beta = \frac{f(\lambda_1)}{f(\lambda_r)}.$$

It is obvious that the ratio β is not less than 1. If $\beta = 1$, the weight matrix $f(\Lambda)$ is equivalent to an identity matrix such that all discriminant vectors of N-LDA are equally weighted. As a consequence, WN-LDA degenerates into N-LDA. Generally speaking, the optimal value of β is database dependent. It depends on the partition of a database, the number of extracted features, and other database-related features. The optimal value of the ratio β can be estimated experimentally. Once the ratio β is fixed, the parameter α can be computed using the formula

$$\alpha = \log(\beta)/\log(\lambda_1/\lambda_r). \tag{5.16}$$

5.2.3 Experimental Evaluation

The proposed facial feature extraction method was evaluated on the benchmark face image database, FERET. WN-LDA was evaluated on a series of subsets of the FERET database. The biggest subset includes 1,400 images of 200 individuals with seven images of each individual.

In all experiments we used the nearest neighbor (NN) classifier with Euclidean distance.

Before comparing the accuracy of WN-LDA with that of state-of-the-art facial feature extraction methods, we first investigate the impact of β, the ratio of the maximum feature weight coefficient to the minimum feature weight coefficient, on the average recognition rate (ARR) of WN-LDA.

5.2.3.1 Impact of the Parameter with Varying Number of Classes

The experiment consists of five tests of ten runs each. In the ith test, three images of each of $40i$ individual are randomly chosen for training, while the remaining

Figure 5.4. ARR curves of WN-LDA over the ratio β with different numbers of classes

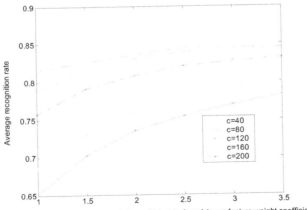

four images are used for testing. Thus, the training sample set size is 120*i* and the testing sample set size is 160*i*, *i* = 1,…,5. In this way, we ran the system ten times and obtained ten different training and testing sample sets for each test. In each run, the ratio β in turn assumes 1, 1.5, 2, 2.5, 3, and 3.5. In addition, in each test, the number of extracted features assumes the maximum value, i.e. the rank of between-class scatter matrix.

Figure 5.4 depicts the ARR curves of WN-LDA over the ratio β when the number of classes *c* is respectively equal to 40, 80, 120, 160, and 200. It can be seen that if all discriminant features are extracted, the larger the number of classes, the more sensitive the accuracy of WN-LDA to the ratio β.

5.2.3.2 Impact of the Parameter with Varying Number of Extracted Features

Seven images of each of 200 individuals were used in the experiment. Three images of each individual were randomly chosen for training, while the remaining four images were used for testing. Thus, the training sample set size was 600 and the testing sample set size was 800. In this way, we ran the system ten times and obtained ten different training and testing sample sets.

Figure 5.5 displays the ARR curves of WN-LDA over the number of extracted features when the ratio β assumes different values. Identifiers WN-LDA2, …, WN-LDA6 in Figure 5.5 stand for WN-LDA with the ratio β being equal to 2, …, 6.

Figure 5.5. The ARR curves of WN-LDA over the number of extracted features when the ratio β assumes different values

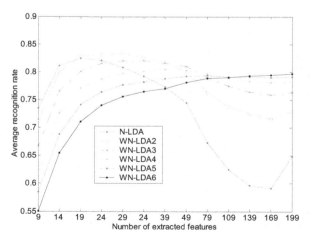

Figure 5.6. Average recognition rate of various methods vs. the number of extracted features

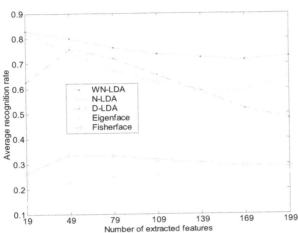

From Figure 5.5 we find that, unlike N-LDA whose ARR is heavily dependent on the number of extracted features, the accuracy of WN-LDA is quite robust. Furthermore, with the increase of the ratio β, the ARR curve of WN-LDA is approaching a monotonically increasing curve. One probable reason for this is that the WN-LDA discriminant vectors corresponding to minor eigenvalues might be incorrect due to roundoff error and poor conditioning of the between-class scatter matrix, and smaller feature weight coefficients properly depress the side effects of these discriminant vectors.

5.2.3.3 Comparison of WN-LDA with Other Facial Feature Extraction Methods

The experimental design is the same as in Section 5.2.3.2. Figure 5.6 shows the ARR curves of WN-LDA (β = 2), N-LDA, D-LDA, Eigenface, and Fisherface. It can be seen that WN-LDA is more accurate than the other four facial feature extraction methods.

5.2.3.4 Experimental Results over Varying Number of Training Samples per Individual

According to Lu, Plataniotis and Venetsanopoulos (2005) the accuracy of D-LDA is heavily dependent on the number of training samples per individual. To fairly

Figure 5.7. Average recognition rates of various feature extraction methods vs. the numbers of training samples per individual

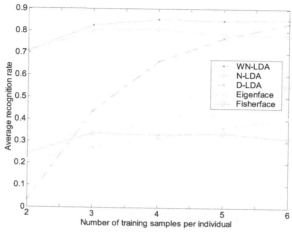

compare WN-LDA with D-LDA and other methods, in this subsection we evaluate the accuracy of WN-LDA (β = 2) with that of N-LDA, D-LDA, Eigenface, and Fisherface when the number of training samples per individual varies from 2 to 6.

The experiment consists of five tests of ten runs each. In each run of the ith test, (i + 1) images of each individual were randomly selected for training and the remaining (6 - i) images for testing. The number of extracted features for WN-LDA, N-LDA, D-LDA, Fisherface, and Eigenface in the ith test were respectively 15i, **15i, 15i, 15i, and** 200i + 199. Figure 5.7 displays the ARR curves of various feature extraction methods over varying number of training samples per individual. It can be seen that WN-LDA is once again the most accurate method among the tested facial feature extraction approaches.

5.3 WEIGHTED LINEAR DISCRIMINANT ANALYSIS IN THE RANGE OF WITHIN-CLASS SCATTER MATRIX

Conventional facial feature extraction methods including Fisherface, N-LDA, and D-LDA perform fairly well in small uniform face image databases such as Yale, UMIST, ORL, and AR. But, if applied to large noisy datasets such as FERET, they suffer from two particular problems. First, they are not very accurate. Second, while their accuracy is heavily dependent on the number of extracted features, the optimal number of extracted features is hard to determine.

To overcome these two drawbacks we propose a novel facial feature extraction method, weighted linear discriminant analysis in the range of the within-class scatter (WLDA-RWS) matrix in this section. We began by first extensively testing simple LDA in the range of the within-class scatter matrix (LDA-RWS) on the FERET benchmark face image database, demonstrating that LDA-RWS generally outperforms N-LDA, D-LDA, and Fisherface. Further tests properly weighting the discriminant vectors of LDA-RWS with feature weight coefficients further improved both its discriminative capability and its stability.

This research also made some discoveries which appear to overturn two very common beliefs about discriminant feature extraction. First, contradicting the prevailing view that, given a small sample size, optimal Fisher discriminant vectors should be derived from the nullspace of the within-class scatter matrix, we found that, when applied to a collection of large scale noisy face images, a set of Fisher discriminant vectors derived from the range of the within-class scatter matrix was more accurate than the set of discriminant vectors of N-LDA. This implies that larger Fisher criterion function values do not guarantee greater accuracy. Second, we discovered that discriminant matrices with the same discriminant criterion value, i.e. they are all the optimal solutions to the model (4.1) are unnecessarily of the same discriminative capability. It is well known that if $W^* \in R^{d \times r}$ is the Fisher discriminant matrix and $\Lambda \in R^{r \times r}$ an arbitrary nonsingular matrix, then the matrix $W^* \Lambda$ is also an optimal solution to the model (4.1). In the past, researchers commonly believed that the matrix Λ had no effect on the discriminative capability of W^* and that thus the matrix $W^* \Lambda$ was equivalent to the matrix W^*. This implied that discriminant vectors (directions) are isotropic. However, our experimental results have shown that proper selection of a weight matrix $\Lambda = diag(f_1, ..., f_r)$ offers the potential to greatly improve the discriminative capability in terms of recognition accuracy. Here, $f_1, ..., f_r$ are feature weight coefficients.

5.3.1 Model and Algorithm

5.3.1.1 The Ideas behind LDA-RWS

Let $N(S_w)$ and $R(S_w)$ be both the nullspace and the range of the within-class scatter matrix. According to linear algebraic theory, the input space R^d can be decomposed as the direct sum of these two subspaces, i.e. $R^d = N(S_W) \oplus R(S_W)$. To avoid the singularity problem, LDA-RWS converts the Fisher discriminant criterion into

$$\max_{W \in R(S_W) \times \cdots \times R(S_W)} J(W) = \frac{\left| W^T S_B W \right|}{\left| W^T S_W W \right|}. \tag{5.17}$$

There always is an optimal solution to the optimization model (5.17). In fact, if P is the matrix comprised of unit eigenvectors of the matrix S_W corresponding to nonzero eigenvalues, and Q_r is the matrix composed of unit eigenvectors of the matrix $(P^T S_W P)^{-1}(P^T S_B P)$ corresponding to the r largest eigenvalues, then PQ_r is an optimal solution to the model (2). Furthermore, here PQ_r is used as the discriminant matrix of LDA-RWS. Let $\lambda_1, ..., \lambda_r$ be the r largest eigenvalues of $(P^T S_W P)^{-1}(P^T S_B P)$. We have $J(PQ_r) = \prod_{i=1}^{r} \lambda_i$. Let W be the discriminant matrix of N-LDA. It follows that $W \in N(S_W) \times \cdots N(S_W)$. Thus, we have $J(W) = \infty > J(PQ_r)$. This is the primary reason why many researchers believe that the optimal Fisher discriminant vectors should be derived from $N(S_W)$ rather than from $R(S_W)$. A detailed discussion of the relevant experimental results can be found in the following subsection.

5.3.1.2 The Concept of Feature Weight

The concept of using feature weights for feature selection, for example in areas such as text representation (Sebastiani, 2002; Gómez, 2003), has been widely investigated. It appears, however, to be new in feature extraction. One reason for this omission may be that many researchers in the field of dimensionality reduction or feature extraction take it for granted that two transformation matrices with the same discriminant criterion value should have the same discriminative capability.

Let W be one discriminant matrix and $f_1, ..., f_r$ to be a set of feature weight coefficients. It is obvious that following equations satisfy

$$J(Wdiag(f_1, ..., f_r)) = \frac{|diag(f_1, ..., f_r)W^T S_B Wdiag(f_1, ..., f_r)|}{|diag(f_1, ..., f_r)W^T S_W Wdiag(f_1, ..., f_r)|} =$$

$$\frac{|W^T S_B W|}{|W^T S_W Wdiag|} = J(W)$$

(5.18)

This would suggest that feature weights should have no impact on the discriminative capability of a discriminant matrix. Yet Song, Liu and Yang (2005) have shown that although orthogonalized Fisher discriminant matrix and Fisher discriminant matrix have the same discriminant criterion value, in terms of recognition accuracy there is a significant difference in their discriminative capabilities.

Further, it is well known that with the increase of number of classes and noise in the data, discriminant vectors with minor eigenvalues become less accurate. As a consequence, average recognition accuracies of various feature extraction methods do not increase with the number of extracted features when associated eigenvalues of newly added discriminant vectors are small enough. This implies that discriminant vectors are anisotropic at least under circumstances with large-scale noisy data.

Let P be the matrix comprised of unit eigenvectors of the matrix S_W corresponding to nonzero eigenvalues, and $\mathbf{q}_1,...,\mathbf{q}_w$ eigenvectors of the matrix $(P^T S_W P)^{-1}(P^T S_B P)$ corresponding to eigenvalues $\lambda_1,...,\lambda_w$ in descending order, the first r ($r \le rank(S_B)$) discriminant vectors of LDA-RWS are $P\mathbf{q}_1,...,P\mathbf{q}_s$. The eigenvalue λ_i reflects the separability of training samples when they are projected onto the discriminant vector $P\mathbf{q}_i$. The larger the eigenvalue λ_i, the better the discriminant vector $P\mathbf{q}_i$. According to the previous assumption, $\lambda_1 \ge ... \ge \lambda_r$, the discriminant vector $P\mathbf{q}_i$ is more important than the discriminant vector $P\mathbf{q}_j$, if $i < j$. Clearly, the discriminative capability of a discriminant matrix will be enhanced if important discriminant vectors are properly emphasized.

5.3.1.3 The WLDA-RWS Algorithm

WLDA-RWS tries to enhance the discriminative ability of LDA-RWS by multiplying its discriminant matrix PQ_r with a diagonal matrix $f(\Lambda) = diag(f(\lambda_1),...,f(\lambda_r))$.

Algorithm 5.2. A general WLDA-RWS algorithm

Input: A group of labeled training samples $\mathbf{x}_1,...,\mathbf{x}_N \in R^d$, the number of extracted features r, and the weight function $f(\cdot)$
Output: WLDA-RWS discriminant matrix $V \in R^{d \times r}$

Step 1. Compute the between-class scatter matrix S_B and the within-class scatter matrix S_W.
Step 2. Calculate the matrix $P \in R^{d \times w}$ of all eigenvectors of S_w corresponding to nonzero eigenvalues using the singular value decomposition theorem. Here w is the rank of S_w.
Step 3. Work out the between- and within-class scatter matrices in the range of S_w using the formulae

$$\tilde{S}_B \leftarrow P^T S_B P,$$

and

$$\tilde{S}_W \leftarrow P^T S_W P.$$

Step 4. Seek the eigenvector- and eigenvalue-matrices $Q = [\mathbf{q}_1,...,\mathbf{q}_w]$ and $\Lambda = diag(\lambda_1,...,\lambda_w)$ of the matrix $\tilde{S}_W^{-1} \tilde{S}_B$.
Step 5. Compute the WN-LDA discriminant matrix V using the formula

$$V \leftarrow P \cdot [\mathbf{q}_1,...,\mathbf{q}_r] \cdot diag(f(\lambda_1),...,f(\lambda_r)).$$

Algorithm 5.3. Algorithm for the pairwise linear weight function

Input: A set of positive eigenvalues $\lambda_1,...,\lambda_r$ in descending order, the ratio of the maximum feature weight coefficient to the minimum feature weight coefficient α, the number of line segments β, and the lift rate of the pairwise linear curve γ

Output: A set of feature weight coefficients $f(\lambda_1),...,f(\lambda_r)$

Step 1. Calculate the slope a_p and the intercept b_p of the previous line segment using the formulae

$$a_p \leftarrow (\alpha - 1)/(\lambda_1 - \lambda_r),$$

and

$$b_p \leftarrow 1 - a_p \lambda_r.$$

Step 2. Compute the *x*- and *y*-coordinates of the right end, and the *x*-coordinate of the left end of the current line segment using the formulae

$$right\_x \leftarrow \lambda_1,$$

$$right\_y \leftarrow \alpha,$$

and

$$left\_x \leftarrow \lambda_r + \frac{\lambda_1 - \lambda_r}{\beta}(\beta-1).$$

Step 3. Derive the slope a_c and the intercept b_c of the current line segment using the formulae

$$left\_y \leftarrow a \cdot left\_x + b,$$

$$left\_y \leftarrow left\_y + \gamma(right\_y - left\_y),$$

$$a_c \leftarrow \frac{right\_y - left\_y}{right\_x - left\_x},$$

and

$$b_c \leftarrow right\_y - a_c \cdot right\_x.$$

Step 4. Work out $f(\lambda)$ for $left\_x \leq \lambda < right\_x$ using the formula

$$f(\lambda) \leftarrow a_c \lambda + b_c.$$

Step 5. Update intermediate variables using the formulae

$$a_p \leftarrow (left\_y - 1)/(left\_x - \lambda_r),$$

$$b_p \leftarrow 1 - a_p \lambda_r,$$

$$right\_x \leftarrow left\_x,$$

$$right\_y \leftarrow left\_y,$$

and

$$left\_x \leftarrow left\_x - \frac{\lambda_1 - \lambda_r}{\beta}.$$

Step 6. Repeat Step 3 to Step 5 until all feature weight coefficients have been obtained.

Here $f(\cdot) \geq 0$ is a monotonically increasing function. We call the matrix $f(\Lambda)$ the weight matrix, and $f(\lambda_1), ..., f(\lambda_r)$ the feature weight coefficients.

The following is a general algorithm for WLDA-RWS which marries the ideas of LDA-RWS and feature weight.

5.3.1.4 Pairwise Linear Weight Functions

Now, the problem is how to properly choose the weight function $f(\cdot)$ such that the discriminative capability of the LDA-RWS discriminant matrix can be enhanced. In this paragraph , we are going to investigate a family of pairwise linear weight functions having three parameters α, β, and γ.

The first parameter α is the ratio of the maximum feature weight coefficient $f(\lambda_1)$ to the minimum feature weight coefficient $f(\lambda_r)$, i.e.

$$\alpha = \frac{f(\lambda_1)}{f(\lambda_r)}.$$

It is obvious that the ratio α is a positive number not less than 1. If $\alpha = 1$, the weight matrix $f(\Lambda)$ is equivalent to an identity matrix such that all discriminant vectors of LDA-RWS are equally weighted. As a consequence, WLDA-RWSM degenerates into LDA-RWS. The second parameter β is the number of line segments in the pairwise linear curve. As a result, β is a positive integer. If $\beta = 1$, the pairwise linear curve degenerates into a line. The third parameter γ is the lift rate of the pairwise linear curve which determines the lift distance of the left end of the current line segment relative to the corresponding point of the previous line segment. γ is a

Figure 5.8. Geometric explanation of the parameters α, β, and γ

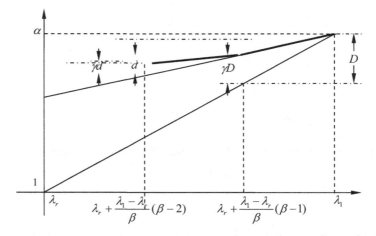

Figure 5.9. Sample pairwise linear curves with varying values of α

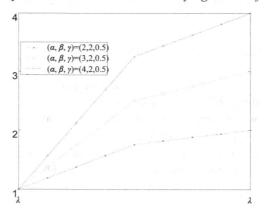

number between zero and one. If $\gamma = 1$, the pairwise linear curve degenerates into a line whereas if $\gamma = 1$, the pairwise linear curve degenerates into a horizontal line. As a consequence, WLDA-RWS degenerates into LDA-RWS. Figure 5.8 gives the geometric explanation of the parameters α, β, and γ.

The detailed algorithm for computing feature weight coefficients of the pairwise linear weight function is as follows.

Figures. 5.9-5.11 plot some sample pairwise linear curves. All these pairwise linear weight functions are monotonically increasing. As a consequence, important discriminant vectors can be endowed with larger weight coefficients.

Figure 5.10. Sample pairwise linear curves with varying values of β

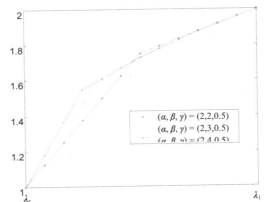

Figure 5.11. Sample pairwise linear curves with varying values of γ

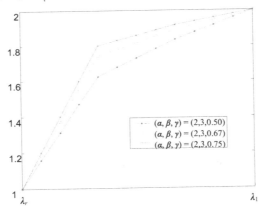

5.3.2 Experimental Evaluation

The proposed facial feature extraction method was evaluated on the benchmark face image database, FERET. WLDA-RWS was evaluated on a subset of the FERET database (please refer to Section 3.4.4). The subset includes 1,400 images of 200 individuals with seven images of each individual.

5.3.2.1 Comparison of WLDA-RWS with Other Facial Feature Extraction Methods

Three images of each individual were randomly chosen for training and the remaining four images were used for testing. Thus, the training sample set size is 600 and the testing sample set size is 800. We ran the system ten times and obtained ten different training and testing sample sets.

Figure 5.12. Average recognition accuracy of various methods vs. the number of extracted features

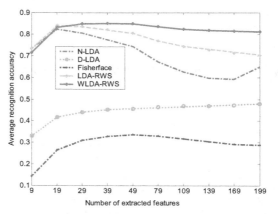

Figure 5.13. Average recognition accuracy of various feature extraction methods vs. the numbers of training samples per individual

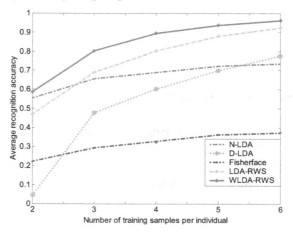

Figure 5.12 shows the average accuracy curves of N-LDA, D-LDA, Fisherface, LDA-RWS, and WLDA-RWS having parameters $(\alpha, \beta, \gamma) = (2, 7, 0.9)$. It can be seen that WLDA-RWS is generally more accurate than the other four facial feature extraction methods.

5.3.2.2 Experimental Results over Varying Number of Training Samples per Individual

As mentioned in Section 5.2.3.4, the accuracy of D-LDA varies with the number of training samples per individual. In this subsection we evaluate the accuracies of WLDA-RWS, N-LDA, D-LDA, Fisherface, and LDA-RWS under the condition that the number of training samples per individual ranges between 2 and 6. This seems to be a fair and reasonable scheme to compare WLDA-RWS with D-LDA and other methods.

The experiment consists of five tests of ten runs. In each run of the ith test, $(i + 1)$ images of each individual were randomly selected for training and the remaining $(6 - i)$ images were retained for testing. There are 199 extracted features for each of N-LDA, D-LDA, Fisherface, LDA- RWS, and WLDA-RWS.

Figure 5.13 shows the average accuracy curves of various feature extraction methods over varying number of training samples per individual. It can be seen that among the tested facial feature extraction approaches, WLDA-RWS is again the most accurate.

5.4 SUMMARY

In this chapter we propose three kinds of parameterized linear discriminant analysis methods. The first is parameterized direct linear discriminant analysis; the second is weighted nullspace linear discriminant analysis; and the third is weighted linear discriminant analysis in the range of within-class scatter matrix. The common points are that they all combine the concept of "feature weight" with existing LDA methods for small sample size problems to further improve their discriminant capability.

REFERENCES

Belhumeur, P. N., Hespanha, J. P., & Kriengman, D. J. (1997). Eigenfaces vs. fisherfaces: recognition using class specific linear projection. *IEEE Trans. on Pattern Anal. Machine Intell.*, *19*(7), 711-720.

Chen, L., Liao, H., Ko, M., Lin, J., & Yu, G. (2000). A new lda-based face recognition system which can solve the small sample size problem. *Pattern Recognition, 33*(10), 1713-1726.

Gómez, J. M. (2003). Text representation for automatic text categorization. *Proceedings of Eleventh Conference of the European Chapter of the Association for Computational Linguistics.*

Huang, R., Liu, Q. S., Lu, H. Q., & Ma, S. D. (2002). Solving the small sample size problem of lda. *Proceedings of International conference on Pattern Recognition,* (pp. 29-32).

Liang, Y. X., Gong, W. G., Pan, Y. J., & Li, W. H. (2005). Generalizing relevance weighted lda. *Pattern Recognition, 38*(11), 2217-2219.

Lotlikar, R., & Kothari, R. (2000). Fractional-step dimensionality reduction. *IEEE Trans. Pattern Anal. Machine Intell., 22*(6), 623-627.

Lu, J., Plataniotis, K., & Venetsanopoulos, A. (2003a). Face recognition using lda-based algorithms. *IEEE Trans. on Neural Networks, 14*(1), 195-200.

Lu, J., Plataniotis, K., & Venetsanopoulos, A. (2003b). Regularized discriminant analysis for the small sample size problem in face recognition. *Pattern Recognition Lett., 24*(16), 3079-3087.

Lu, J., Plataniotis, K., & Venetsanopoulos, A. (2003c). Face recognition using kernel direct discriminant analysis algorithms. *IEEE Trans. on Neural Networks, 14*(1), 117-126.

Lu, J., Plataniotis, K., & Venetsanopoulos, A. (2005). Regularization studies of linear discriminant analysis in small sample size scenarios with application to face recognition. *Pattern Recognition Letter, 26*(2), 181-191.

Lu, J., Plataniotis, K., Venetsanopoulos, A., & Li, S. (2006). Ensemble-based discriminant learning with boosting for face recognition. *IEEE Trans. on Neural Networks, 17*(1), 166- 178.

Qin, A. K., Suganthan, P. N., & Loog, M. (2006). Generalized null space uncorrelated Fisher discriminant analysis for linear dimensionality reduction. *Pattern Recognition, 39*(9), 1805-1808.

Sebastiani, F. (2002). Machine learning in automated text categorization. *ACM Computing Surveys, 34*(1), 1-47.

Song, F. X., Liu, S. H., & Yang, J. Y. (2005). Orthogonalized Fisher Discriminant. *Pattern Recognition, 38*(2), 311-313.

Song, F. X., Zhang, D., Wang, J. Z., Liu, H., & Tao, Q. (2007). A parameterized direct LDA and its application to face recognition. *Neurocomputing*, *71*(1-3), 191-196.

Turk, M., & Pentland, A. (1991). Face recognition using Eigenfaces. *Proc. IEEE Conf. Computer Vision and Pattern Recognition*, (pp. 586-591).

Yang, J., Zhang, D., Frangi, A. F., & Yang, J. Y. (2004). Two-dimensional pca: a new approach to appearance-based face representation and recognition. *IEEE Trans. on Pattern Anal. Machine Intell.*, *26*(1), 131-137.

Yu, H., & Yang, J. (2001). A direct lda algorithm for high-dimensional data—with application to face recognition. *Pattern Recognition*, *34*(10), 2067-2070.

Zhao, H. T., Yuen, P. C., & Yang, J. Y. (2005). Optimal subspace analysis for face recognition. *International Journal of Pattern Recognition and Artificial Intelligence*, *19*(3), 375- 393.

Zheng, W. M., Zhao, L., & Zou, C. R. (2004). An efficient algorithm to solve the small sample size problem for lda. *Pattern Recognition*, *37*(5), 1077-1079.

Chapter VI
Two Novel Facial Feature Extraction Methods

ABSTRACT

In this chapter, we introduce two novel facial feature extraction methods. The first is multiple maximum scatter difference (MMSD) which is an extension of a binary linear discriminant criterion, i.e. maximum scatter difference. The second is discriminant based on coefficients of variances (DCV) which can be viewed as a generalization of N-LDA. At last, we give a summery of the chapter.

6.1 MULTIPLE MAXIMUM SCATTER DIFFERENCE

The maximum scatter difference (MSD) discriminant criterion (Song, Zhang, Chen, & Wang, 2007) presented in Section 3.4 is a binary discriminant criterion for pattern classification. Because MSD utilizes the generalized scatter difference rather than the generalized Rayleigh quotient as a class separability measure, it avoids the singularity problem when addressing the SSS problems that trouble the Fisher Discriminant Criterion. Further, experimental studies demonstrated that MSD classifiers based on this discriminant criterion have been quite effective on face recognition tasks (Song et al., 2007). The drawback of the MSD classifier is that, as a binary classifier, it cannot be applied directly to multiclass classification problems such as face recognition. This means that multiple recognition tasks have to be divided into a series of binary classification problems using one of three implementation strategies: one-vs-rest, one-vs-one, or directed-acyclic-graph (Hsu

& Lin, 2002). Experiments have shown that MSD classifiers are not very effective when using the first strategy, while using the latter two strategies requires the training of $l(l-1)/2$ MSD classifiers for a l-class recognition problem. The efficiency of such an approach will greatly be affected by any increase in the number of classes. Ultimately, then, like all binary classifiers, MSD classifiers are not suitable for large-scale pattern recognition problems.

To address the problem, this section generalizes the classification-oriented binary criterion to its multiple counterpart—multiple maximum scatter difference (MMSD) discriminant criterion for facial feature extraction (Song, Liu, & Yang, 2006; Song, Zhang, Mei, & Guo, 2007). The MMSD feature extraction method based on this novel discriminant criterion is a new subspace-based feature extraction method. Unlike most conventional subspace-based feature extraction methods that derive their discriminant vectors either in the range of the between-class scatter matrix or in the null space of the within-class scatter matrix, MMSD computes its discriminant vectors in both subspaces. MMSD is theoretically elegant and easy to calculate. Extensive experimental studies conducted on the benchmark database, FERET, show that MMSD outperforms many state-of-the-art facial feature extraction methods including nullspace LDA (N-LDA) (Chen, Liao, Ko, Lin, & Yu, 2000), direct LDA (D-LDA) (Yu & Yang, 2001), Eigenface (Turk & Pentland, 1991), Fisherface (Belhumeur, Hespanha, & Krieqman, 1997), and complete LDA (Yang, Frangi, Yang, Zhang, & Jin, 2005).

6.1.1 Related Works

Almost all facial feature extraction methods have been developed from Fisher linear discriminant (FLD). FLD seeks an optimal linear transformation $W^* \in R^{d \times r}$ from a high-dimensional input space R^d into a low-dimensional feature space R^r, by observing the following Multiple Fisher Discriminant Criterion,

$$\max_{W \in R^{d \times r}} \frac{\left|W^T S_B W\right|}{\left|W^T S_W W\right|}. \tag{6.1}$$

Here S_B and S_W are respectively the between- and within-class scatter matrices. The transformation matrix W^* is called the Fisher discriminant matrix and its column vectors are called Fisher discriminant vectors. It has been proved that the matrix whose ith column vector is an eigenvector of $S_W^{-1} S_B$ corresponding to the ith largest eigenvalue is an optimal solution for the model (6.1) when S_W is nonsingular. Unfortunately, in SSS problems such as face recognition, the dimension of an input space d is usually greater than the number of training samples N. As a result, the within-class scatter matrix S_W degenerates into a singular matrix. In such a case, model (6.1) is ill-posed and therefore FLD cannot be directly applied to face recognition.

Various facial feature extraction methods have been proposed based on one or another modification of FLD. These methods fall roughly into two groups: computation-oriented and subspace-based. Computation-oriented methods seek an approximate substitute for the inverse of the within-class scatter matrix when it is singular. Well known computation-oriented methods include the pseudo inverse (Tian, Barbero, Gu, & Lee, 1986), singular value disturbation (Hong & Yang, 1991), and regularization (Zhao, Chellappa, & Phillip, 1999). Because computation-oriented approaches incur a heavy burden of calculation and are not effective they are no longer the focus of studies.

Subspace-based approaches compress the feasible region of discriminant vectors from the total input space into one subspace such that discriminant matrices can be easily derived in this subspace. Early examples include Fisherface (Belhumeur et al., 1997), the nullspace LDA (N-LDA) (Chen et al., 2000), and direct LDA (D-LDA) (Yu & Yang, 2001). Fisherface calculates its discriminant vectors in the subspace spanned by a set of several major eigenvectors of the total scatter matrix. N-LDA seeks its discriminant vectors in the null space of the within-class scatter matrix, $N(S_W)$ whereas D-LDA tries to find its discriminant vectors in the range of the between-class scatter matrix, $R(S_B)$. Subspace-based feature extraction methods have flourished in recent years. Numerous studies have shown that both $N(S_W)$ and $R(S_B)$ contain important discriminant information so feature extraction methods that derive discriminant vectors in both subspaces should perform better. Based on this belief, Yang et al. proposed complete LDA (C-LDA) (Yang et al., 2005) and experimental studies have shown that C-LDA does outperform other subspace-based facial feature extraction methods.

6.1.2 Model and Algorithm

6.1.2.1 The MMSD Discriminant Criterion

The goal of discriminant criteria for feature extraction is to seek r discriminant vectors $\mathbf{w}_1, ..., \mathbf{w}_r$ such that training samples from a high-dimensional input space are farthest apart after they are projected on these vectors. In order to eliminate the influences of lengths of discriminant vectors and linear dependences between these vectors we usually require them to be orthonormal. That is, discriminant vectors should satisfy the constraints $\mathbf{w}_i^T \mathbf{w}_j = \delta_{ij}, i, j = 1, ..., r$.

Let $W = [\mathbf{w}_1, ..., \mathbf{w}_r] \in R^{d \times r}$ be the discriminant matrix. The projection of a sample $\mathbf{x}$ on discriminant vectors $\mathbf{w}_1, ..., \mathbf{w}_r$ is $W^T\mathbf{x}$. The between- and within-class scatter matrices of projected training samples $W^T \mathbf{x}_1, ..., W^T \mathbf{x}_N$ are $\tilde{S}_B = W^T S_B W$ and $\tilde{S}_W = W^T S_W W$ respectively.

The trace of the between-class scatter matrix of projected training samples, $tr(W^T S_B W)$ reflects the scatter of projected training samples between categories whereas the trace of the within-class scatter matrix of projected training samples, $tr(W^T S_W W)$ reflects the scatter of projected training samples within each category. The larger the $tr(W^T S_B W)$, the more separable the projected data; the smaller the $tr(W^T S_W W)$, the more separable the projected data. Thus, we wish to achieve two distinct objectives:

$$\max tr(W^T S_B W), \tag{6.2}$$

$$\min tr(W^T S_W W), \tag{6.3}$$

satisfying the orthonormal constraints:

$$\mathbf{w}_i^T \mathbf{w}_j = \delta_{ij}, \, i, j = 1, 2, ..., r. \tag{6.4}$$

The problem of seeking a set of discriminant vectors is then translated into a problem of solving a multi-objective programming model which is defined by (6.2-6.4). It is well known that a multi-objective programming model cannot be solved directly. It has to first be converted into a single-objective programming model. There are two main ways to convert a multi-objective programming model into a single-objective model: The first is the goal programming approach in which one of the objectives is optimized while the remaining objectives are converted into constraints. The second is the combining objective approach in which all objectives are combined into one scalar objective. When using a combining objective approach there are two major rules: the multiplicative and the additive. By utilizing the multiplicative rule to combine objectives (6.2) and (6.3), we gain a discriminant criterion that is similar to the generalized Fisher discriminant criterion (Guo, Li, Yang, Shu, & Wu, 2003). If using the additive rule to combine the two objectives, we obtain the multiple maximum scatter difference (MMSD) discriminant criterion. The single-objective optimization model corresponding to the MMSD discriminant criterion is as follows:

$$\max_{\mathbf{w}_i^T \mathbf{w}_j = \delta_{ij}, i,j=1,2,...,r} tr\{[\mathbf{w}_1, \mathbf{w}_2, ..., \mathbf{w}_r]^T (S_B - c \cdot S_W)[\mathbf{w}_1, \mathbf{w}_2, ..., \mathbf{w}_r]\}. \tag{6.5}$$

It can further be transformed into

$$\max_{\mathbf{w}_i^T \mathbf{w}_j = \delta_{ij}, i, j = 1, 2, \dots, r} \sum_{i=1}^{r} \mathbf{w}_i^T (S_B - c \cdot S_W) \mathbf{w}_i. \tag{6.6}$$

Here $S_B - c \cdot S_W$ is a generalized scatter difference matrix and c a nonnegative parameter.

Obviously, model (6.6) is an extension of the model (3.28).

According to Theorem 4 in (Guo et al., 2003), we can conclude that the ortho-normal eigenvectors $\varphi_1, \dots, \varphi_r$ of the matrix $S_B - c \cdot S_W \mathbf{v}$ corresponding to the r largest eigenvalues make of an optimal solution of model (6.6). We call these orthonormal eigenvectors MMSD discriminant vectors. It should be pointed out that a similar discriminant criterion—differential scatter discriminant criterion has been inves-tigated in Fukunaga (1990) and extended to tensor minimax probability machines (Tao, Li, Hu, Maybank, & Wu, 2005) and general tensor discriminant analysis (Tao, Li, Maybank, & Wu, 2006) .

6.1.2.2 The MMSD-Based Feature Extraction Algorithm

It is expensive both in time and memory to directly perform eigen decomposition on the matrix $S_B - c \cdot S_W$ when the dimensionality of the input space d is large enough. It is the key of the MMSD-based feature extraction algorithm how to decompose the matrix $S_B - c \cdot S_W$ quickly. Fortunately, however, with the following lemma and theorem we can always compute the eigenvectors of $S_B - c \cdot S_W$ by performing ei-gen-decomposition on a much smaller matrix whose dimension is equal to or less than $(N-1) \times (N-1)$.

Lemma 6.1. Let S_B and S_W be respectively the between- and within-class scatter matrices. Let P be the matrix of all unit eigenvectors of the total scatter matrix S_T $(= S_B + S_W)$ corresponding to nonzero eigenvalues. Then it follows that

(1) $PP^T S_B = S_B$,

(2) $PP^T S_W = S_W$.

Proof: Let $Q = [\mathbf{q}_1, \dots, \mathbf{q}_s]$ be the matrix of all unit eigenvectors of the total scatter matrix corresponding to zero eigenvalues. It is obvious that $V = [P \ Q]$ is a unitary matrix.

Since $\mathbf{q}_i (i = 1, 2, \dots, s)$ is an eigenvector of S_T corresponding to zero eigenvalue, it follows that $S_T \mathbf{q}_i = \mathbf{0}$. Thus we have $\mathbf{q}_i^T S_B \mathbf{q}_i + \mathbf{q}_i^T S_W \mathbf{q}_i = \mathbf{0}$. In consideration of the fact that S_B and S_W are both semi-positive matrices, it can be concluded that $\mathbf{q}_i^T S_B \mathbf{q}_i = \mathbf{0}$

and $\mathbf{q}_i^T S_W \mathbf{q}_i = \mathbf{0}$. Using the Theorem 2 in Liu, Cheng and Yang (1992a) it follows that $\mathbf{q}_i^T S_B = \mathbf{0}$ and $\mathbf{q}_i^T S_W = \mathbf{0}$. As a consequence, we have

$$S_B = VV^T S_B = PP^T S_B + QQ^T S_B = PP^T S_B + Q \begin{pmatrix} \mathbf{q}_1^T S_B \\ \vdots \\ \mathbf{q}_s^T S_B \end{pmatrix} = PP^T S_B,$$

and

$$S_W = VV^T S_W = PP^T S_W + QQ^T S_W = PP^T S_W + Q \begin{pmatrix} \mathbf{q}_1^T S_W \\ \vdots \\ \mathbf{q}_s^T S_W \end{pmatrix} = PP^T S_W.$$

Theorem 6.1. Let $P \in R^{d \times t}$ be the matrix of all unit eigenvectors of the total scatter matrix S_T corresponding to nonzero eigenvalues and $\varphi \in R^{t \times 1}$ to be the eigenvector of the matrix $P^T(S_B - c \cdot S_W)P$ corresponding to the eigenvalue λ. Then $P\varphi$ is the eigenvector of the matrix $S_B - c \cdot S_W$ corresponding to the eigenvalue λ.

Proof: Since φ is the eigenvector of the matrix $P^T(S_B - c \cdot S_W)P$ corresponding to the eigenvalue λ, we have

$$P^T(S_B - c \cdot S_W)P\varphi = \lambda\varphi \Rightarrow PP^T(S_B - c \cdot S_W)P\varphi = \lambda P\varphi$$
$$\Rightarrow (PP^T S_B - c \cdot PP^T S_W)P\varphi = \lambda P\varphi \qquad .$$

From Lemma 6.1, it follows that $(S_B - c \cdot S_W)P\varphi = \lambda P\varphi$.
Thus, we complete the proof of the theorem.

According to Theorem 6.1, we can calculate the MMSD discriminant vectors in a high-dimensional input space in three major steps: First, we calculate the matrix of

Algorithm 6.1. Facial feature extraction algorithm based on MMSD

Input: Training samples $\mathbf{x}_1, \mathbf{x}_2, ..., \mathbf{x}_N$, class labels of these samples $l(\mathbf{x}_1), ..., l(\mathbf{x}_N)$, parameter value c, and the number of extracted features r
Output: The discriminant matrix of MMSD V

1. Compute the between-class scatter matrix S_B, the with-class scatter matrix S_W, and the total scatter matrix S_T.
2. Calculate the matrix P of all unit eigenvectors of S_T corresponding to nonzero eigenvalues using the singular value decomposition theorem.
3. Work out the matrix U of the first r unit eigenvectors of $P^T(S_B - c \cdot S_W)P$ corresponding to the largest eigenvalues.
4. Compute the discriminant matrix of MMSD using the formula $V = PU$.

all unit eigenvector of the total scatter matrix corresponding nonzero eigenvalues, P using singular value decomposition theorem; second, we map the high-dimensional input space into the range of the total scatter matrix using $P^T : R^d \rightarrow R^t, \mathbf{x} \mapsto P^T \mathbf{x}$; and third, we perform eigen decomposition on the matrix $P^T (S_B - c \cdot S_W) P$. Algorithm 6.1 is a detailed description of the novel facial feature extraction algorithm based on MMSD.

6.1.3 Theoretical Analyses of MMSD Feature Extraction Method

To further investigate MMSD feature extraction method we explored its relationship to other feature extraction approaches. Section 6.1.3.1 reveals the relation between MMSD and Principal Component Analysis. Section 6.1.3.2 reveals the relation between MMSD and Karhunen-Loève expansion. Section 6.1.3.3 reveals the relation between MMSD and N-LDA. And Section 6.1.3.4 discusses the physical meaning of the parameter of MMSD.

6.1.3.1 Connection to Principal Component Analysis

Although MMSD is a supervised feature extraction method, it is closely related to a well-known unsupervised feature extraction approach, PCA. When the parameter c assumes the value of -1, the generalized scatter difference matrix is $S_B - (-1) \cdot S_W = S_B + S_W = S_T$, i.e. the total scatter matrix. This implies that when c = -1 MMSD discriminant vectors are in fact principal component directions.

In facial feature extraction, we can obtain eigenfaces of MMSD by reverting MMSD discriminant vectors to images. Figure 6.1 displays the first seven eigenfaces of MMSD when the parameter c assumes the values of -1, 1, 10, 100, and 1000. These eigenfaces are calculated on the training set, which consists of the first five images of each individual from the ORL face image database. As shown earlier, the eigenfaces of MMSD are actually Eigenface (Belhumeur et al., 1997) when the parameter c assumes the value of -1 and as can be seen in Figure 6.1, the details in the MMSD eigenfaces increases with the value of the parameter c.

6.1.3.2 Connection to K-L Expansion Based on the Between-Class Scatter Matrix

When the parameter c assumes the value of 0, MMSD degenerates into a feature extraction method which derives its discriminant vectors in the range of the between-class scatter matrix. In fact, MMSD is equivalent to the Karhunen-Loève (K-L) expansion whose generation matrix is the between-class scatter matrix S_B. Here discriminant vectors of MMSD are orthonormal eigenvectors of the matrix

Figure 6.1. The first seven eigenfaces of MMSD when the parameter c are -1, 1, 10, 100, and 1000, respectively

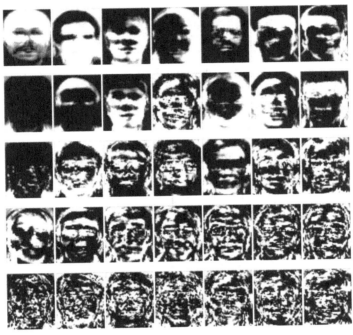

S_B corresponding to the r largest eigenvalues. It implies that discriminant vectors of MMSD are solely dependent on the objective (6.2) in this case.

6.1.3.3 Asymptotic Property of MMSD

The asymptotic property of MMSD is revealed by the following theorem.

Theorem 6.2 If S_W is singular, discriminant vectors of MMSD are approaching discriminant vectors of N-LDA when the value of the parameter c is approaching infinity.

Proof: We only prove that the first discriminant vector of MMSD is approaching the first discriminant vector of N-LDA when the value of the parameter c is approaching infinity. Other proofs are similar.

Let $\mathbf{w}_b$, $\mathbf{w}_c$ be the unit eigenvectors of matrices S_B, $(S_B - c \cdot S_W)$ corresponding to the largest eigenvalues λ_b, λ_c respectively. Since S_W is a singular matrix, there exists a nonzero unit vector $\mathbf{w}_0$ such that $S_W \mathbf{w}_0 = 0$. Considering the fact that S_B is a semi-positive matrix, we have

$$\lambda_c = \max_{\|\mathbf{w}\|=1} \mathbf{w}^T (S_b - C \cdot S_w) \mathbf{w} \geq \mathbf{w}_0^T S_b \mathbf{w}_0 - C \cdot \mathbf{w}_0^T S_w \mathbf{w}_0 = \mathbf{w}_0^T S_b \mathbf{w}_0 \geq 0.$$

$$(6.7)$$

From the meaning of λ_c and $\mathbf{w}_c$ the following equation is always true for any positive real number c:

$$(S_B - c \cdot S_W) \mathbf{w}_c = \lambda_c \mathbf{w}_c. \tag{6.8}$$

By combining equality (6.8), inequality (6.7) and the meaning of λ_b we obtain:

$$\mathbf{w}_c^T S_W \mathbf{w}_c = \frac{1}{c}(\mathbf{w}_c^T S_B \mathbf{w}_c - \lambda_c) \leq \frac{1}{c} \mathbf{w}_c^T S_B \mathbf{w}_c \leq \frac{1}{c} \lambda_b. \tag{6.9}$$

Since the matrix S_W is also semi-positive, the following inequality holds:

$$\mathbf{w}_c^T S_W \mathbf{w}_c \geq 0. \tag{6.10}$$

By combining inequalities (6.9) and (6.10) we can conclude that

$$\lim_{c \to \infty} \mathbf{w}_c^T S_W \mathbf{w}_c = 0. \tag{6.11}$$

Thus we complete the proof of the theorem. From the theorem it is easy to understand that N-LDA is in fact an asymptotic form of MMSD.

6.1.3.4 The Physical Meaning of the Parameter

From previous discussions we find that, like C-LDA, MMSD derives its discriminant vectors both in the range of the between-class scatter matrix and in the null space of the within-class scatter matrix. But MMSD is much more flexible than C-LDA. The parameter c can be used to adjust the balance between the two subspaces. When $c = 0$, the discriminant vectors of MMSD are solely from the range of the between-class scatter matrix .With the increase of the value of c from zero to infinite, the discriminant vectors of MMSD are more and more from the null space of the within-class scatter matrix. When the parameter c is approaching infinity, the discriminant vectors of MMSD are solely from the null space of the within-class scatter matrix.

6.1.4 Experimental Evaluation

MMSD was evaluated on the same subset of the FERET database as shown in Section 3.4.4. Similarly, all images were resized to 80×80 pixels and preprocessed by histogram equalization. In all experiments we used the nearest neighbor (NN) classifier with Euclidean distance.

6.1.4.1 Accuracy of MMSD vs. No. of Extracted Features and the Parameter Value

Three images of each individual were randomly chosen for training, while the remaining four images were used for testing. Thus, the training sample set size was 600 and the testing sample set size was 800. In this way, we ran the system ten times and obtained ten different training and testing sample sets. Figure 6.2 demonstrates average recognition rates of MMSD over various numbers of extracted features and different values of the parameter c. From Figure 6.2 we find two facts: First, the effectiveness of MMSD is quite robust on the number of extracted features; second, the effectiveness of MMSD is sensitive to the value of the parameter c.

6.1.4.2 Comparison of MMSD with Other Facial Feature Extraction Methods

The experimental design is the same as in Section 6.1.4.1. To make N-LDA applicable, PCA is first used to compress a high-dimensional image space into the range

Figure 6.2. Average recognition rate of MMSD over the number of extracted features and the value of the parameter c

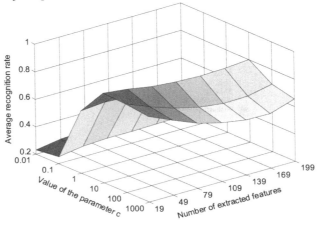

of the total scatter matrix. Figure 6.3 displays curves of average recognition rates of MMSD ($c = 10$), NSM, D-LDA, Eigenface, and Fisherface. From Figure 6.3 we find that MMSD is much more effective than the other four facial feature extraction methods and Fisherface achieve its maximum value at 49.

6.1.4.3 Further Comparison of MMSD with Fisherface and Other Methods

According to Yang et al. (2005) the accuracy of Fisherface is heavily dependent on the number of principal components used in the PCA stage. In this subsection we compare MMSD with N-LDA, D-LDA, and Fisherface in the cases where the number of principal components used in the PCA stage varies from 50 to 400. The experimental design is the same as in Section 6.14.1. The number of extracted feature for each method is 49. The value of the parameter c of MMSD is 10. Figure 6.4 displays curves of average recognition rates of various feature extraction methods over varying number of principal components. We can see that MMSD outperforms the other three feature extraction methods when there are more than 100 principal components.

6.1.4.4 Experimental Results over Varying Number of Training Samples per Individual

Taking into account the statement that the accuracy of D-LDA is heavily dependent on the number of training samples per individual as mentioned in Section 5.2.3.4,,we

Figure 6.3. Average recognition rates of various methods vs. the number of extracted features

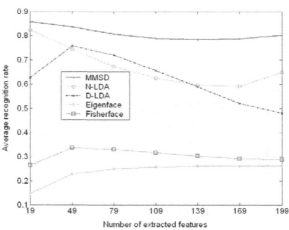

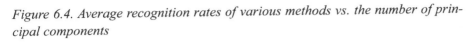

Figure 6.4. Average recognition rates of various methods vs. the number of principal components

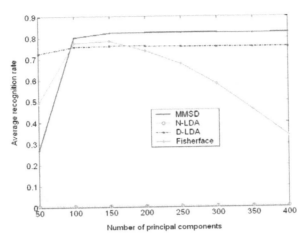

compare the effectiveness of MMSD with that of N-LDA, D-LDA, Eigenface, Fisherface, and C-LDA when the number of training samples per individual varies from 2 to 6. The experiment consisted of five tests of seven runs each. In each run of the ith test, $(i + 1)$ images of each individual were used for training and the remaining $(6 - i)$ images for testing. Images of each individual numbered 1 to $(i + 1)$, 2 to $(i + 2)$, ..., 7 to i were used as training samples in the first, second,..., seventh run respectively. The number of extracted features for MMSD, N-LDA, D-LDA, Fisherface, Eigenface, and C-LDA in the ith test are respectively 199, 199, 199, 199, $200i + 199$, and 398. Figure 6.5 displays curves of average recognition rates of various feature extraction methods over varying number of training samples per individual. MMSD is again the most effective of the facial feature extraction approaches that were tested.

6.1.4.5 Comparison of MMSD with MSD

The comparison of effectiveness of MMSD with effectiveness of MSD is conducted on a small database, ORL (please refer to Section 3.2.3). In each of the ten runs, we use five images of each person for training and the remaining five for testing. The images of each person numbered 1 to 5, 2 to 6, ..., 10 to 4 are used as training samples for the first, second,..., and the tenth run respectively. In the experiment, the number of features extracted by MMSD is 39 and the classifier used in combination with MMSD is the nearest neighbor. Table 6.1 lists the means and standard

Figure 6.5. Average recognition rates of various feature extraction methods vs. the numbers of training samples per individual

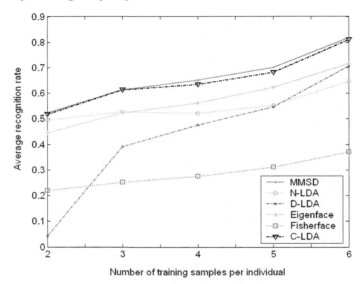

Number of training samples per individual

Table 6.1. Means and standard deviations of recognition rates of MMSD and MSD

Parameter c		10	100	1000
MMSD	Mean	0.9605	0.9625	0.9630
	Std	0.0140	0.0153	0.0140
MSD	Mean	0.9505	0.9525	0.9515
	Std	0.0192	0.0186	0.0197

deviations of recognition rates of MMSD and MSD using various values of the parameter c. Experimental results indicate that MMSD is more effective than MSD on the ORL face image database.

6.1.4.6 Efficiencies of MMSD and MSD on the ORL Database

The chief motivation for extending MSD to MMSD is to promote efficiency. In this subsection we compare the efficiency of an MSD classifier with that of MMSD in combination with a NN classifier on the ORL database. The experimental design is the same as in Section 6.1.4.5. Figure 6.6 displays the time (seconds) taken by the MSD classifier and MMSD in combination with a NN classifier for pattern clas-

Figure 6.6. Comparison of the efficiencies of MSD classifiers with MMSD + NN classifiers on the ORL face image database

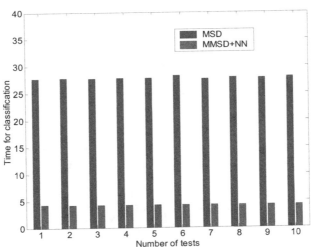

sification in each run on the ORL database. MMSD in combination with an NN classifier is much faster than an MSD classifier.

6.1.4.7 Efficiency Comparison of MMSD and Other Methods on the FERET Database

In this subsection we compare the efficiency of MMSD with that of N-LDA, D-LDA, Fisherface, and C-LDA on the FERET database. The experimental design is the same as in Section 6.1.4.4. Figure 6.7 displays the average time (seconds) taken by various methods used for feature extraction in each test on the FERET database. Although slower than D-LDA and Fisherface, MMSD is faster than N-LDA and C-LDA.

6.2 FEATURE EXTRACTION BASED ON COEFFICIENTS OF VARIANCES

PCA and LDA are two popular feature extraction techniques in statistical pattern recognition field. It is generally believed that PCA extracts the most representative features whereas LDA extracts the most discriminative features. Theoretically speaking, LDA features should be more suitable for classification than PCA features but PCA does outperform LDA for face recognition in certain circumstances (Martinez & Kak, 2001).

Figure 6.7. Efficiency comparison of MMSD with those of N-LDA, D-LDA, Fisherface, and C-LDA on the FERET database

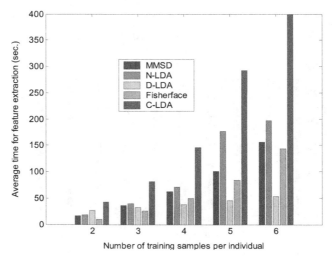

Extensive experimental results show that nullspace LDA (N-LDA) is one of the most effective techniques for face recognition. N-LDA tries to find a set of discriminant vectors which maximize the between-class scatter in the null space of the within-class scatter matrix. The calculation of its discriminant vectors involves performing singular value decomposition on a high-dimensional matrix. It is generally memory- and time-consuming.

One of the key ideas of the N-LDA is to calculate discriminant vectors in the null space of the within-class scatter matrix. Its main advantage is that projections of training samples from each class are exactly the same when they are projected on discriminant vectors. Thus, the difference between the projection of a test sample and projections of training samples from a certain class is a good metric of its pertinence to this class. Borrowing the idea in N-LDA and the concept of coefficient of variance in statistical analysis we present a novel facial feature extraction method, i.e. discriminant based on coefficient of variance (DCV) in this section.

6.2.1 Dimensionality Reduction Based on Coefficient of Variation

In this subsection, at first we introduce the concept of the minimum coefficient of variance (MCV) direction, then present calculation methods for this direction, and last propose a feature extraction method based on MCV directions for each class of training samples.

6.2.1.1 Definition of the MCV Direction

Before defining the concept of the MCV direction, let us briefly review the term of coefficient of variation of a dataset.

Let $y_1,...,y_n$ be a set of scalars, $\bar{y} = \frac{1}{n}\sum_{i=1}^{n} y_i$ and $\sigma^2 = \frac{1}{n}\sum_{i=1}^{n}(y_i - \bar{y})^2$ be its sample mean and sample variance respectively. The coefficient of variation (CV) of the dataset $y_1,...,y_n$ is defined as follows:

$$CV = \frac{\sigma}{\bar{y}}. \tag{6.12}$$

CV is a measure of scatter of a dataset. The smaller the CV score of a dataset the less disperse the dataset.

Suppose that $x_1,...,x_n$ is a group of d-dimensional samples from a certain class. When they are projected on a one-dimensional subspace spanned by a direction $\mathbf{w} \in R^{d \times 1}$ ($\mathbf{w} \neq \mathbf{0}$), a set of scalars $\mathbf{w}^T x_1,...,\mathbf{w}^T x_n$ is obtained and the corresponding CV score, i.e. the CV score of the class of samples along the direction, $CV(\mathbf{w})$ can be calculated.

Definition 6.1 A direction is called a MCV direction of a class of samples, if the absolute value of the CV score of the set of samples from the class along this direction is the smallest.

The definition of MCV direction means that when a d-dimensional dataset is projected on its MCV direction the density of the projected dataset is the highest and the square of the mean of the projected dataset is synchronously the largest. If a direction is used to judge whether an unknown sample comes from a certain class according to projections of samples on it, the MCV direction of training samples from the class is out of question the best choice.

Fig 6.8 shows the MCV direction and the PCA direction for a two-dimensional dataset. From the figure we find that: 1. While the PCA direction $\mathbf{w}_{PCA}$ achieves the maximum variance of the projected dataset, the MCV direction $\mathbf{w}_{MCV}$ achieves the minimum coefficient of variance of the projected dataset; 2. The direction $\mathbf{w}_{MCV}$ is slightly different from the direction $\mathbf{w}_0$ which achieves the minimum variance of the projected dataset and is perpendicular to the PCA direction $\mathbf{w}_{PCA}$; 3. We can conclude that the sample $\mathbf{x}$ is an outlier of the dataset with enough confidence since the projection of $\mathbf{x}$ on $\mathbf{w}_{MCV}$ is apart from projections of samples from the dataset.

6.2.1.2 Calculation of a MCV Direction

When dataset $\mathbf{x}_1,...,\mathbf{x}_n$ is projected on a one-dimensional subspace spanned by a direction $\mathbf{w}$, the CV score of the dataset along this direction is

$$CV(\mathbf{w}) = \frac{\sqrt{\frac{1}{n}\mathbf{w}^T\left[\sum_{i=1}^{n}(\mathbf{x}_i-\mathbf{m})(\mathbf{x}_i-\mathbf{m})^T\right]\mathbf{w}}}{\mathbf{w}^T\mathbf{m}}$$

$$= \frac{\sqrt{\mathbf{w}^T S\mathbf{w}}}{\mathbf{w}^T\mathbf{m}}. \tag{6.13}$$

Here $\mathbf{m} = \frac{1}{n}\sum_{i=1}^{n}\mathbf{x}_i$ is the mean sample, and $S = \frac{1}{n}\sum_{i=1}^{n}(\mathbf{x}_i-\mathbf{m})(\mathbf{x}_i-\mathbf{m})^T$ the scatter

matrix. Thus, the MCV direction is a solution of the following optimization model,

$$\min\frac{\sqrt{\mathbf{w}^T S\mathbf{w}}}{|\mathbf{w}^T\mathbf{m}|}, \tag{6.14}$$

which is equivalent to the following one,

$$\min\frac{\mathbf{w}^T S\mathbf{w}}{\mathbf{w}^T\mathbf{m}\mathbf{m}^T\mathbf{w}}. \tag{6.15}$$

From model (6.15) we find that if $\mathbf{w}^*$ is a MCV direction, $k\mathbf{w}^*$ is a MCV direction as well. Here k is an arbitrary nonzero real number. Since they span the same one-dimensional subspace they are viewed as one direction in this subsection. Thereafter we assume that MCV directions are unit vectors for simplicity.

Theorem 6.3 and Theorem 6.4 give a solution of the optimization model (6.15) when S is nonsingular or singular respectively.

Theorem 6.3 If S is nonsingular, the eigenvector of the matrix $S^{-1}\mathbf{m}\mathbf{m}^T$ corresponding to the largest eigenvalue is a MCV direction.

Proof. The Lagrangian Function of $f(\mathbf{w}) = \dfrac{\mathbf{w}^T S\mathbf{w}}{\mathbf{w}^T\mathbf{m}\mathbf{m}^T\mathbf{w}}$ is

$$L(\mathbf{w}) = \mathbf{w}^T S \mathbf{w} - \lambda \cdot (\mathbf{w}^T \mathbf{mm}^T \mathbf{w} - c).$$

Let $\dfrac{\partial L}{\partial \mathbf{w}} = 0$, we have $S^{-1} \mathbf{mm}^T \mathbf{w} = \dfrac{1}{\lambda} \mathbf{w}$.

Suppose $\mathbf{w}^*$ be an eigenvector of matrix $S^{-1} \mathbf{mm}^T$ corresponding to the largest eigenvalue ν. We have $\dfrac{\mathbf{w}^{*T} S \mathbf{w}^*}{\mathbf{w}^{*T} \mathbf{mm}^T \mathbf{w}^*} = \dfrac{1}{\nu}$.

It means that the function $f(\mathbf{w})$ achieves its minimum at $\mathbf{w}^*$. Thus, $\mathbf{w}^*$ is a MCV direction.

□

If S is singular, there might exist infinite different directions whose corresponding CV values are zero. Thus, the MCV direction can not be properly calculated. In this case, a MCV direction is defined as one unit vector which is in the null space of S and maximizes the square of the mean of projected dataset. That is, a MCV direction is a solution of the following optimization model:

$$\max_{\substack{\mathbf{w} \in N(S) \\ \|\mathbf{w}\|=1}} \mathbf{w}^T \mathbf{mm}^T \mathbf{w}. \tag{6.16}$$

Here $N(S) = \{\mathbf{x} \in R^d \mid S\mathbf{x} = \mathbf{0}\}$ is the null space of S.

Theorem 6.4 Suppose $\varphi_1, ..., \varphi_k$ be an orthonormal basis for $N(S)$. The unit vector $\Phi\Phi^T \mathbf{m} / \|\Phi\Phi^T \mathbf{m}\|$ is a MCV direction. Here $\Phi = [\varphi_1, ..., \varphi_k]$, and $\|\Phi\Phi^T \mathbf{m}\|$ is the 2-norm of $\Phi\Phi^T \mathbf{m}$.

Proof For any vector $\mathbf{w}$ in $N(S)$, there exists a group of scalars $a_1, ..., a_k$ such that

$$\mathbf{w} = \sum_{i=1}^{k} a_i \varphi_i = \Phi \mathbf{a}.$$

Here $\mathbf{a} = [a_1, ..., a_k]^T$. Since $\Phi^T \Phi$ is an identity matrix, the optimization model (6.16) can be transformed into:

$$\max_{\mathbf{a}^T \mathbf{a}=1} \mathbf{a}^T \Phi^T \mathbf{mm}^T \Phi \mathbf{a}. \tag{6.17}$$

By using Lagrange multiplier, it is easy to conclude that vector $\mathbf{a} = \Phi^T \mathbf{m} / \|\Phi^T \mathbf{m}\|$ is one solution of above optimization problem. Thus, the unit vector $\Phi\Phi^T \mathbf{m} / \|\Phi\Phi^T \mathbf{m}\|$ is a MCV direction.

When *d*, the dimensionality of a dataset, is very large the calculation of an orthonormal basis for *N(S)* is not a simple task. It will consume a large amount of memory and computing time to find a MCV direction. Handy calculating method should be considered. Theorem 6.5 provides a simple approach to calculate a MCV direction when *S* is singular.

Before presenting the theorem a lemma is introduced first.

Lemma 6.2 (Liu, Cheng, & Yang, 1992b) Let $A \in R^{n \times n}$ be a real symmetric matrix, $\mathbf{w} \in R^{n \times 1}$ a real column vector. It can be concluded that $A\mathbf{w} = \mathbf{0}$ if and only if $\mathbf{w}^T A \mathbf{w} = \mathbf{0}$.

Theorem 6.5 A MCV direction for a dataset $\mathbf{x}_1, ..., \mathbf{x}_n$ can be calculated using the formula

$$\mathbf{w}_{MCV} = (X^T)^+ \mathbf{1}_n / \left\| (X^T)^+ \mathbf{1}_n \right\|.$$

Here $X = \mathbf{x}_1, ..., \mathbf{x}_n$ is the data matrix, A^+ is the Moore-Penrose inverse of A, $\mathbf{1}_n$ is a column vector with all *n* elements being ones.

Proof: From the definition of the scatter matrix S ($S = \frac{1}{n} \sum_{i=1}^{n} (\mathbf{x}_i - \mathbf{m})(\mathbf{x}_i - \mathbf{m})^T$), we have

$$\mathbf{w}^T S \mathbf{w} = \mathbf{0} \Leftrightarrow \frac{1}{n} \sum_{i=1}^{n} [\mathbf{w}^T (\mathbf{x}_i - \mathbf{m})]^2 = 0 \Leftrightarrow \forall i \in [1, ..., n], \mathbf{w}^T \mathbf{x}_i = \mathbf{w}^T \mathbf{m}.$$

Since *S* is a real symmetric matrix, from Lemma 1 we know that

$$\mathbf{w} \in N(S) \Leftrightarrow \mathbf{w}^T S \mathbf{w} = \mathbf{0} \Leftrightarrow \forall i \in [1, ..., n], (\frac{\mathbf{w}}{\mathbf{w}^T \mathbf{m}})^T \mathbf{x}_i = 1.$$

Let **v** denote $\mathbf{w} / \mathbf{w}^T \mathbf{m}$. The constrain of the optimization model (6.16) is converted into $\mathbf{v}^T \mathbf{x}_i = 1, i = 1, ..., n$ and $\|\mathbf{w}\| = 1$.

Since the objective of the optimization model (6.16) is max $\mathbf{w}^T \mathbf{m} \mathbf{m}^T \mathbf{w} = \frac{\mathbf{w}^T \mathbf{w}}{\mathbf{v}^T \mathbf{v}}$, which can be rewritten as min $\frac{\mathbf{v}^T \mathbf{v}}{\|\mathbf{w}\|^2}$, the optimization model (6.16) can be transformed into

$$\min_{\mathbf{v}^T \mathbf{x}_i = 1,\, i=1,\dots,n} \mathbf{v}^T \mathbf{v}, \tag{6.18}$$

and

$$\mathbf{w} = \mathbf{v}/\|\mathbf{v}\|. \tag{6.19}$$

The constraint of the optimization model (6.18) can be written in the following matrix form $\mathbf{v}^T \begin{bmatrix} \mathbf{x}_1 & \cdots & \mathbf{x}_n \end{bmatrix} = \begin{bmatrix} 1 & \cdots & 1 \end{bmatrix}$ which can be further converted into $X^T \mathbf{v} = \mathbf{1}_n$. In a point of view of matrix theory the optimization model (6.18) tries to find the minimum norm minimum square error solution for a system of linear equations. Thus, the unique solution of the optimization model (6.18) can readily be computed by

$$\mathbf{v} = (X^T)^+ \mathbf{1}_n. \tag{6.20}$$

□

6.2.1.3 Discriminant Based on Coefficient of Variance

Assume $\mathbf{x}_1,\dots,\mathbf{x}_N$ be a set of training samples from l classes, with N_i samples from the ith class. For class i $(i = 1,\dots,l)$ there is a MCV direction $\mathbf{w}_i$ corresponding to training samples from that class. Due to similarities between samples from different classes, MCV vectors $\mathbf{w}_1,\dots,\mathbf{w}_l$ are generally dependent. In order to eliminate linear dependency among them, the Gram-Schmidt orthogonalization and normalization procedure is performed here.

Let

$$\mathbf{u}_1 = \mathbf{w}_1/\|\mathbf{w}_1\|, \tag{6.21}$$

$$\mathbf{v}_i = \mathbf{w}_i - \sum_{j=1}^{i-1}(\mathbf{u}_j^T \mathbf{w}_i)\mathbf{u}_j, \tag{6.22}$$

$$\mathbf{u}_i = \mathbf{v}_i/\|\mathbf{v}_i\|,\ 2 \leq i \leq l. \tag{6.23}$$

We call $\mathbf{u}_1,\dots,\mathbf{u}_l$ the discriminant vectors based on coefficient of variance.

Once discriminant vectors $\mathbf{u}_1,\dots,\mathbf{u}_l$ are calculated, the d-dimensional input space can be mapped into a l-dimensional feature space by the discriminant matrix $U = \mathbf{u}_1,\dots,\mathbf{u}_l$. We call this dimensionality reduction method discriminant based on coefficient of variance (DCV). The feature extraction procedure of DCV is illustrated in Figure 6.9. The physical meaning, advantages and disadvantages of DCV will be discussed in some detail in Section 6.2.4.

6.2.2 Experimental Evaluation

We applied DCV to face recognition in order to test its accuracy and compared it with six famous facial feature extraction methods: Fisherface, the orthogonal complimentary space method, Eigenface, N-LDA, uncorrelated linear discriminant analysis (U-LDA), and D-LDA on two benchmark face image databases, i.e. the FERET and AR (please refer to Section 3.4.4) face image database. The FERET dataset is used to evaluate the performance of DCV under conditions where the pose, sample size, and number of classes are varied. The AR dataset is employed to test the performance of DCV under conditions where there is a variation in facial expressions. In all experiments, the nearest neighbor decision rule is used in classification.

Figure 6.8. Illustration of the MCV direction and the PCA direction for a two-dimensional dataset

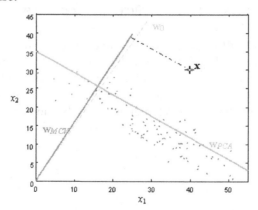

Figure 6.9. Flowchart of DCV

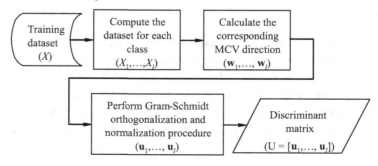

6.2.2.1 Experiment on the FERET Database

The same subset of the FERET database as shown in Section 3.4.4 is used in the experiment. All images are also resized and pre-processed by histogram equalization as shown in Section 3.4.4. In the experiment the number of classes, i.e. the number of individuals, k is varied from 100 to 200 with an interval 10. For a given number of classes there are seven tests for each feature extraction method. In each test, three images of each person are used for training and the remaining four images for testing. Thus the total amount of training samples and testing samples are $3 \times k$ and $4 \times k$ respectively. Three training samples are taken in turn, i.e. face images numbered 1 to 3, 2 to 4, ..., 7 to 2 for each individual are used as training samples respectively.

Figure 6.10 illustrates the tendencies of average recognition rates of each facial feature extraction method when the number of classes varies from 100 to 200. Partial experimental results are shown in Table 6.2. From Table 6.2 and Figure 6.10 we find that: 1. As other facial feature extraction method, the average recognition rate of DCV decreases with the increase of number of classes; 2. The proposed method always outperforms Fisherface, Eigenface, U-LDA, and D-LDA; 3. DCV is slightly inferior to N-LDA and OCS when the number of classes is small and is superior to them when the number of classes is large enough. An interesting fact is that OCS is as effective as N-LDA.

Figure 6.11 displays average times consumed by various feature extraction methods on this subset of FERET database. All results are derived from experiments performed on a PC with a P4 3.0GHz CPU and 1GB main memory running Microsoft Windows XP Professional. Here PCA, N-LDA, and FLD stand for the feature extraction methods Eigenface, nullspace LDA, and Fisherface respectively. From Figure 6.11 we find that DCV is much more efficient than N-LDA and OCS.

6.2.2.2 Experiment on the AR Database

The 119 individuals each having 26 face images taken in two sessions of the AR face database were involved in the experiment. For each individual, eight image samples taken under different lighting conditions (Please refer to Figure 3.10 (a), 3.10 (e), 3.10 (f), 3.10(g), 3.10 (n), 3.10 (r), 3.10 (s), and 3.10 (t)) were employed in the experiment. All images were also normalized and pre-processed using the same approch as shown in Section 3.4.4. For each individual, a sample from the first section and a sample from the second section are used as training samples and the remaining six samples are used for testing. Thus, the total numbers of training and test samples are 240 and 720 respectively. Since there are 16 (= 4×4) choices in the selection of training samples for each individual, the experiment contains 16 tests.

Figure 6.10. Average recognition rates of various feature extraction methods vs. No. of classes

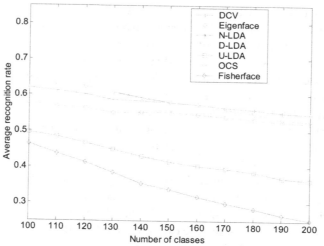

Table 6.2. The average recognition rates and standard deviations with varying number of classes on FERET database for various methods

		Number of classes (k)					
		100	120	140	160	180	200
Fisherface	mean	0.4636	0.4128	0.3538	0.3174	0.2837	0.2518
(k-1)	std	0.1019	0.0960	0.0859	0.0896	0.0834	0.0833
OCS	mean	0.6486	0.6229	0.5901	0.5703	0.5478	0.5282
(k-1)	std	0.1051	0.1142	0.1220	0.1261	0.1296	0.1326
Eigenface	mean	0.5779	0.5631	0.5515	0.5460	0.5317	0.5211
(3×k-1)	std	0.0664	0.0641	0.0725	0.0727	0.0716	0.0704
N-LDA	mean	0.6486	0.6229	0.5923	0.5703	0.5478	0.5282
(k-1)	std	0.1051	0.1142	0.1226	0.1261	0.1296	0.1326
U-LDA	mean	0.4957	0.4658	0.4291	0.4031	0.3865	0.3636
(k-1)	std	0.1017	0.0990	0.0956	0.0929	0.0891	0.1003
D-LDA	mean	0.5182	0.4911	0.4653	0.4379	0.4115	0.3914
(k-1)	std	0.1148	0.1084	0.1189	0.1118	0.1048	0.1068
DCV	mean	0.6200	0.6018	0.5842	0.5734	0.5595	0.5463
(k)	std	0.0718	0.0707	0.0724	0.0698	0.0667	0.0663

Figure 6.11. Average times for feature extraction of various methods on FERET database

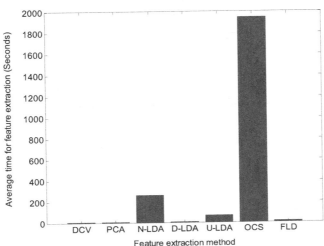

Table 6.3 reports the average recognition rates and standard deviations of various facial feature extraction methods on this subset of AR database.

From Table 6.3 we can conclude that DCV is superior to all feature extraction methods except OCS and N-LDA. Figure 6.12 displays average times consumed by various feature extraction methods on this subset of AR database. Here PCA and FLD stand for Eigenface and Fisherface respectively. From Figure 6.12 we find that DCV is again much more efficient than N-LDA and OCS.

6.2.3 Discussion on DCV

6.2.3.1 Necessity for Orthnormalization of the Matrix of MCV Vectors

In comparison to MCV vectors which are nature representatives for corresponding individuals' face images, DCV discriminant vectors emphasize deliberately different parts of face images for different individuals. Figure 6.13 and 6.14 show the two-dimensional displays of MCV vectors for some individuals in the FERET database and their corresponding DCV discriminant vectors, respectively.

Table 6.3. The average recognition rates and standard deviations of various methods on a subset of AR database with variances in facial expression

	Facial Feature Extraction Method						
	Fisherface (119)	OCS (119)	Eigenface (239)	N-LDA (119)	U-LDA (119)	D-LDA (119)	DCV (120)
mean	0.8761	0.9477	0.9189	0.9477	0.9082	0.2244	0.9270
std	0.0272	0.0174	0.0204	0.0174	0.0206	0.0174	0.0192

Figure 6.12. Average times for feature extraction of various methods on AR database

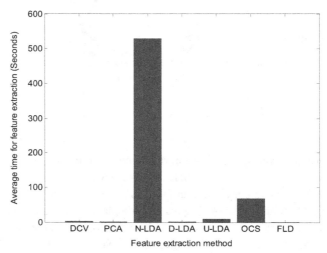

6.2.3.2 General Properties of the DCV Transform

Similar to LDA transforms, the DCV transform maps high-dimensional input spaces into low-dimensional feature spaces such that the samples from the same classes are as close as possible and the samples from the different classes are as apart as possible. Unlike most LDA algorithms which synchronously achieve the two goals—minimizing the within-class distances and maximizing the between-class distances, DCV achieves these two goals in two phases: First, it tries to minimize the within-class distances by projecting samples along MCV directions; second, it tries to maximize the between-class distances by eliminating the linear dependences among the MCV vectors. The discrimination process of DCV quite resembles that

Figure 6.13. Two-dimensional displays of MCV vectors for some individuals in FERET face image database

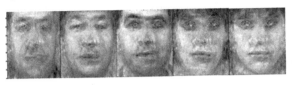

Figure 6.14. Two-dimensional displays of the DCV discriminant vectors corresponding to above individuals

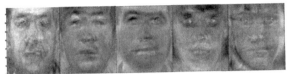

of human beings. When we discriminate different objects we first try to capture the chief characteristics of each object and then attempt to distinguish the differences between these characteristics.

Since the DCV calculates its discriminant vectors in two phases, it is much scalable for large-scale face recognition tasks in the following sense: When samples from new classes successively pool in the training dataset there is no need to recalculate all discriminant vectors but the MCV vectors and the corresponding DCV discriminant vectors of the newly added classes.

6.3 SUMMARY

In this chapter we introduce two novel facial feature extraction methods. The first is multiple maximum scatter difference (MMSD) which is an extension of a binary linear discriminant criterion, i.e. maximum scatter difference. The second is discriminant based on coefficients of variances (DCV) which can be viewed as a generalization of N-LDA. Experimental studies demonstrate that these two methods are both promising. Especially, MMSD outperforms almost all state-of-the-art facial feature extraction methods in terms of recognition accuracy.

REFERENCES

Belhumeur, P. N., Hespanha, J. P., & Krieqman, D. J. (1997). Eigenfaces vs. Fisher-faces: recognition using class specific linear projection. *IEEE Trans. Pattern Anal. Machine Intell.*, *19*(7), 711-720.

Chen, L., Liao, H., Ko, M., Lin, J., & Yu, G. (2000). A new lda-based face recognition system which can solve the small sample size problem. *Pattern Recognition*, *33*(10), 1713-1726.

Fukunaga, K. (1990). *Introduction to statistical pattern recognition* (2nd ed.). Boston: Academic Press.

Guo, Y. F., Li, S. J., Yang, J-Y., Shu, T. T., & Wu, L. D. (2003). A generalized Foley-Sammon transform based on generalized Fisher discriminant criterion and its application to face recognition. *Pattern Recognition Letters*, *24*(1-3), 147-158.

Hong, Z. Q., & Yang, J-Y. (1991). Optimal discriminant plane for a small number of samples and design method of classifier on the plane. *Pattern Recognition*, *24*(4), 317-324.

Hsu, C., & Lin, C. (2002). A comparison of methods for multiclass support vector machines. *IEEE Trans. Neural Networks*, *13*(2), 415-425.

Liu, K., Cheng, Y. Q., & Yang, J-Y. (1992a). A generalized optimal set of discriminant vectors. *Pattern Recognition*, *25*(7), 731-739.

Liu, K., Cheng, Y. Q., & Yang, J-Y. (1992b). An efficient algorithm for Foley-Sammon optimization set of discriminant vectors by algebraic method. *International Journal of Pattern Recognition and Artificial Intelligence*, *6*(5), 817-829.

Martinez, A. M., & Kak, A. C. (2001). PCA versus lda. *IEEE Trans. Pattern Anal. Machine Intell.*, *23*(2), 228-233.

Song, F. X., Liu, S. H., & Yang, J-Y. (2006). Face representation based on the multiple-class maximum scatter difference. *Acta Automatica Sinica (in Chinese)*, *32*(3), 378-385.

Song, F. X., Zhang, D., Chen, Q. L., & Wang, J. Z. (2007). Face recognition based on a novel linear discriminant criterion. *Pattern Analysis & Applications*, *10*(3), 165-174.

Song, F. X., Zhang, D., Mei, D. Y., & Guo, Z. W. (2007). A multiple maximum scatter difference discriminant criterion for facial feature extraction. *IEEE Trans. System, Man and Cybernetics, Part B*, *37*(6), 1599-1606.

Tao, D. C., Li, X. L., Hu, W. M., Maybank, S. J., & Wu, X. D. (2005). Supervised tensor learning. *Proc. IEEE Int'l Conf. Data Mining* (pp. 450-457).

Tao, D. C., Li, X. L., Maybank, S. J., & Wu, X. D. (2006). Human carrying status in visual surveillance. *Proc. IEEE Conf. Computer Vision and Pattern Recognition* (pp. 1670-1677).

Tian, Q., Barbero, M., Gu, Z. H., & Lee, S. H. (1986). Image classification by the Foley- Sammon transform. *Optical Engineering, 25*(7), 834-840.

Turk, M., & Pentland, A. (1991). Face Recognition Using Eigenfaces. *Proc. IEEE Conf. Computer Vision and Pattern Recognition* (pp. 586-591).

Yang, J., Frangi, A. F., Yang, J-Y., Zhang, D., & Jin, Z. (2005). KPCA plus lda: a complete kernel Fisher discriminant framework for feature extraction and recognition. *IEEE Trans. Pattern Anal. Machine Intell., 27*(2), 230-244.

Yu, H., & Yang, J. (2001). A direct LDA algorithm for high-dimensional data—with application to face recognition. *Pattern Recognition, 34* (10), 2067-2070.

Zhao, W., Chellappa, R., & Phillip, P. J. (1999). *Subspace linear discriminant analysis for face recognition* (Technical Report CAR-TR-914). Baltimore, MD: Center for Automatic Research, University of Maryland.

Section II
Tensor Technology

Chapter VII
Tensor Space

ABSTRACT

In this chapter, we first give the background materials for developing tensor discrimination technologies in Section 7.1. Section 7.2 introduces some basic notations in tensor space. Section 7.3 discusses several tensor decomposition methods. Section 7.4 introduces the tensor rank.

7.1 BACKGROUND

Matrix decompositions, such as the singular value decomposition (SVD), are ubiquitous in numerical analysis. One usual way to think of the SVD is that it decomposes a matrix into a sum of rank-1 matrices. In other words, an $I_1 \times I_2$ matrix A can be expressed as a minimal sum of rank-1 matrices:

$$A = u_1 \circ v_1 + u_2 \circ v_2 + \cdots + u_r \circ v_r, \tag{7.1}$$

where $u_i \in \mathfrak{R}^{I_1}$ and $v_i \in \mathfrak{R}^{I_2}$ for all $i = 1, \cdots, r$. The operator $\circ$ denotes the outer product. Thus the ijth entry of the rank-1 matrix $a \circ b$ is the product of the ith entry of a and the jth entry of b, denoted by $(a \circ b)_{ij} = a_i b_j$. Such decompositions provide possibilities to develop fundamental concepts such as the matrix rank and the approximation theory and gain a range of applications including WWW searching and mining, image processing, signal processing, medical imaging, and principal component analysis. The decompositions are well-understood mathematically, numerically, and computationally.

A tensor is a higher order generalization of a vector or a matrix. In fact, a vector is a first-order tensor and a matrix is a tensor of order two. Furthermore speaking, tensors are multilinear mapping over a set of vector spaces. If we have data in three or more dimensions, then we mean to deal with a higher-order tensor. In tensor analysis, higher-order tensor (also known as multidimensional, multiway, or n-way array) decompositions (Martin, 2004; Comon, 2002) are used in many fields and also have received considerable theoretical interest.

Different from some classical matrix decompositions, extending matrix decompositions such as the SVD to higher-order tensors has proven to be quite difficult. Familiar matrix concepts such as rank become ambiguous and more complicated. One goal of the tensor decomposition is the same as for a matrix decomposition: to rewrite the tensor as a sum of rank-1 tensors. Consider, for example, an $I_1 \times I_2 \times I_3$ tensor A. We would like to express A as the sum of rank-1 third-order tensors, that is,

$$A = u_1 \circ v_1 \circ w_1 + u_2 \circ v_2 \circ w_2 + \cdots + u_r \circ v_r \circ w_r, \qquad (7.2)$$

where, $u_i \in \mathfrak{R}^{I_1}$, $v_i \in \mathfrak{R}^{I_2}$, and $w_i \in \mathfrak{R}^{I_3}$ for all $i = 1, \cdots, r$. Note that if a, b, c are vectors, then $(a \circ b \circ c)_{ijk} = a_i b_j c_k$.

7.2 BASIC NOTATIONS

In this section, we introduce some elementary notations and definitions needed in the later chapter.

If A is an $I_1 \times \cdots \times I_N$ tensor, then the order of A is N. The nth mode, way, or dimension of A is of size $I_n (n = 1, \cdots, N)$.

7.2.1 Tensors as Vectors

First, let us define the operators. Let $B \in \mathfrak{R}^{I_1 \times I_2}$. Then vec($B$) is defined as

$$vec(B) = \begin{bmatrix} B(:,1) \\ \vdots \\ B(:,I_2) \end{bmatrix} \in \mathfrak{R}^{I_1 I_2}, \qquad (7.3)$$

where $B(:,i)$ denotes the ith column of matrix B.

In other words, the vec operator is to transform a matrix into a vector by stacking columns of matrix B.

Let $b \in \mathfrak{R}^{I_1 \times I_2}$. Then reshape($b, I_1 \times I_2$ is defined as

$$\text{reshape}(b, I_1 \times I_2 = \left[b(1:I_1) \big| b(I_1+1:2I_1) \big| \cdots \big| b((I_2-1)I_1 + 1 : I_1 I_2) \right] \in \mathfrak{R}^{I_1 \times I_2}.$$
(7.4)

In other words, reshape($b, I_1 \times I_2$ produces an $I_1 \times I_2$ matrix from b. In fact, the operators vec and reshape are related. It is straightforward to obtain

$$b = \text{vec}(\text{reshape}(b, I_1 \times I_2)), \tag{7.5}$$

$$\text{vec}(B) = \text{reshape}(B, I_1 \times I_2, 1. \tag{7.6}$$

Similarly, for, $A \in \mathfrak{R}^{I_1 \times I_2 \times I_3}$ then vec(A) is defined as

$$vec(A) = \begin{bmatrix} vec(A(:,:,1)) \\ \vdots \\ vec(:,:,I_3) \end{bmatrix} \in \mathfrak{R}^{I_1 \times I_2 \times I_3}. \tag{7.7}$$

For example: for $A \in \mathfrak{R}^{I_1 \times I_2 \times I_3}, I_1 = I_2 = I_3 = 2$

$$vec(A) = \begin{bmatrix} a_{111} \\ a_{211} \\ a_{121} \\ a_{221} \\ a_{112} \\ a_{212} \\ a_{122} \\ a_{222} \end{bmatrix}.$$

7.2.2 Tensors as Matrices

In real applications, it is often necessary to represent tensors as matrices. Typically, all the columns along a certain mode are rearranged to form a matrix. Transforming a tensor into a matrix in this way is referred as flattening, matricizing, or matrix unfolding. In general, there are multiple ways to order the columns. More than often not, the mode-n matricizing or matrix unfolding of an Nth-order A ($I_1 \times \cdots \times I_N$) is the set of vectors in $\mathfrak{R}^{I_n}$ obtained by keeping the index I_n fixed and varying the other indices. Therefore, the mode-n matricizing of an Nth-order tensor is a matrix $A_{(n)} \in \mathfrak{R}^{I_n \times \bar{I}_n}$, where

$$\bar{I}_n = \prod_{i \neq n} I_i .$$

In other words, the matrix unfolding $A_{(n)} \in \mathfrak{R}^{I_n \times (I_{n+1} \cdots I_N I_1 \cdots I_{n-1})}$ contains the elements $a_{i_1 \cdots i_N}$ at the position with row number i_n and column number equal to $(i_{n+1} - 1)I_{n+2} \cdots I_N I_1 \cdots I_{n-1} + (i_{n+2} - 1)I_{n+3} \cdots I_N I_1 \cdots I_{n-1} + \cdots + (i_N - 1)I_1 \cdots I_{n-1} + (i_1 - 1)I_2 \cdots I_{n-1} + (i_2 - 1)I_3 \cdots I_{n-1} + \cdots + i_{n-1}$.

For a third-order tensor, there are three possible flattening matrices. Figure 7.1 shows three possible cuts for a $2 \times 2 \times 2$ tensor.

As a result, there are three possible flattening matrices for a $2 \times 2 \times 2$ tensor A, denotes A as follows:

Figure 7.1. An illustration of a 2 × 2 × 2 tensor that is cut in three ways

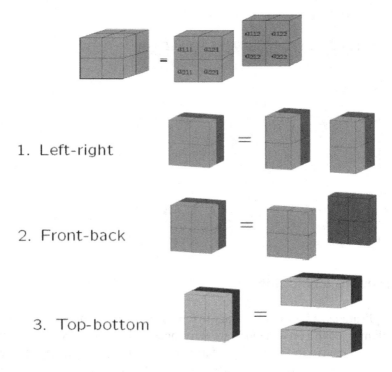

1. Left-right

2. Front-back

3. Top-bottom

Figure 7.2. Three flattening matrices of a third-order tensor

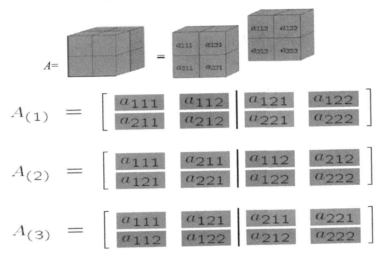

$$A_{(1)} = \begin{bmatrix} a_{111} & a_{112} & a_{121} & a_{122} \\ a_{211} & a_{212} & a_{221} & a_{222} \end{bmatrix}$$

$$A_{(2)} = \begin{bmatrix} a_{111} & a_{211} & a_{112} & a_{212} \\ a_{121} & a_{221} & a_{122} & a_{222} \end{bmatrix}$$

$$A_{(3)} = \begin{bmatrix} a_{111} & a_{121} & a_{211} & a_{221} \\ a_{112} & a_{122} & a_{212} & a_{222} \end{bmatrix}$$

7.2.3 Norms and Inner Products, Outer Product

If $A, B \in \mathfrak{R}^{I_1 \times I_2 \times I_3 \dots \times I_N}$, then the inner product is

$$\langle A, B \rangle = \sum_{i_1=1}^{I_1} \sum_{i_2=1}^{I_2} \sum_{i_3=1}^{I_3} \cdots \sum_{i_N=1}^{I_N} a_{i_1 \dots i_N} b_{i_1 \dots i_N} = vec(A)^T vec(B). \tag{7.8}$$

If $x \in \mathfrak{R}^{I_1}, y \in \mathfrak{R}^{I_2}$, then the outer product, yx^T, is a rank-1 matrix. Note that

$$vec(yx^T) \Leftrightarrow x \otimes y. \tag{7.9}$$

More generally, if x, y, z are vectors, $x \otimes y \otimes z$ is a rank-1 tensor.
If $A = U\Sigma V^T$, $U = [u_1, \dots u_n]$, and $V = [v_1, \dots v_n]$, then

$$A = \sum_{i=1}^{n} \sum_{j=1}^{n} \sigma_{ij} u_i v_j^T. \tag{7.10}$$

Further, it is easy to verify

$$vec(A) = \sum_{i=1}^{n}\sum_{j=1}^{n}\sigma_{ij}v_j \otimes u_i = V \otimes U)vec(\Sigma). \qquad (7.11)$$

When A is a three-order tensor, we have

$$vec(A) = \sum_{i=1}^{n}\sum_{j=1}^{n}\sum_{k=1}^{n}\sigma_{ijk}w_k \otimes v_j \otimes u_i.$$
$$= (W \otimes V \otimes U)vec(\Sigma). \qquad (7.12)$$

where $U = [u_1,\cdots,u_n]$, $V = [v_1,\cdots,v_n]$, and $W = [w_1,\cdots,w_n]$.
From Eq. (7.12), we have

$$A_{(1)} = U\Sigma_{(1)}(V \otimes W)^T,$$

$$A_{(2)} = V\Sigma_{(2)}(W \otimes U)^T,$$

$$A_{(3)} = W\Sigma_{(3)}(U \otimes V)^T.$$

7.2.4 N-Mode Multiplication

To multiply a tensor by a matrix, one needs to specify which mode of the tensor is multiplied by the columns of the matrix. Let us first have a look at the matrix product $G = U \cdot F \cdot V^T$, involving three matrices $F \in \mathfrak{R}^{I_1 \times I_2}$, $U \in \mathfrak{R}^{J_1 \times I_1}$ and $V \in \mathfrak{R}^{J_2 \times I_2}$. Note that the relationship between U and F and the relationship between V and F are completely similar: in the same way that U makes linear combinations of the rows of F, V makes linear combinations of the column of the column of F. In other words, the columns of F are multiplied by U and the rows of F are multiplied by V. Moreover, one can see that the columns of U are associated with the column space of G and the columns of V are associated with the row space of G. This typical relationship will be denoted by means of the $\times_n$ symbol $G = F \times_1 U \times_2 V$.

In general, the following definition (Lathauwer, Moor, & Vandewalle, 1994, 1996a, 1996b)for the n-mode product of a tensor is given.

Definition 7.1. The n-mode product of a tensor $A \in \mathfrak{R}^{I_1 \times I_2 \times I_3 \cdots \times I_N}$ by a matrix $U \in \mathfrak{R}^{J_n \times I_n}$, denoted by $A \times_n U$ is an $(I_1 \times I_2 \times \cdots \times I_{n-1} \times J_n \times I_{n+1} \cdots \times I_N)$-tensor of which the entries are given by

$$(A \times_n U)_{i_1 \cdots i_{n-1} j_n i_{n+1} \cdots i_N} = \sum_{i_n} a_{i_1 \cdots i_{n-1} i_n i_{n+1} \cdots i_N} u_{j_n i_n}. \tag{7.13}$$

Based on the definition of the *n*-mode product, one can obtain

Property 7.2. Given the tensor $A \in \mathfrak{R}^{I_1 \times I_2 \times I_3 \cdots \times I_N}$ and the matrices $F \in \mathfrak{R}^{J_n \times I_n}$ and $G \in \mathfrak{R}^{J_m \times I_m}$, one has

$$(A \times_n F) \times_m G = (A \times_m G) \times_n \cdot F = A \times_n F) \times_m G. \tag{7.14}$$

Property 7.3. Given the tensor $A \in \mathfrak{R}^{I_1 \times I_2 \times I_3 \cdots \times I_N}$ and the matrices $F \in \mathfrak{R}^{J_n \times I_n}$ and $G \in \mathfrak{R}^{K_n \times I_n}$, one has

$$(A \times_n F) \times_n G = (A \times_n (G \cdot F)). \tag{7.15}$$

Often the following simplified notations are used in the case of the *n*-mode product of a tensor by some researchers.

$$A \times_1 U_1 \times_2 U_2 \times \cdots \times_N U_N \stackrel{def}{=} A \prod_{k=1}^{N} \times_k U_k, \tag{7.16}$$

and

$$A \times_1 U_1 \times_2 U_2 \times \cdots \times_{i-1} U_{i-1} \times_{i+1} U_{i+1} \cdots \times_N U_N \stackrel{def}{=} A \prod_{k=1, k \neq i}^{N} \times_k U_k \stackrel{def}{=} A \bar{\times}_i U_i, \tag{7.17}$$

where $U_i (i = 1, \cdots, N)$ are matrices.

Figure 7.3 shows the equation $A = B \times_1 U_1 \times_2 U_2 \times_3 U_3$ for the third-order tensors $A \in \mathfrak{R}^{J_1 \times J_2 \times J_3}$, and $B \in \mathfrak{R}^{I_1 \times I_2 \times I_3}$. Different from the classical way to visualize the second-order matrix product, U_2 has not been transposed for reasons of symmetry. Multiplication with U_1 needs linear combinations of the horizontal matrices (index i_1 fixed) in B. Multiplication of B with U_1 means that every column of B (index i_2 and i_3) has to be multiplied from the left with U_1. In a similar way, multiplication with U_2 needs linear combinations of the horizontal matrices (index i_2 fixed) in B and multiplication with U_3 needs linear combinations of the horizontal matrices (index i_3 fixed) in B. Figure 7.3 further provides the insight for understanding the tensor technology. In fact, the *n*-mode product of a tensor and a matrix is a special case of the inner product in multilinear algebra and tensor analysis. In the previous literature, it is often used in the form of an Einstein summation.

Figure 7.3. Visualization of the multiplication of a third tensor $B \in \Re^{J_n \times I_n} B \in$ $\Re^{I_1 \times I_2 \times I_3}$ with matrices $U_1 \in \Re^{J_1 \times I_1}$, $U_2 \in \Re^{J_2 \times I_2}$ and $U_3 \in \Re^{J_3 \times I_3}$.

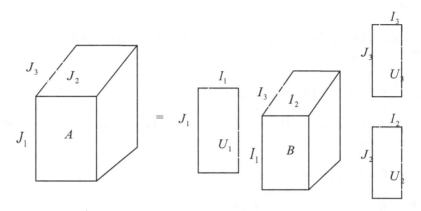

7.3 TENSOR DECOMPOSITION

There are two types of decompositions used most in real applications. The first decomposition is the CANDECOMP-PARAFAC (CP) model (Carroll & Chang, 1970; Harshman, 1970) and the second decomposition is refereed to as the TUCKER model (Tucker, 1966). These two models are widely used in three-order tensors and in fact they can be extended to arbitrary ordered tensors.

7.3.1 CANDECOMP-PARAFAC Decomposition

For the sake of simplicity, let us consider three-order tensors. Given an $I_1 \times I_2 \times I_3$ tensor, A, the CP model has a decomposition of the form

$$A = \sum_{i=1}^{R} u_i \circ v_i \circ w_i, \qquad (7.18)$$

where $u_i \in \Re^{I_1}$, $v_i \in \Re^{I_2}$ and $w_i \in \Re^{I_3}$ for $i = 1, \cdots, R$.

Without loss of generality, the vectors are assumed to be real. However, the model is also valid for the complex-valued vectors. Note that there are no constraints (such as orthogonality) on the vectors $u_i \in \Re^{I_1}$, $v_i \in \Re^{I_2}$ and $w_i \in \Re^{I_3}$. However, one can impose the constraints such as orthogonality, nonnegativity, or unimodality when needed. Note that a CP decomposition always exists (take R to be the product of the sizes of each mode and take outer products of scaled standard basis vectors). Ideally, R is chosen to be the minimal number of terms needed to sum to A. When R is minimal, then R is known as the tensor rank and is discussed in Section 7.4.

7.3.2 TUCKER Decomposition

In this subsection, we first consider three-order tensors. Given an $I_1 \times I_2 \times I_3$ tensor, A, the TUCKER model has a decomposition of the form

$$A = \sum_{i=1}^{R_1}\sum_{j=1}^{R_2}\sum_{k=1}^{R_3}\sigma_{ijk}(u_i \circ v_i \circ w_i),$$ (7.19)

where $R_1 \leq I_1, R_2 \leq I_2, R_3 \leq I_3, u_i \in \mathfrak{R}^{R1}, v_i \in \mathfrak{R}^{R2}$ and $w_i \in \mathfrak{R}^{R3}$ for i, j, k.

The tensor, $S = (\sigma_{ijk})$, is called the core tensor. Note that the core tensor does not always need to have the same dimensions as A. From Eq. (7.19), one can see that the CP decomposition is a special case of the TUCKER decomposition. Note that there are no constraints on the vectors $u_i \in \mathfrak{R}^{I_1}$, $v_i \in \mathfrak{R}^{I_2}$ and $w_i \in \mathfrak{R}^{I_3}$ in the TUCKER decomposition. However, one may impose constraints when needed. If the $u_i \in \mathfrak{R}^{I_1}$, $v_i \in \mathfrak{R}^{I_2}$ and $w_i \in \mathfrak{R}^{I_3}$ are columns from orthogonal matrices U, V, W, then the TUCKER model is referred to as the Higher-Order Singular Value Decomposition, or HOSVD.

Futher research showed Higher-Order Singular Value Decomposition by the following theorem (Lathauwer, 1997; Lathauwer, Comon, Moor, & Vandewalle, 1995; Lathauwer, Moor, & Vandewalle, 1997, 2000).

Theorem 7.4. (*n*th order SVD). Every $A \in \mathfrak{R}^{I_1 \times I_2 \times I_3 \dots \times I_N}$ can be written as the product

$$A = S \times_1 U_1 \times_2 U_2 \times \dots \times_N U_N$$ (7.20)

in which

1. $U_n = (u_1^n, \dots u_{I_n}^n)$ is a unitary $I_n \times I_n$ matrix,
2. S is an $I_1 \times \dots \times I_N$ tensor of which the subtensor $S_{i_n=\alpha}$, obtained by fixing the *n*th index to α, have the properties of
    (i) all-orthogonality: two subtensors $S_{i_n=\alpha}$ and $S_{i_n=\beta}$ are orthogonal for all possible values of n, α and β subject to $\alpha \neq \beta$: $\langle S_{i_n=\alpha}, S_{i_n=\beta}\rangle=0$ when $\alpha \neq \beta$.

Figure 7.4. Visualization of HOSVD for a third-order tensor

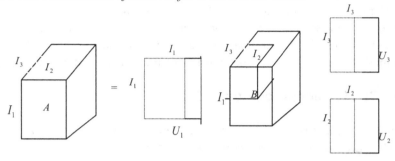

(ii) ordering: $\| S_{i_n=1} \| \geq \| S_{i_n=2} \| \geq \cdots \geq \| S_{i_n=I_n} \| \geq 0$ for all possible values of n.

The Frobenius-norm $\| S_{i_n=i} \| \geq 0$, symbolized by σ_i^n are n-mode singular values of A and the vector u_i^n is an ith n-mode singular vector.

For a tensor $A \in \Re^{I_1 \times I_2 \times I_3}$, Figure 7.4 shows HOSVD for a third-order tensor. Theorem 7.4 says that it is always possible to find orthogonal transformations of the column, row, and 3-mode space such that $S = A \times_1 (U_1)^T \times_2 (U_2)^T \times_3 (U_3)^T$ is all-orthogonal and ordered. Note that the new basis vectors are the columns of U_1, U_2 and U_3. All-orthogonality means that the different horizontal matrices of S (the first index i_1 kept fixed, while the two other indices, i_2 and i_3 are free) are mutually orthogonal with respect to the scalar product of matrices (i.e., the sum of the products of the corresponding entries vanishes). At the same time, the different frontal matrices (i_2 fixed) and the different vertical matrices (i_3 fixed) should be mutually orthogonal as well. The ordering constraint imposes that the Frobenius-norm of the horizontal (frontal, resp., vertical) matrices does not increase as the index i_1 (i_2, resp., i_3) is increased. While the orthogonality of U_1, U_2 and U_3, and the all-orthogonality of S are the basic assumptions of the model, the ordering condition should be regarded as a convention, meant to fix a particular ordering of the columns of U_1, U_2 and U_3 (or the horizontal, frontal, and vertical matrices of S, stated otherwise).

There are some similar characteristics between the matrix decomposition and the tensor decomposition. First, the role of the singular values in tensor decomposition is taken over by the Frobenius-norms of the $(N-1)$th-order subtensors of the core tensor S. Second, the left and right singular vectors of a matrix are generalized as the n-mode singular vectors in tensor decomposition. Note at this point that in the matrix case, the singular values also correspond to the Frobenius-norms of the rows and the columns of the core matrix S. For Nth order tensors, N (possibly different) sets of n-mode singular values are defined. In this respect, an Nth-order tensor can also have N different n-rank values. The essential difference is that S is in general a full tensor, instead of being pseudodiagonal (this would mean that nonzero elements could only occur when the indices $i_1 = i_2 = \cdots i_N$). Instead, S obeys the condition of all-orthogonality. Here notice that in the matrix case S is all-orthogonal as well due to the diagonal structure and the scalar product of two different rows or columns also vanishes. We also observe that, by definition, the n-mode singular values are positive and real, like in the matrix case. On the other hand the entries of S are not necessarily positive in general. They can even be complex, when A is a complex-valued tensor.

In addition, we say that a tensor is diagonalizeable if the HOSVD yields a diagonal core tensor. Note that if the core is diagonal, we can write the HOSVD as a PARA-FAC with orthogonality constraints. In general a tensor cannot be diagonalized. Up till now, it is not clear under what conditions permit a diagonalizeable core.

7.4 TENSOR RANK

Tensor rank (Kruskal, 1989; Hastad, 1990) is also an important problem in tensor analysis. There are major differences between matrices and higher-order tensors when rank properties are concerned. The differences may directly affect the way that an SVD generalization could look. As a matter of fact, there is not a unique way to generalize the rank concept in general. First, it is easy to generalize the notion of column and row rank. If we refer in general to the column and row vectors of an Nth-order tensor $A \in \Re^{I_1 \times I_2 \times I_3 \cdots \times I_N}$ as its n-mode vectors, defined as the I_n-dimensional vectors obtained from A by varying the index i_n and keeping the other indices fixed, then the following definition is given.

Definition 7.5. The n-rank of A, denoted by $R_n = rank_n(A)$, is the dimension of the vector space spanned by the n-mode vectors.

The n-rank of a given tensor can be analyzed by means of matrix techniques.

Property 7.6. The n-mode vectors of A are the column vectors of the matrix unfolding $A_{(n)}$ and

$$rank_n(A) = rank(A_{(n)}). \tag{7.21}$$

A major difference with the matrix case, however, is the fact that the different n-ranks of a higher-order tensor are not necessarily the same, as can easily be verified by checking some examples in the following.

The rank of a higher-order tensor is usually defined in analogy with the fact that a rank-R matrix can be decomposed as a sum of R rank-1 terms.

Definition 7.7. An Nth-order tensor A has rank 1 when it equals the outer product of N vectors, i.e.

$$a_{i_1 \cdots i_N} = u^1_{i_1} \cdots u^N_{i_N}, \qquad\qquad (7.22)$$

for all values of the indices.

The rank of an arbitrary Nth-order tensor A, denoted by R =rank(A), is the minimal number of rank-1 tensors that yield A in a linear combination.

From the definition of a rank-1 tensor, a remark on the notation has to be made. For matrices, the vector-vector outer product of a and b is denoted as ab^T. To avoid an ad hoc notation based on "generalized transposes", one will further denote the outer product of $u_1, \cdots u_N$ by $u_1 \otimes \cdots \otimes u_N$.

Another difference between matrices and higher-order tensors is the fact that the rank is not necessarily equal to an n-rank, even when all the n-ranks are the same. From the definitions it is clear that we always have $R_n \leq R$. In general, there is no known method to compute tensor rank. It is shown in Hastad (1990) that tensor rank is NP-complete.

In the following, some examples are shown with the context of comparing matrix rank to tensor rank and complexity of understanding tensor rank.

Example 7.1 Let the field of scalars be $\mathfrak{R}$, and suppose that

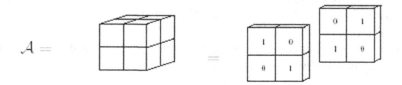

Then rank(A)=2:

$$A = \frac{1}{2}\begin{bmatrix}1\\1\end{bmatrix} \circ \begin{bmatrix}1\\1\end{bmatrix} \circ \begin{bmatrix}1\\1\end{bmatrix} + \frac{1}{2}\begin{bmatrix}1\\-1\end{bmatrix} \circ \begin{bmatrix}1\\-1\end{bmatrix} \circ \begin{bmatrix}1\\-1\end{bmatrix}$$

Example 7.2 Let the field of scalars be $\Re$, and suppose that

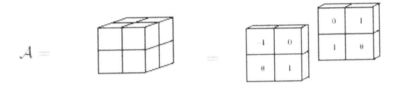

Then rank(A)=3:

$$A = \frac{1}{2}\begin{bmatrix}1\\1\end{bmatrix}\circ\begin{bmatrix}1\\1\end{bmatrix}\circ\begin{bmatrix}1\\1\end{bmatrix} + \frac{1}{2}\begin{bmatrix}1\\-1\end{bmatrix}\circ\begin{bmatrix}1\\-1\end{bmatrix}\circ\begin{bmatrix}1\\-1\end{bmatrix} - 2\begin{bmatrix}1\\0\end{bmatrix}\circ\begin{bmatrix}1\\0\end{bmatrix}\circ\begin{bmatrix}1\\0\end{bmatrix}$$

Example 7.3 Let the field of scalars be C, and suppose that

Then rank(A)=2:

$$A = \frac{1}{2}\begin{bmatrix}-i\\1\end{bmatrix}\circ\begin{bmatrix}-i\\1\end{bmatrix}\circ\begin{bmatrix}1\\i\end{bmatrix} + \frac{1}{2}\begin{bmatrix}i\\1\end{bmatrix}\circ\begin{bmatrix}i\\1\end{bmatrix}\circ\begin{bmatrix}1\\-i\end{bmatrix}.$$

Examples 7.2 and 7.3 illustrate that the rank depends on the field of scalars. In general, the maximum rank of a 2×2×2- tensor over R is 3 but the maximum rank over C is 2.

Example 7.4 Consider the (2×2×2)-tensor A defined by

$$\begin{cases} a_{111} = a_{221} = a_{112} = 1 \\ a_{211} = a_{121} = a_{212} = a_{122} = a_{222} = 0, \end{cases}$$

It follows that $R_1 = R_2 = 2$ but $R_3 = 1$.

Example 7.5. Consider the (2×2×2)-tensor A defined by

$$\begin{cases} a_{211} = a_{121} = a_{112} = 1 \\ a_{111} = a_{122} = a_{212} = a_{221} = a_{222} = 0 \end{cases}$$

The 1-rank, 2-rank, and 3-rank are equal to 2. The rank, however, equals 3, since

$$\begin{cases} a_{111} = a_{221} = a_{112} = 1 \\ A = X_2 \circ Y_1 \circ Z_1 + X_1 \circ Y_2 \circ Z_1 + X_1 \circ Y_1 \circ Z_2 . \\ a_{211} = a_{121} = a_{212} = a_{122} = a_{222} = 0 \end{cases}$$

in which

$$X_1 = Y_1 = Z_1 = \begin{pmatrix} 1 \\ 0 \end{pmatrix}, X_2 = Y_2 = Z_2 = \begin{pmatrix} 0 \\ 1 \end{pmatrix}.$$

is a decomposition in a minimal linear combination of rank-1 tensors.

Example 7.6. Let the field of scalars be $\mathfrak{R}$, and suppose that

Then rank(A)=2:

$$A = \begin{bmatrix} 1 \\ 1 \end{bmatrix} \circ \begin{bmatrix} 1 \\ 1 \end{bmatrix} \circ \begin{bmatrix} 1 \\ 1 \end{bmatrix} + \begin{bmatrix} 1 \\ 0 \end{bmatrix} \circ \begin{bmatrix} 1 \\ 0 \end{bmatrix} \circ \begin{bmatrix} 1 \\ 0 \end{bmatrix}.$$

Example 7.6 shows that the minimal tensor decomposition is not always orthogonal. In other words, it is impossible to write A as the sum of two orthogonal tensors (i.e., $u_1 \perp u_2 \ v_1 \perp v_2 \ w_1 \perp w_2$).

In addition, if the field of scalars is $\mathfrak{R}$, then the following results are known:

(a) The maximum rank of an 2×2×2 tensor is 3,
(b) The maximum rank of an 3×3×3 tensor is 5,
(c) The maximum rank of an 8×8×8 tensor is 11.

REFERENCES

Carroll, J. D., & Chang, J. (1970). Analysis of individual differences in multidimensional scaling via an n-way generalization of "Eckart-Young" decomposition. *Psychometrika, 35*(3), 283-319.

Comon, P. (2002). Tensor decompositions. In J. G. McWhirter & I. K. Proudler (Eds.), *Mathematics in signal processing V.* Oxford: Clarendon Press.

Harshman, R. A. (1970). Foundations of the PARAFAC procedure: model and conditions for an explanatory multi-mode factor analysis". *UCLA Working Papers in phonetics, 16*(1), 1-84.

Hastad, J. (1990). Tensor rank is NP-complete. *J. Algorithms, 11*(4), 644-654.

Kruskal, J. B. (1989). Rank, decomposition, and uniqueness for 3-way and n-way arrays. In R. Coppi & S. Bolasco (Eds.), *Multiway data analysis.* Amsterdam: Elsevier.

Lathauwer, L. (1997). *Signal processing based on multilinear algebra.* Ph.D thesis, K.U. Leuven, Belgium.

Lathauwer, L., Comon, P., Moor, B., & Vandewalle, J. (1995). Higher-order power method-application in independent component analysis. *Proceedings of the International Symposium on Nonlinear Theory and Its Applications* (pp. 91-96).

Lathauwer, L., Moor, B., & Vandewalle, J. (1994). Blind source separation by higher order singular value decomposition. *Proc. of the 7th European Signal Processing Conference* (pp. 175-178).

Lathauwer, L., Moor, B., & Vandewalle, J. (1996a). Blind source separation by simultaneous third-order tensor diagonalization. *Proc. of the 8th European Signal Processing Conference* (pp. 2089-2092).

Lathauwer, L., Moor, B., & Vandewalle, J. (1996b). Independent component analysis based on higher-order statistics only. *Proceedings of the IEEE Signal Processing Workshop on Statistical Signal and Array Processing* (pp. 356-359).

Lathauwer, L., Moor, B., & Vandewalle, J. (1997). Dimensionality reduction in higher order only ICA. *Proceedings of the IEEE Signal Processing Workshop on HOS* (pp. 316-320).

Lathauwer, L., Moor, B., & Vandewalle, J. (2000). A multilinear singular value decomposition. *J. Matrix Anal. Appl., 21*(4), 1253-1278.

Martin, C. D. (2004). *Tensor decompositions workshop discussion notes.* American Institute of Mathematics (AIM).

Tucker, L. R. (1966). Mathematical notes of three-mode factor analysis. *Psychometrika, 31*(3), 279-311.

Chapter VIII
Tensor Principal Component Analysis

ABSTRACT

Tensor principal component analysis (PCA) is an effective method for data reconstruction and recognition. In this chapter, some variants of classical PCA are introduced and the properties of tensor PCA are analyzed. Section 8.1 gives the background and development of tensor PCA. Section 8.2 introduces tensor PCA. Section 8.3 discusses some potential applications of tensor PCA in biometrics. Finally, we summarize this chapter in Section 8.4.

8.1 INTRODUCTION

Principal component analysis (Turk & Pentland, 1991; Penev & Sirovich, 2000), also known as Karhunen-Loève (K-L) transform, is a classical statistical technique that has been widely used in various fields, such as face recognition, character recognition, and knowledge representation. The aim of PCA is to reduce the dimensionality of the data so that the extracted features are representative as possible. In general, the key idea of PCA is to project data to an orthogonal subspace, which can transform correlated variables into a smaller number of uncorrelated variables. The first principal component can capture variance of the data along some direction as possible, and consequent components capture as much of the remaining variability as possible. Up to now, there are a number of theoretical analyses and discussion for PCA in the literature and PCA is one of the most popular methods for data representation.

In recent years, some researchers (Yang, Zhang, Frangi, & Yang, 2004; Ye, 2004) noted that classical PCA often runs up against computational limits due to the high time and space complexity for dealing with large image matrices, especially for images and videos. In applying PCA, data must be converted to a vector form. This results in the difficulty in eigen-decomposition in a high dimensional vector space. To overcome this limitation, a novel idea is developed. This novel idea lies in dealing with image matrices or video data directly rather than converting them into vectors prior to dimensionality reduction. Based on this, Yang, Zhang, Frangi and Yang (2004) proposed a two-dimensional PCA for image representation, whose idea is that 2D image matrices are used to directly construct the image covariance matrix. This improves the computational efficiency. Moreover, the projection of sample on each principal orthogonal vector is a vector. A drawback of 2DPCA is that it needs more coefficients than PCA for image representation and costs more time to calculate distance in classification phase. In order to address this problem, Ye (2004) proposed a new algorithm called generalized low rank approximations of matrices (GLRAM) to reduce the computational cost. Then some researchers proposed a non-iterative algorithm for GLRAM (Liang & Shi, 2005; Liang, Zhang, & Shi, 2007). Moreover, they reveal the optimal property of GLRAM and show that the reconstruction errors of GLRAM are not smaller than those of PCA when considering the same dimension. Likewise, their method is proved to have much less computational time than the traditional singular value decomposition (SVD) technique. In addition, researchers also developed a number of variants of 2DPCA (Xu et al., 2005; Nhat & Lee, 2005; Xu, Jin, Jiang, & Guo, 2006; Hou, Gao, Pan, & Zhang, 2006; Vasilescu & Terzopoulos, 2002; Wang & Ahuja, 2004; Zuo Wang, & Zhang, 2005a, 2005b). In fact, the methods mentioned above belong to the framework proposed by Lathauwer and his partners (Lathauwer, 1997; Lathauwer, Moor, & Vandewalle, 2000a). In 2000, a multilinear generalization of the singular value decomposition was further proposed (Lathauwer, Moor, & Vandewalle, 2000b). Moreover, they also analyzed some properties of the matrix and the higher-order tensor decompositions. Yu and Bennamoun (2006) also proposed nD-PCA algorithm which exploits higher-order singular value decomposition. All the methods contribute to the development of the tensor PCA.

8.2 BASIC ALGORITHMS

8.2.1 Classical PCA

Assume that $x_1, \ldots x_M$ are M data points in $\Re^N$. Without loss of generality, we assume that the data are centered, which shows that the mean of all data is zero. In fact, they can be easily achieved by performing a translation of data. Generally speaking, PCA extracts the desired number of principal components for data. In other words, PCA is to find a matrix W that maps these M points to another set of points $y_1, \ldots, y_M$ in R^d, where d < N.

From the viewpoint of data reconstruction, PCA can be considered to find the matrix $W = (w_1, \ldots, w_d)$ by minimizing the average L_2 reconstruction errors for all data, denoted by

$$\varepsilon(x) = \frac{1}{M} \sum_{i=1}^{M} \left\| x_i - \sum (w_i^T x_i) x_i \right\|^2. \tag{8.1}$$

The transformation matrix W can be obtained in the following way. Let X be an $N \times M$ matrix whose columns consist of $x_1, \ldots x_M$. Then the matrix W is obtained by the eigen-decomposition of $C = XX^T / M$ whose columns consist of the eigenvectors corresponding to the first m largest eigenvalues of C. It is not difficult to verify that the ith eigenvalue is the variance of the data projection on w_i. In addition, another good property of PCA is that it decorates the data.

8.2.2 Two-Dimensional PCA

Since it involves image matrices in 2DPCA, it is useful to introduce image projections before we begin. Let $\{A_1, \ldots, A_M\}$ be M image matrices, where A_i is an $m \times n$ matrix. Then the image A is projected onto a n-dimensional vector v. That is, the following transformation is adopted: $Y_i = A_i v$. It is obvious that the projection vector Y_i is an m-dimensional vector. In order to measure the discriminatory power of vector v, the total scatter of the projected vectors is introduced. In Yang, Zhang, Frangi and Yang (2004), the total scatter of the projected samples is defined by the trace of the covariance matrix of the projected feature vectors, which is denoted as follows:

$$J(X) = trace(S_x), \tag{8.2}$$

where S_x denotes the covariance matrix of the projected feature vectors of training samples.

Using the definition of the image covariance matrix, one can obtain

$$J(X) = v^T \left(\frac{1}{M} \sum_{i=1}^{M} (A_i - \overline{A})^T (A_i - \overline{A}) \right) v = v^T G_t v, \tag{8.3}$$

where $\overline{A}$ denotes the average image of all training samples.

In general, the optimal projected vector v is the eigenvector corresponding to the largest eigenvalue of G_t. In some cases, only a projected vector is not enough. It is necessary to obtain a set of the projected vectors $v_1,...,v_d$ which can maximize the criterion function $J(X)$. In such a case, the optimal projected vectors $v_1,...,v_d$ are the orthogonal eigenvectors of G_t corresponding to the first d largest eigenvalues.

8.2.3 Generalized Low Rank Approximations of Matrices

Consider a $p \times q$-dimensional space $L \otimes R$, where $\otimes$ denotes the tensor product, L is spanned by $\{u_1,...,u_p\}$, and R is spanned by $\{v_1,...,v_q\}$. Then the following matrices are defined: $L = [u_1,...,u_p]$ and $R = [v_1,...,v_q]$. The GLRAM method is to find L and R so that LD_iR^T is a good approximation of $A_i (i = 1,...,s)$, where $D_i \in \Re^{p \times q}$. In other words, the GLRAM method is to solve the following optimization problem:

$$\min_{\substack{L \in \Re^{r \times p} : L^T L = I_p \\ R \in \Re^{c \times q} : R^T R = I_q \\ D_i \in \Re^{p \times q}}} \frac{1}{M} \sum_{i=1}^{M} \left\| A_i - LD_iR^T \right\|_F^2. \tag{8.4}$$

Compared with the optimization problem in Ye (2004), we add a constant in Eq. (8.4). However, this does not affect the following discussion.

It has theoretically proved that the minimization problem of Eq. (8.4) is equivalent to the following maximization problem:

$$\max_{\substack{L \in \Re^{r \times p} : L^T L = I_p \\ R \in \Re^{c \times q} : R^T R = I_q}} \frac{1}{M} \sum_{i=1}^{M} \left\| L^T A_i R \right\|_F^2. \tag{8.5}$$

Ye noticed that there is no closed solution of Eq. (8.5). To this end, the following theorem which is very useful for obtaining the solution of Eq. (8.5) is proposed.

Theorem 8.1 Let L, R and $\{D_i\}_{i=1}^{M}$ be the optimal solution to the minimization problem in Eq. (8.4). Then

1. For a given R,L consists of the p eigenvectors of the matrix

$$D_L = \frac{1}{M} \sum_{i=1}^{M} A_i RR^T A_i^T \text{ corresponding to the largest } p \text{ eigenvalues.}$$

2.   For a given L,R consists of the q eigenvectors of the matrix

$$D_R = \frac{1}{M} \sum_{i=1}^{M} A_i^T LL^T A_i \text{ corresponding to the largest } q \text{ eigenvalues.}$$

By virtue of the idea of Theorem 8.1, an iterative procedure is proposed for obtaining L and R. A much more detailed discussion for the iterative procedure can be found in Ye (2004).

8.2.4 Non-Iterative GLRAM

Before non-iterative GLRAM is developed, it is necessary to introduce lemma 8.2 and its corollary.

Lemma 8.2 (Schott, 1997)**:** Let B be an $N \times N$ symmetric matrix and H be an $N \times h$ matrix which satisfies $H^T H = I_h$, where I_h is a $h \times h$ identity matrix. Then, for $i = 1,...,h$, we have

$$\lambda_{N-h+i} \leq \lambda_i(H^T BH) \leq \lambda_i(B), \tag{8.6}$$

where $\lambda_i(B)$ denotes the *ith* largest eigenvalue of the matrix B.
From Lemma 8.2, it is obvious that the following corollary can be obtained.

Corollary 8.3 Let w_i be the eigenvector corresponding to the ith largest eigenvalue λ_i of B and H be an $N \times h$ matrix which satisfies $H_T H = I_h$. Then

$$\lambda_{N-h+1} + \cdots + \lambda_m \leq trace(H^T BH) \leq \lambda_1 + \cdots + \lambda_h, \tag{8.7}$$

the second equality holds if $H = WQ$, where $W = (w_1,...,w_h)$ and Q is any $h \times h$ orthogonal matrix.
From corollary 8.3, it is not difficult to obtain the following theorem.

Theorem 8.4 Let w_i be the eigenvector corresponding to the ith largest eigenvalue λ_i of $C = XX^T / M$ ($i = 1,...,mn$). Then

$$\lambda_{r \times c-p \times q+1} + \cdots + \lambda_{m \times n} \le \frac{1}{M} \sum_{i=1}^{M} \left\| L^T A_i R \right\|_F^2 \le \lambda_1 + \cdots + \lambda_{p \times q}. \tag{8.8}$$

Proof:

$$\sum_{i=1}^{M} \left\| L^T A_i R \right\|_F^2 = \sum_{i=1}^{M} \left\| vec(L^T A_i R) \right\|_2^2, \tag{8.9}$$

where vec denotes the vec operator which can convert the matrix to a vector by stacking the columns of matrix.

Note that $vec(L^T A_i R) = (R^T \otimes L^T)vecA_i$. For the sake of notational simplicity, let $W^T = (R^T \otimes L^T)$. In such a case, Eq. (8.9) is further represented as

$$\sum_{i=1}^{M} \left\| vec(L^T A_i R) \right\|_2^2 \sum_{i=1}^{M} tr(W^T vec(A_i)vec(A_i)^T W) = tr(W^T XX^T W).$$

That is

$$\frac{1}{M} \sum_{i=1}^{M} \left\| L^T A_i R \right\|_F^2 = \frac{1}{M} tr(W^T XX^T W).$$

Note that $W^T W = (R^T \otimes L^T)(R \otimes L) = (R^T R) \otimes (L^T L) = I_q \otimes I_p = I_{pq}$. In such a case, applying Corollary 8.3, we can obtain

$$\lambda_{m \times n-p \times q+1} + \cdots + \lambda_{m \times n} \le \frac{1}{M} \sum_{i=1}^{M} \left\| L^T A_i R \right\|_F^2 \le \lambda_1 + \cdots + \lambda_{p \times q}. \tag{8.10}$$

This completes the proof of the theorem.

Theorem 8.4 demonstrates the bound for the objective function in Eq. (8.5). However, it does not provide the solution for GLRAM. It is obvious that the objective function obtains the optimal value when W consists of the eigenvectors of C corresponding to the first pq largest eigenvalues. To our knowledge, it is easy to compute the Kronecker product of two matrices. It is, however, very difficult or impossible to decompose a large matrix into the form of the Kronecker product of two matrices. In addition, it is straightforward to verify that the second equality in Eq. (8.5) holds if A_i ($i = 1,...,M$) are $m \times 1$ matrices, namely, vectors. It is clear that this is the form of classical PCA. Therefore, in some sense, PCA is a special case of GLRAM when the objective function achieves the optimal value. From the viewpoint of data reconstruction, we can see that the reconstruction errors obtained by GLRAM are not smaller than those obtained by PCA when the same dimensionality which has reduced is considered.

To further develop the theory, the following matrix is defined (Liang et al., 2007):

$$G_{s1} = \frac{1}{M} \sum_{i=1}^{M} (A_i)^T (A_i), \; G_{s2} = \frac{1}{M} \sum_{i=1}^{M} (A_i)(A_i)^T. \tag{8.11}$$

Assume that F_1 consists of the eigenvectors of G_{s1} corresponding to the first q largest eigenvalues and F_2 consists of the eigenvectors of G_{s2} corresponding to the first p largest eigenvalues. Let

$$D_{L1} = \frac{1}{M} \sum_{i=1}^{M} A_i F_1 F_1^T A_i^T, \; D_{R1} = \frac{1}{M} \sum_{i=1}^{M} A_i^T F_2 F_2^T A_i. \tag{8.12}$$

Assume that K_1 consists of the eigenvectors of D_{L1} corresponding to the first largest eigenvalues and K_2 consists of the eigenvectors of D_{R1} corresponding to the first q largest eigenvalues.

Applying Corollary 8.3 in such a case, it is not difficult to obtain the following theorem.

Theorem 8.5 Let $d1$ be the sum of the first p largest eigenvaules of D_{L1} and $d2$ be the sum of the first q largest eigenvaules of D_{R1}. In such a case, the maximal value of Eq. (8.5) is equal to max{$d1$, $d2$}.

Proof: (a) Note that L and R maximize

$$\frac{1}{M} \sum_{i=1}^{M} \left\| L^T A_i R \right\|_F^2. \tag{8.13}$$

Equation (8.13) is further represented as

$$\frac{1}{M} \sum_{i=1}^{M} \left\| L^T A_i R \right\|_F^2 = \frac{1}{M} \sum_{i=1}^{M} trace(L^T A_i R R^T A_i^T L)$$

$$= trace(L^T \sum_{i=1}^{M} \frac{1}{M}(A_i RR^T A_i^T)L) = trace(L^T D_L L).$$

Applying Corollary 8.3, we have

$$trace(L^T D_L L) \leq trace(D_L)_p. \tag{8.14}$$

Since $trace(D_L) = trace(\sum_{i=1}^{M} \frac{1}{M}(A_i RR^T A_i^T)) = trace(R^T G_{s1} R)$, we have

$$trace(R^T G_{s1} R) \leq trace(G_{s1})_q. \tag{8.15}$$

From Eq. (8.14) and Eq. (8.15), we obtain

$$trace(L^T G_{s1} L) \leq trace(G_{s1})_q.$$

From Eq. (8.15) and corollary 8.3, it is not difficult to obtain R, denoted as,

$$R = F_1 Q_{q \times q}^2, \tag{8.16}$$

where $Q_{q \times q}^2$ is any orthogonal matrix.
Substituting Eq. (8.16) into D_L, we obtain D_{L1} in Eq. (3.12).
From Eq. (8.14) and Corollary 8.3, it is not difficult to obtain L, denoted as,

$$L = K_1 Q_{p \times p}^1, \tag{8.17}$$

where $Q_{p \times p}^1$ is any orthogonal matrix.
Furthermore, it is straightforward to verify that the maximal value of Eq. (8.5) is equal to $d1$

(b) $\frac{1}{M} \sum_{i=1}^{M} \left\| L^T A_i R \right\|_F^2 = \frac{1}{M} \sum_{i=1}^{M} trace(R^T A_i^T LL^T A_i R) \; trace(R^T D_R R)$

Applying Corollary 8.3, we have

$$trace(R^T D_R R) \leq trace(D_R)_q. \tag{8.18}$$

Since $trace(D_R) = trace\sum_{i=1}^{M}\frac{1}{M}(L^T A_i A_i^T L)= trace(L^T G_{s2} L)$, we have

$$trace(L^T G_{s2} L) \leq trace(G_{s2})_p. \tag{8.19}$$

From Eq. (8.17) and Eq. (8.18), we obtain $trace(R^T D_L R) \leq trace(G_{s2})_p$.

From Eq. (8.18) and Corollary 8.3, it is not difficult to obtain L, denoted as,

$$L = F_2 Q_{p\times p}^1, \tag{8.20}$$

Substituting Eq. (8.19) into D_R, we obtain D_{R1} in Eq. (8.12). Similarly, we can obtain R, denoted as

$$R = K_2 Q_{q\times q}^2, \tag{8.21}$$

where $Q_{q\times q}^2$ is any orthogonal matrix.

In such a case it is straightforward to verify that the maximal value of Eq. (8.5) is equal to *d2.*

From (a) and (b), this completes the proof of the theorem.

From the proof of Theorem 8.4, it is not difficult to find the algorithm for GL-RAM. Finally, the method is summarized as follows.

The non-iterative GLRAM algorithm

Step 1: Assume that p,q are given. Compute the matrices G_{s1} and G_{s2}.

Step 2: Compute the eigenvectors of G_{s1} and G_{s2}, let $R = K_2 Q_{q\times q}^2$ and $L = F_2 Q_{p\times p}^1$

Step 3: Compute the eigenvectors of D_{L1} and D_{R1}, and obtain $L = K_1 Q_{p\times p}^1$ corresponding to R in step 2, and $R = F_1 Q_{q\times q}^2$ corresponding to L in step 2, and compute d1 and d2.

Step 4: Choose R, L corresponding to max{d1, d2}, and compute $D_i = L^T A_i R$.

In addition, for the non-iterative algorithms, the following remarks are given.

1. We can see from the proof of Theorem 8.5 that two different solutions are obtained. Note that although $A_i^T A_i$ and $A_i A_i^T$ have the same nonzero eigenvalues, G_{s1} and G_{s2} may have different nonzero eigenvalues. But $traceG_{s1}$ and $traceG_{s2}$ are equal. Therefore, the objective values corresponding to different solutions are different in general cases. In other words, d1 and d2 are not in general equal. To this end, we choose the bigger value in order to obtain smaller reconstruction errors. Meanwhile, we notice that d1 and d2 are equal if $A_i(i = 1,...,s)$ are symmetric square matrices.

2. We can also notice that the reconstruction errors obtained by the non-iterative algorithm for GLRAM are not bigger than those obtained by Ye's iterative algorithm (2004) because Ye's solution may be locally optimal. Likewise, the reconstruction errors obtained by non-iterative algorithm are not smaller than those obtained by PCA.

3. We can see that L and R are not unique. However, the solutions subject to an orthogonal transformation. In general, for the sake of simplicity, $Q^2_{q \times q}$ and $Q^1_{p \times p}$ are chosen as identity matrices in real applications.

4. It is straightforward to verify that $\min\{p,q\}$ affects the performance of generalized low rank approximations of matrices. In general, the bigger $\min\{p,q\}$ is, the better the approximation performance is. However, it increases the computational cost. Hence, we must make a compromise between the reconstruction errors and the computational cost. Meanwhile, we also notice that a simple strategy for choosing $\{p,q\}$ is provided. That is, assume that the ratio of lost information in the second step of the algorithm is smaller than the threshold value. Then we choose $\{p,q\}$. In a similar way, we can choose another corresponding dimensionality by setting another threshold value. In such a case, we can choose the solution with smaller dimensions.

5. It is of interest to note that the above algorithm is related to 2DPCA. Assume that $E(A) = 0_{r \times c}$, $L = I_{r \times r}$, and $R = V$. It is clear that the method for generalized low rank approximations of matrices is equivalent to 2DPCA in such a case. In other words, the method for generalized low rank approximations of matrices is a generalization of 2DPCA. In addition, we can know that the distributions of eigenvalues have a similar characteristic of those of PCA (see Theorem 8.4).

6. Compared with Ye's iterative algorithm (2004), the non-iterative algorithm for GLRAM has smaller computational complexity. However, it is not superior to 2DPCA in terms of the computational efficiency because the non-iterative algorithm for GLRAM needs to run several times (each time corresponds to a 2DPCA algorithm). It is obvious that the non-iterative algorithm for GLRAM has lower computational cost than PCA since the non-iterative algorithm for GLRAM needs to solve a small eigenvalue problem.

8.2.5 Higher-Order PCA

Lathauwer et al. (2000a) developed a higher-order tensor based the singular value decomposition, which provides the basis for developing some variants of higher-order PCA. Based on their theories, it is easy to use the ideas of tensors to represent higher dimensional datasets.

For the sake of clarity, we restate this Nth-order SVD as shown in Chapter VII.

Theorem 8.6 (Lathauwer et al., 2000a) Each complex $(I_1 \times I_2 ... \times I_N)$-tensor A can be written as the product

$$A = S \times_1 U^{(1)} \times_2 U^{(2)} ... \times_N U^{(N)}, \text{ in which}$$

1. $U^{(n)} = (U_1^{(n)} U_2^{(n)} \cdots U_{I_n}^{(n)})$ is a unitary $(I_n \times I_n)$-matrix,
2. S is a complex $(I_1 \times I_2 ... \times I_N)$-tensor of which the subtensor $S_{i_n=\alpha}$, obtained by fixing the nth index to α, have the properties of

i. all-orthogonality: two subtensors $S_{i_n=\alpha}$ and $S_{i_n=\beta}$ are orthogonal for all possible of n, α β subject to $\alpha \neq \beta$:

$$<S_{i_n=\alpha}, S_{i_n=\beta}>=0 \text{ when } \alpha \neq \beta,$$

ii. ordering: $\left\|S_{i_n=1}\right\| \geq \left\|S_{i_n=2}\right\| \geq \cdots \geq \left\|S_{i_n=I_n}\right\| \geq 0$ for all possible values of n.

The Frobenious-norms $\left\|S_{i_n=i}\right\|$ are n-mode singular values of A and the vector $U_i^{(n)}$ is an ith n-mode singular vector.

Note that the mode-n multiplication in theorem 8.6 is first implemented by unfolding the tensor A along the given mode-n to generate its model-n matrix form $A_{(n)}$, and then performing the matrix multiplication. After that, the resulting matrix $B_{(n)}$ is folded back to the tensor form. Lathauwer et al. (2000a) pointed out that it is not impossible to reduce the higher-order tensors to a pseudodiagnonal form by means of the orthogonal transformation.

Yu and Bennamoun (2006) constructed a different tensor as follows: $D = ((X_1 - \bar{X}), \cdots, (X_N - \bar{X}))$ where $X_i \in R^{I_1 \times \cdots \times I_N}$. It is obvious that D is a tenor. In such a case, applying Theorem 8.6 to D will produce a mode-n singular vector contained in $U^{(n)}, n = 1, \cdots, N$. After that, one can determine the desired principal orthogonal vectors for each mode of the tensor D in terms of the mode-n singular values. Then the projection of sample X onto the mode-n principal vector $U_k^{(n)}$ is expressed as

$$Y_n = (X - \bar{X}) \times_n (U_k^{(n)})^T.$$

It is straightforward to verify that the projection Y_n is still an N-order tensor. Projecting X onto a principal vector $u_i^{(n)}$ of $U_k^{(n)}$ will produce $Y_{n,i} = (X - \bar{X}) \times_n (u_k^{(n)})^T, i \leq k$.

The projection $Y_{n,i}$ is a $(N-1)$-order tensor. The final construction of X can be obtained by $\tilde{X} = \bar{X} + Y_n \times_n U_k^{(n)}$. For classification, the Forbenious-norms between two mode-n principal component tensors, Y_n^i and $Y_n^j (i \neq j)$ are adopted as follows.

$$d(Y_n^i, Y_n^j) = \left\| Y_n^i - Y_n^j \right\|_F.$$

8.3 APPLICATIONS TO BIOMETRIC VERIFICATION

In this section, experiments on face images and handwritten characters are made to test PCA and its several variants. From the discussion in section 8.2, we can see that two important parameters p and q are involved in GLRAM. For the sake of simplicity, p and q are set to the common value d in the following experiments. As pointed out in Ye (2004), this choice is a good strategy for obtaining good classification performance. In addition, when the classification performance is involved, it is necessary to use a classifier for evaluation. To this end, the nearest neighbor classifier is adopted due to its simplicity.

8.3.1 Experiments on the ORL Face Database

Each face image of the ORL database (please refer to Section 3.2.3) is downsampled to 28×23 pixels to reduce the computational complexity. First, we perform experiments to check the distributions of eigenvalues of the non-iterative algorithm for GLRAM. Figure 8.1(a) denotes the distributions of eigenvalues of Eq. (8.11) and Figure 8.1 (b) denotes the distributions of eigenvalues of Eq. (8.12) when F_1 chooses different dimensions. As observed in Figure 8.1, the magnitude of eigenvalues decreases quickly. The first several eigenvalues contain most information (energy) of the original image. As a result, it is very reasonable to choose the first several eigenvectors to approximate the original image so that the dimensions of images can be drastically reduced, which is very useful for image retrieval and recognition.

In the following, experiments are made to obtain the reconstructed images. Figure 8.2 shows the reconstructed images of four methods, namely PCA, 2DPCA, GLRAM, and the non-iterative algorithm for GLRAM (NGLRAM), by adding the dimensions of features. It should be noted that the dimension of 2DPCA is $28 \times d$, while the dimensions of other three methods are $d \times d$. As can be seen from Figure 8.2, the visual quality of the reconstructed images is improved with the increase of features. It is obvious that the reconstructed images obtained by the non-iterative algorithm for GLRAM have slightly better visual quality than those obtained by GLRAM, while they are not superior to those obtained by PCA. When the first

Figure 8.1 (a). The distributions of eigenvalues in q, (b) the distributions of eigenvalues in p.

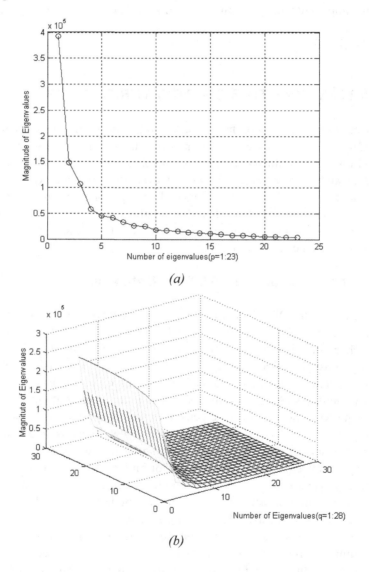

(a)

(b)

several eigenvectors are used to reconstruct the images, PCA shows the contours of images, whereas other three methods cannot show the contours of images.

This set of experiments was used to compare non-iterative GLRAM with 2DPCA, PCA and GLRAM in terms of the reconstruction errors and the recogni-

Figure 8.2. The reconstruction images of four methods (d=1:23)

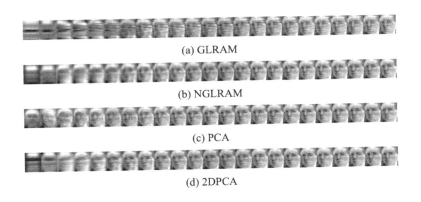

(a) GLRAM

(b) NGLRAM

(c) PCA

(d) 2DPCA

tion performance. We use a tenfold cross-validation to evaluate the classification performance. Note that the reconstruction errors are defined as a square root of Eq. (8.5). Figure 8.2 (a) denotes the reconstruction errors obtained by four methods with the change of features and Figure 8.3 (b) denotes the recognition performance obtained by four methods with the change of features. As can be seen from Figure 8.3 (a), the reconstruction errors decrease with the increase of features. The PCA method obtains the smallest reconstruction errors in all methods. It is clear that the non-iterative algorithm for GLRAM is superior to 2DPCA or GLRAM in terms of the reconstruction errors. When the dimension is small, GLRAM obtains smaller reconstruction errors than 2DPCA. However, with the increase of features, the reconstruction errors of 2DPCA are smaller than those of GLRAM. Here, we also explain this reason. When the dimension $m = p \times q$ is small, p is a constant in 2DPCA. Therefore, q is smaller, and thus results in large information lost. However, for GLRAM and our method, we make $p = q$. In such a case, we can obtain bigger p and q. Consequently, the information is lost in two stages in GLRAM. As discussed in Ye (2004), GLRAM may obtain locally optimal solutions, which helps us to explain this phenomenon. As observed in Figure 8.3 (b), in most cases, the recognition performance increases with the increase of features. When the number of features is small, the 2DPCA method is not superior to other three methods in terms of the recognition performance. However, with the increase of features, these four methods can obtain similar results, which show the matrix-based methods have potential applications for image recognition.

In addition, we also conduct the experiments to compare the classification performance of non-iterative GLRAM with those of 2DPCA, PCA and GLRAM, under

Figure 8.3 (a) reconstruction errors obtained by four methods with the change of features. (b) recognition performance obtained by four methods with the change of features.

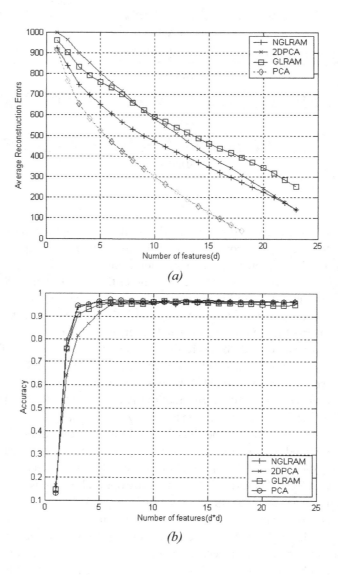

(a)

(b)

the conditions where the number of training samples is varied. To reduce variation, the experimental results reported in this experiment are obtained by 20 runs. Figure 8.4 denotes the recognition performance of four methods with the change of the

Figure 8.4. Recognition performance of four methods with the change of the number of training samples

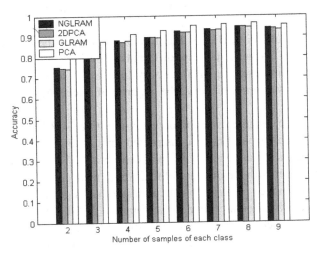

number of training samples. Here we set the number of features to 28×7 (14×14). From Figure 8.4, we can see that PCA obtains the best classification performance in all methods, which shows the matrix-based methods are not always superior to PCA. However, we know that the matrix-based methods are superior to PCA in terms of the computational efficiency in dealing with large image matrices (Yang et al., 2004). It is also observed that the non-iterative algorithm for GLRAM obtains slightly better classification performance than 2DPCA or GLRAM.

8.3.2 Experiments on Handwritten Numeral Character Database

The handwritten numeral characters are obtained from the UCI data set repository. This data set consists of 5620 handwritten numeral characters. The original image of each character has the size of 32×32 pixels. In order to reduce the size of the image, we obtain the size of 16×16 pixels where each pixel is obtained from the average of the block of 2×2 pixels in the original images. In other words, the number of features of each character image is 256. In our experiments, we only choose 100 samples from each class to constitute training samples and others are used for testing. As a result, the number of training samples is 1000 and the number of testing samples is 4620. To enhance the accuracy of performance evaluation, the classification performance reported in our experiments is averaged over ten times. In other words, 10 different training and testing sets are used for evaluating the performance.

As discussed in the ORL experiments in Section 8.3.1, the first experiment is made to show the distributions of eigenvalues. Figure 8.5 (a) denotes the distributions of eigenvalues of Eq. (8.11) and Figure 8.5 (b) denotes the distributions of eigenvalues of Eq. (8.12) when F_1 chooses different dimensions. As can be seen from Figure 8.5, the magnitudes of eigenvalues also decrease. It shows that extracting the first several eigenvectors to preserve the majority of information of the original images is enough.

Then we conduct experiments to compare non-iterative GLRAM with 2DPCA, PCA and GLRAM in terms of the reconstructed images. Figure 8.6 denotes the reconstruction images of handwritten numeral character "2". It is obvious that the images become clearer with the increase of features in most cases. We can see that the reconstruction images obtained by the non-iterative algorithm for GLRAM have slightly better visual quality than those obtained by GLRAM. As discussed in Section 8.3.1, PCA achieves the best reconstructed images in all methods.

In addition, experiments are performed to compare the non-iterative GLRAM with 2DPCA, PCA and GLRAM in terms of the reconstruction errors and the classification performance. Figure 8.7 (a) denotes the reconstruction errors obtained by four methods with the change of features and Figure 8.7 (b) denotes the recognition performance obtained by four methods with the change of features. From Figure 8.7 (a), it is clear that the reconstructed errors of four methods decrease with the increase of features. The PCA method obtains the smallest reconstruction errors in all methods. Like experiments in Section 8.3.1, GLRAM obtains smaller reconstruction errors than 2DPCA when the number of features is small. However, with the increase of features, the reconstruction errors between 2DPCA and GLRAM make no remarkable difference. It is different from experimental results in Section 8.3.1. Probably, a relatively large number of samples are used as training samples in this experiment. But it is clear that the non-iterative algorithm for GLRAM is superior to 2DPCA or GLRAM in terms of the reconstruction errors. Note that the reconstruction errors obtained by the non-iterative algorithm for GLRAM approach those obtained by PCA in this experiment. This may come from the fact that the rank of the covariance matrix is relatively big compared with the dimensions of samples. As observed in Figure 8.7 (b), the classification performance is improved with the increase of features in most cases. However, 2DPCA still obtains higher recognition rates even when the number of features is 2. But there is no remarkable difference in the classification performance for four methods when the number of features is big. Therefore, since matrix-based methods are more efficient than PCA in terms of the computational time, matrix-based methods such as 2DPCA and GLRAM can be used to recognize images even when a number of training samples are available.

Figure 8.5 (a) The distributions of eigenvalues in q, (b) the distributions of eigen-values in p.

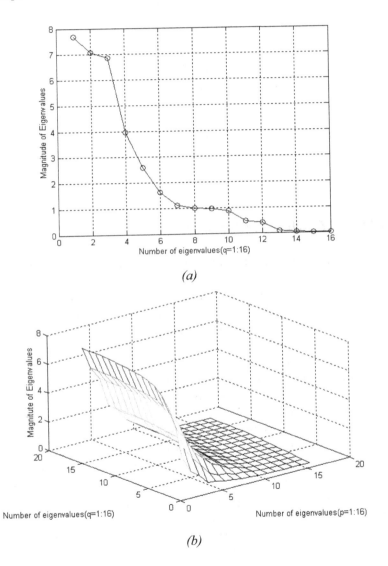

(a)

(b)

Figure 8.6. The reconstructions images of four methods (d=1:16)

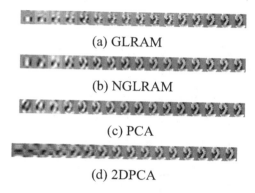

(a) GLRAM

(b) NGLRAM

(c) PCA

(d) 2DPCA

8.4 SUMMARY AND DISCUSSION

Tensor PCA is an effective method for data reconstruction and recognition. However, tensor PCA adopts an iterative procedure to extract features. In this chapter, we discuss the properties of tensor PCA. It is of interest to note that the optimal value of tensor PCA is closely related to classical PCA. We theoretically show the reconstruction errors obtained by GLRAM (a special of tensor PCA) are not smaller than those obtained by PCA when the same number of dimensionality is considered. We also show that the reconstruction errors obtained by non-iterative GLRAM method are still not bigger than those obtained by Ye's iterative algorithm (2004) when considering the same dimensionality. In the meantime, a simple strategy for choosing dimensions is provided.

A possible explanation that PCA has smaller reconstruction errors than matrix-based methods even high-order methods is that the covariance matrix of classical PCA is positive semi-definite, especially for the small sample-size problem, which makes the data information tight, while the image (tensor) covariance matrix in the matrix (tensor)-based methods is positive definite in general cases, which results in information lost as long as the dimension is reduced.

Experimental results on face images and handwritten numerical characters demonstrate that tensor PCA is still competitive with other existing methods such as classical PCA in terms of the classification performance or the reconstructed errors.

However, there are still several aspects needed to be pointed out. On the one hand, the computational complexity is still a challenging problem in the case of tensor PCA due to the high dimension arrays. Consequently, how to improve the

Figure 8.7 (a). reconstruction errors obtained by four methods with the change of features. (b) Recognition performance obtained by four methods with the change of features.

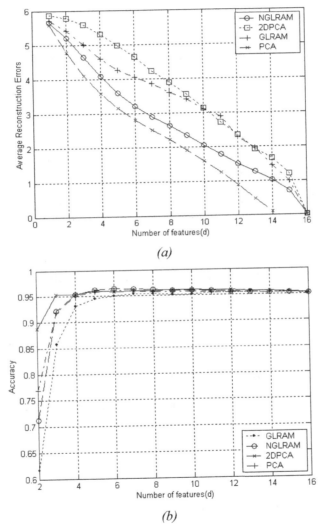

(a)

(b)

computational speed needs to be further considered. One the other hand, whether there exists the condition such that the reconstruction errors of tensor PCA are equal to those of PCA is unclear up till now and whether the solution obtained by the iterative algorithm is optimal needs to be further investigated. But we expect that the insights in this chapter will pave the way for building close relationship between classical PCA and tensor PCA.

REFERENCES

Hou, J., Gao, Q. X., Pan, Q., & Zhang, H. C. (2006). Essence of 2DPCA and modification method for face recognition. *Proceedings of the International Conference on Machine learning and Cybernetic* (pp. 3351-3353).

Lathauwer, L. D. (1997). *Signal processing based on multilinear algebra*. Ph.D thesis, K.U. Leuven, Belgium.

Lathauwer, L., Moor, B., & Vandewalle, J. (2000a). A multilinear singular value decomposition. *J. Matrix Anal. Appl.*, *21*(4), 1253-1278.

Lathauwer, L., Moor, B., & Vandewalle, J. (2000b). On the best of rank-1 and rank-$(R_1,R_2,...R_N)$ approximation of high-order tensors. *J. Matrix Anal. Appl.*, *21*(4), 1324-1342.

Liang, Z. Z., & Shi, P. F. (2005). An analytical method for generalized low rank approximation matrices. *Pattern Recognition*, *38*(11), 2213-2216.

Liang, Z. Z., Zhang, D., & Shi, P. F. (2007). The theoretical analysis of GRLDA and its applications. *Pattern Recognition*, *40*(3), 1032-1041.

Nhat, V. D., & Lee, S. Y. (2005). Two-dimensional weighted PCA algorithm for face recognition. *Proceedings of the IEEE Symposium on Computational intelligence in Robotics and Automation* (pp. 219-223).

Penev, P. S., & Sirovich, L. (2000). The global dimensionality of face space. *Proc. fourth IEEE Int'l Conference Automatic face and Gesture Recognition* (pp. 264-270).

Schott, J. R. (1997). *Matrix analysis for statistics*. New York: Wiley InterScience publication.

Turk, M., & Pentland, A. (1991). Eigenface to recognition. *J. cognitive Neurosience*, *3*(1), 71-86.

Vasilescu, M. A., & Terzopoulos, D. (2002). Multilinear image analysis for facial recognition. *Proceedings of the 16th International Conference on Pattern Recognition (ICPR)* (pp. 511-514).

Wang, H. C., & Ahuja, N. (2004). Compact representation of multidimensional data using tensor rank-one decomposition. *Proceedings of the 17th International Conference on Pattern Recognition (ICPR)* (pp. 44-47).

Xu, A. B., Jin, X., Jiang, Y. G., & Guo, P. (2006). Complete two-dimensional PCA for face recognition. *Proceedings of the 18th International Conference on Pattern Recognition (ICPR)* (pp. 481-484).

Xu, D., Yan, S. C., Zhang, L., Li, M. J., Ma, W. Y., & Liu, Z. K., et al. (2005). Parallel image matrix compression for face recognition. *Proceedings of the 11th International Conference on Multimedia Modeling* (pp. 232-238).

Yang, J., Zhang, D., Frangi, A. F., & Yang, J-Y. (2004). Two-dimensional PCA: a new approach to appearance-based face representation and recognition. *IEEE Trans. Pattern Anal. Machine Intell.*, *26*(1), 131-137.

Ye, J. P. (2004). Generalized low rank approximations of matrices. *International Conference on Machine Learning Conference Proceedings* (pp. 887–894).

Yu, H., & Bennamoun, M. (2006). 1D-PCA, 2D-PCA to nD-PCA. *Proceedings of the 18th International Conference on Pattern Recognition (ICPR)* (pp. 181-184).

Zuo, W. M., Wang, K. Q., & Zhang, D. (2005a). Assembled matrix distance metric for 2DPCA-based face and palmprint recognition. *Proceedings of the International Conference on Machine Learning and Cybernetics* (pp. 4870-4875).

Zuo, W. M., Wang, K. Q., & Zhang, D. (2005b). Bi-directional PCA with assembled matrix distance metric. *Proceedings of the International Conference on Image Processing* (pp. 958-961).

Chapter IX
Tensor Linear Discriminant Analysis

ABSTRACT

Linear discriminant analysis is a very effective and important method for feature extraction. In general, image matrices are often transformed into vectors prior to feature extraction, which results in the curse of dimensionality when the dimensions of matrices are huge. In this chapter, classical LDA and its several variants are introduced. In some sense, the variants of LDA can avoid the singularity problem and achieve computational efficiency. Experimental results on biometric data show the usefulness of LDA and its variants in some cases.

9.1 INTRODUCTION

Linear discriminant analysis is a popular technique for feature extraction, which has been successfully applied in many fields such as face recognition and character recognition. Linear discriminant analysis seeks to find the direction which maximizes between-class scatter and minimizes the within-class scatter. Based on linear discriminant analysis, Foley and Sammon (1975) proposed optimal discriminant vectors for two-class problems. Duchene and Leclercq (1988) further presented a set of discriminant vectors to solve multi-class problems. Although Foley-Sammon optimal discriminant vectors (FSODV) are orthogonal and perform well in some cases, the features which are obtained by optimal orthogonal discriminant vectors are statistically correlated. To avoid this problem, Jin, Yang, Hu, and Luo (2001) proposed a new set of uncorrelated discriminant vectors(UDV) which is proved to be more powerful than that of optimal orthogonal discriminant vectors in some cases. Then Jing, Zhang, and Jin (2003) further stated improvements on uncorrelated optimal discriminant vectors. Subsequently, Xu, Yang, and Jin (2003) studied the relationship between the Fisher criterion values of FSODV and UDV. Then Xu, Yang, and Jin (2004) developed a new model for Fisher discriminant analysis, which applies the maximal Fisher criterion and the minimal statistical correlation between features. Since the methods mentioned above are based on vectors rather than matrices, these methods face the computational difficulty when the dimension of data is too huge. To overcome this problem, Liu, Cheng, and Yang (1993) firstly proposed a novel linear projection method, which performs linear discriminant analysis in terms of image matrices. However, feature vectors using Liu's method could be statistically correlated. In order to effectively deal with this problem, Yang, Yang, Frangi, and Zhang (2003) proposed a set of two-dimensional (2D) projection vectors which satisfy conjugate orthogonal constraints. Most importantly, feature vectors obtained by Yang's method are statically uncorrelated. Then Liang, Shi, and Zhang (2006) proposed a new technique for 2D Fisher discriminant analysis. In their algorithm, the Fisher criterion function is directly constructed in terms of image matrices. Then they utilize the Fisher criterion and statistical correlation between features to construct an objective function. Then discriminant vectors are obtained in terms of the objection function. At the same time, they theoretically analyze that the proposed algorithm is equivalent to uncorrelated two-dimensional discriminant analysis in some condition. In Xiong, Swam and Ahmad (2005), one-sided 2DLDA is developed for classification tasks. Ye, Janardan, Park, and Park (2004) further developed generalized 2DLDA, which can overcome the singularity problem and achieves the computational efficiency. In Liang (2006; Yan et al., 2005), a multilinear generalization of linear discriminant analysis is discussed and an iterative algorithm is developed for solving multilinear linear discriminant analysis. Meanwhile, a non-iterative algorithm is also proposed in Liang (2006). In addition, multilinear LDA provides a unified framework for classical LDA and 2DLDA.

9.2 BASIC ALGORITHMS

Notations: Let $\{A_1,...,A_M\}$ denote a set of images, $A_i \in \mathfrak{R}^{m \times n}$. Each image belongs to exactly one of c object class $\{l_1,...,l_c\}$. The number of images in class l_i is denoted by n_i and $\sum n_i = M$. Let $x_i = vec(A_i)$, where vec denotes the vector operator which can convert the matrix by stacking the column of the matrix. $x_i \in \mathfrak{R}^N$, $N = m \times n$.

9.2.1 Classical Linear Discriminant Analysis

In discriminant analysis, the within-class and between-class scatter matrices are defined as follows:

$$S_b = \sum_{i=1}^{c} n_i (m_i - m)(m_i - m)^T = H_b H_b^T, \tag{9.1}$$

$$S_w = \sum_{i=1}^{c} \sum_{x \in l_i} (x - m_i)(x - m_i)^T = H_w H_w^T, \tag{9.2}$$

where the precursors H_b and H_w of the between-class and within-class scatter matrices in (9.1) and (9.2) are

$$H_b = [\sqrt{n_1}(m_1 - m), \cdots, \sqrt{n_c}(m_c - m)], \tag{9.3}$$

$$H_w = [X_1 - m_1 e_1^T, \cdots, X_c - m_c e_c^T], \tag{9.4}$$

$e_i = (1, \cdots, 1)^T \in \Re^{n_i}$, X_i is the data matrix for class l_i, m_i is the centroid of the ith class and m is the global centroid of the data set.

Classical LDA is to compute a linear transformation $G \in \Re^{N \times d}$ that maps x_i in the N-dimensional space to a vector $\hat{x}_i$ in the d-dimensional space by $\hat{x}_i = G^T x_i$. Applying the linear transformation matrix G, one can obtain the within-class and between-class distance in the projected space. Then one can maximize the between-class distance and minimize the within-class distance in the projection space. Often, the optimization criterion in classical LDA can be defined as follows:

$$J(G) = \max trace(\frac{G^T S_b G}{G^T S_w G}) \tag{9.5}$$

The optimization problem can be solved by applying the eigen-decomposition on the matrix $S_w^{-1} S_b$ if S_w is nonsingular. In general, there are at most $c - 1$ eigenvectors corresponding to nonzero eigenvalues since the rank of the matrix S_b is not bigger than $c - 1$. In the case of singularity, some effective methods (Ye, 2005; Ye & Li, 2005) have been developed in recent years.

9.2.2 Two-Dimensional LDA

Without loss of generality, let the image A be an $m \times n$ matrix. Then the image A is projected onto an n-dimensional vector X. That is, the following transformation is adopted:

$$Y = AX. \tag{9.6}$$

It is obvious that the projection vector Y is an m-dimensional vector. In this case, the image A is transformed into an m-dimensional vector Y and each image corresponds to a vector.

Let A_{ij} denote the ith image in the jth class. Then we project the image onto X and obtain the following form:

$$Y_{ij} = A_{ij}X, i = 1, 2, \cdots, n_j, j = 1, 2, \cdots, c. \tag{9.7}$$

Let

$$m_j = \frac{1}{n_j}\sum_{i=1}^{n_j} Y_{ij} \text{ and } P_j = n_j / M,$$

where M is the total number of training samples, m_j denotes the mean projection vector of class j and P_j is a prior probability of class j. Then the between-class scatter matrix S_b, within-class matrix S_w, and total population scatter matrix S_t are defined as

$$S_b = \sum_{j=1}^{c} P_j[m_j - E(Y)][m_j - E(Y)]^T, \tag{9.8}$$

$$S_w = \sum_{j=1}^{c} P_j E[(Y - m_j)(Y - m_j)^T |_j], \tag{9.9}$$

$$S_t = E\{[Y - E(Y)][Y - E(Y)]^T\} = S_b + S_w, \tag{9.10}$$

where $E(\ )$ denotes the expectation value of vectors or matrices.

In order to construct the criterion function for class separability, we need to transform the above matrices to numbers. The criteria should be larger when the between-class scatter is larger or the within-class scatter is smaller. To this end, the following function is constructed from Eqs. (9.8) and (9.10), which is a generalization of classical linear discriminant analysis:

$$J = \frac{tr(S_b)}{tr(S_t)}, \tag{9.11}$$

where $tr()$ denotes the trace of matrices.

According to Eq. (9.8), one obtains the following equation:

$$tr(S_b) = \sum_{j=1}^{c} P_j[m_j - E(Y)]^T[m_j - E(Y)]. \tag{9.12}$$

Substituting Eq. (9.7) into Eq. (9.12), one obtains

$$tr(S_b) = \sum_{j=1}^{c} P_j [A_j X - E(A)X]^T [A_j X - E(A)X]$$

$$= X^T \sum_{j=1}^{c} P_j [A_j - E(A)]^T [A_j - E(A)] X, \qquad (9.13)$$

where A_j is the average image matrix of class j.

Define the matrix below

$$S_{b1} = \sum_{j=1}^{c} P_j [A_j - E(A)]^T [A_j - E(A)]. \qquad (9.14)$$

The matrix S_{b1} is called image between-class scatter matrix. It is obvious that S_{b1} is an $n \times n$ matrix. In a similar way, we can define the following two matrixes:

$$S_{w1} = \sum_{j=1}^{c} P_j E[(A - A_j)^T (A - A_j)|_j], \qquad (9.15)$$

$$S_{t1} = E\{[A - E(A)]^T [A - E(A)]\}. \qquad (9.16)$$

The matrix S_{w1} is called image within-class scatter matrix and the matrix S_{t1} is called image total population scatter matrix. Accordingly, it is easy to verify that S_{w1} and S_{t1} are $n \times n$ matrices. In such a case, we transform Eq. (9.11) into the following form:

$$J(X) = \frac{X^T S_{b1} X}{X^T S_{t1} X}. \qquad (9.17)$$

In general, the problem of Eq. (9.17) can be solved by the following generalized eigenvalue problem:

$$S_{b1} X = \lambda S_{t1} X. \qquad (9.18)$$

It should be pointed out that the matrix S_{t1} is nonsingular unless there is only one sample for each class. As discussed in Yang, Yang, Frangi and Zhang (2003), the eigenvector corresponding to maximum eigenvalue of Eq. (9.18) is taken as the first uncorrelated discriminant vector. According to Jing's theory, the $(d+1)$th uncorrelated discriminant vector X_{d+1} is the eigenvector corresponding to maximum eigenvalue of the following eigenequation:

$$PS_{b1}X = \lambda S_{t1}X, \tag{9.19}$$

where $P = I - S_{t1}D^T(DS_{t1}D^T)^{-1}D$, $D = (X_1\ X_2 \cdots X_r)^T$, and $I = diag(1,1,...,1)$.

In the following, an effective method for two-dimensional linear discriminant analysis is described, which applies the Fisher criterion and statistical correlation between extracted features. Assume that optimal 2D projection vectors $X_1, X_2,...,X_d$ are used for feature extraction. Let $Y_k = AX_k (i = 1,\cdots,d)$. Thus, the image space is transformed into the feature space. Let Y_i and Y_j be any two features. Then the covariance between them is defined as

$$\text{cov}(Y_i,Y_j) = E\left[(Y_i - E(Y_i))(Y_j - E(Y_j))\right] = X_i^T S_{t1} X_j \tag{9.20}$$

Accordingly, the correlation coefficient between Y_i and Y_j is defined as

$$\rho(Y_i,Y_j) = \frac{\text{cov}(Y_i,Y_j)}{\sqrt{\text{cov}(Y_i,Y_i)}\sqrt{\text{cov}(Y_j,Y_j)}} = \frac{X_i^T S_{t1} X_j}{\sqrt{(X_i^T S_{t1} X_i)}\sqrt{(X_j^T S_{t1} X_j)}}.$$

$$\tag{9.21}$$

For the sake of discussion, let $\rho(Y_i,Y_j) = f(X_i,X_j)$. In a similar way, we select the vector corresponding to the maximum value of Eq. (4.17) as the first discriminant vector. Then the following optimization model is used to obtain the $(d+1)$th discriminant vector, denoted as

max $J(X)$,

min $f_1^2(X,X_1)$

min $f_d^2(X,X_d)$,

where $f_i(X,X_i) = \dfrac{X_i^T S_{t1} X}{\sqrt{X_i^T S_{t1} X_i}\sqrt{X^T S_{t1} X}}$, $i = 1,...,d.$ \hfill (9.22)

It is obvious that the correlation between X and $X_i(i = 1,...,d)$, namely Y and $Y_i(i = 1,...,d)$, is the lowest when $f_i^2(X,X_r)$ $i = 1,...,d$ are zero. This new model shows that the feature vector extracted by the $(d+1)$th discriminant vector has the lowest correlation with those extracted by previous d discriminant vectors.

In order to deal with the above model, the model is further transformed into the following equation:

$$G(X) = s_0 J(X) - \sum_{i=1}^{d} s_i f_i^2(X, X_i),$$ (9.23)

where $s_i \geq 0 (i = 0, \cdots, r)$ are weighting factors and $\sum_{i=0}^{d} s_i = 1$.

From Eq. (9.23), we can see that the smaller $f_i^2(X, X_r)$ is and the bigger $J(X)$ is, the bigger $G(X)$ is. Therefore, it is necessary to obtain the $(d+1)$th discriminant vector corresponding to the maximal value of $G(X)$.

Substituting Eqs. (9.17) and (9.21) into Eq. (9.23), one can obtain

$$G(X) = s_0 \frac{X^T S_{b1} X}{X^T S_{t1} X} - \sum_{i=1}^{d} s_i \frac{(X_i^T S_{t1} X)^2 / (X_i^T S_{t1} X_i)}{X^T S_{t1} X}.$$ (9.24)

From Eq. (9.24), it is straightforward to verify that for any nonzero constant μ, $G(\mu X) = G(X)$. In such a case, one adds the constraint to $G(X)$ and the corresponding model is denoted as

$$\max G(X),$$
$$X^T S_{t1} X = 1.$$ (9.25)

In order to further deal with Eq. (9.25), one can construct the following Lagrange function in terms of the Lagrange multiplier λ, denoted by

$$L(X) = G(X) - \lambda (X^T S_{t1} X - 1).$$ (9.26)

Setting the partial derivative of $L(X)$ with respect to X equal to zero, one obtains

$$2 s_0 S_{b1} X - 2\lambda S_{t1} X - 2 \sum_{i=1}^{d} s_i S_{t1} X_i (X_i^T S_{t1} X) / (X_i^T S_{t1} X_i) = 0.$$ (9.27)

Then one can obtain the following equation:

$$(s_0 S_{b1} - \sum_{i=1}^{d} s_i S_{t1} (X_i X_i^T) S_{t1} / (X_i^T S_{t1} X_i)) \; X = \lambda S_{t1} X,$$ (9.28)

From the above discussion, we obtain the following theorem.
Theorem 9.1 The $(d + 1)$th discriminant vector is the vector corresponding to maximum eigenvalue of the following generalized eigenequation:

$$PX = \lambda S_{t1} X,$$ (9.29)

where $P = s_0 S_{b1} - \sum_{i=1}^{d} s_i S_{t1}(X_i X_i^T) S_{t1} / (X_i^T S_{t1} X_i)$, $\sum_{i=0}^{d} s_i = 1$, $s_i \geq 0 (i = 0,...,d)$.

Compared with Eq. (9.19), we can see that it is not necessary to use the matrix inverse in Eq. (9.29). Moreover, we can directly apply previous results to compute P in Eq. (9.28). Therefore, performing the 2DLDA method costs less computational time than performing uncorrelated discriminant analysis. Applying Eq. (9.29), we can obtain optimal discriminant vectors $\{X_1,...,X_r\}$. Then corresponding Fisher criterion values can be obtained by Eq. (9.17). As is pointed out in Xu,Yang and Jin (2003), the Fisher criterion value of Liu's method (1993) corresponding to each discriminant vectors is not smaller than that of the corresponding uncorrelated discriminant vector. One asks: does there exist a relationship of Fisher criterion values between the 2DLDA method and UIDA. To answer this question, we firstly give some related knowledge on generalized eigenvalue problems. Assume that $X_1,...,X_n$ are linear independent eigenvectors of $S_{t1}^{-1} S_{b1}$ corresponding to the eigenvalues $\lambda_1 \geq \cdots \geq \lambda_n$. Let $W_1 = span\{X_{r+1}, \cdots, X_n\}$ and $W_2 = span\{X_1, \cdots, X_r\}$. Then we obtain

$$\lambda_{r+1} = \max\{J(X)|0 \neq X \in W_1\}, \tag{9.30}$$

$$\lambda_r = \min\{J(X)|0 \neq X \in W_2\}. \tag{9.31}$$

According to the above theories, we can obtain the following proposition.

Proposition 9.2 Let $J_y(X_i)(i = 1,...,n)$ be Fisher criterion values obtained by uncorrelated image discriminant analysis and $J_l(X_i)(i = 1,...,n)$ be Fisher criterion values obtained by the 2DLDA method. Then we obtain

$$J_l(X_i) \geq J_y(X_i) \ (i = 1,...,n). \tag{9.32}$$

Proof. According to the theories of generalized eigenvalue problems, it is sure that $J_y(X_i) = \lambda_i (i = 1,...,n)$. However, the discriminant vectors $\{X_1,...,X_n\}$ using the 2DLDA method may not be a basis of R^n. Assume that the rth discriminant vector X_{r1} is obtained using the 2DLDA method. If $X_{r1} \in W_2$, $J_l(X_{r1}) \geq \lambda_r = J_y(X_r)$; if $X_{r1} \in W_1$, $J_l(X_{r1}) \leq \lambda_{r+1} = J_y(X_r) \leq \lambda_r = J_y(X_r)$. Therefore, the proposition holds.

Proposition 9.2 states that Fisher criterion values of the 2DLDA algorithm must not be smaller than those of corresponding uncorrelated discriminant vectors.

Since Fisher criterion and statistical correlation are applied to construct the evaluation function, one guesses there exists the relationship between the 2DLDA method and uncorrelated discriminant analysis. To this end, we further analyze the proof of uncorrelated discriminant analysis which can be found in Jin, Yang, Tang and Hu (2001). In deducing Eq. (4.19), the following equation is applied:

$$2S_{b1}X - 2\lambda S_{t1}X - \sum_{i=1}^{d} S_{t1}X_i\; \mu = 0, \tag{9.33}$$

where $\mu_i = 2X_i^T S_{b1} X /(X_i^T S_{t1} X_i)$.

Substituting μ_i into Eq. (9.33), one can obtain

$$S_{b1}X - \sum_{i=1}^{d} S_{t1}X_i X_i^T S_{b1} X /(X_i^T S_{t1} X_i) = \lambda S_{t1}X. \tag{9.34}$$

In what follows, the relationship between Eq. (9.34) and Eq. (9.29) is further discussed.

Let

$$c_i = S_{t1}X_i X_i^T S_{b1} /(S_{t1}X_i X_i^T S_{t1}),$$

then one transforms Eq. (9.34) into the following form:

$$(S_{b1} - \sum_{i=1}^{d} c_i S_{t1}X_i X_i^T S_{t1} /(X_i^T S_{t1} X_i))X = \lambda S_{t1}X. \tag{9.35}$$

Let

$$s_0 = \frac{1}{1+\sum_{i=1}^{r} c_i} \text{ and } s_i = \frac{c_i}{1+\sum_{i=1}^{r} c_i}(i=1,\ldots,r).$$

In such a case, it is obvious that $\sum_{j=0}^{r} s_j = 1$, which satisfies the constraint in Eq. (9.29). Therefore, Eq. (9.29) is a generalization of Eq. (9.19). In other words, if we choose suitable parameters in Eq. (9.28), the solutions to Eq. (9.28) is equivalent to the solutions to Eq. (9.19). As a result, one builds a bridge between the 2DLDA algorithm and UIDA. That is, the relationship between Eq. (9.29) and Eq. (9.19) is revealed. From the above discussion, we also find an efficient method for computing the matrix P in Eq. (9.19), which doesn't need to use the matrix inverse.

9.2.3 Two-Dimensional LPP (2DLPP)

A. One-Sided 2DLPP

Since we focus on dealing with image matrices, it is useful to introduce image projections before we begin. Let $A_1 = A_M$ be M image matrices, where A_i is an $m \times n$ matrix. Then the image A is projected onto an n-dimensional vector u. That is, the following transformation is adopted: $Y_i = A_i u$. It is obvious that the projection vector Y_i is an m-dimensional vector.

As discussed in the standard spectral theory (Chung, 1997) for data representation vectors, a reasonable criterion for choosing a good map is to minimize the following objective function $\sum_{i,j}(y_i - y_j)^2 W_{ij}$ under approximate constraints. If neighbor points are mapped far apart, the objective function suffers from a heavy penalty by the weights. Applying the ideas, one can develop the following objective function for image matrices, denoted by

$$f_1(u) = \sum_{i,j} \left\| A_i u - A_j u \right\|_2^2 W_{ij} / 2. \tag{9.36}$$

Applying some algebra operations, we deal with $f_1(u)$.

$$f_1(u) = \sum_{i,j} \left\| A_i u - A_j u \right\|_2^2 W_{ij} / 2 = \frac{1}{2} \sum_{i,j} (A_i u - A_j u)^T (A_i u - A_j u) W_{ij}$$

$$= \frac{1}{2} u^T \sum_{i,j} (A_i - A_j)^T W_{ij} (A_i - A_j) u.$$

For the sake of simplicity, let us define the following matrix

$$G_w = \frac{1}{2} \sum_{i,j} (A_i - A_j)^T W_{ij} (A_i - A_j).$$

It is obvious that G_w is an $n \times n$ matrix. It is easy to obtain the matrix G_w if W is known.

G_w is further presented by

$$G_w = \frac{1}{2} \sum_{i,j} (A_i)^T W_{ij} A_i + \frac{1}{2} \sum_{i,j} (A_j)^T W_{ij} A_j - \frac{1}{2} \sum_{i,j} (A_i)^T W_{ij} A_j$$

$$= F_1 (D \otimes I_m) F_1^T - F_1 (W \otimes I_m) F_1^T$$

where $F_1 = [A_1^T \cdots A_s^T]$, D is a diagonal matrix whose diagonal elements is the column sum of W, that is, $D_{ii} = \sum_j W_{ij}$, I_m is an $m \times m$ identity matrix, $\otimes$ denotes Kronecker product. In such a case, let us define the following matrix: $L = D \otimes I_m - W \otimes I_m$, then L is a generalized Laplacian matrix.

As discussed in He and Niyogi (2003), we add the constraint on the objective function $f_1(u)$. The corresponding constraint is denoted as follows:

$$u^T F_1 (D \otimes I_m) F_1^T u = 1.$$

In all, the optimization problem can be transformed into

$$\min f_1(u) = u^T F_1 L F_1^T u, \tag{9.37}$$

subject to $u^T F_1 (D \otimes I_m) F_1^T u = 1$.

The vector u which minimizes Eq. (9.37) can be obtained by solving the following generalized eigenvalue problems $F_1 L F_1^T u = \lambda F_1 (D \otimes I_m) F_1^T u$. It is straightforward to verify that the optimal u is the eigenvector corresponding to the smallest eigenvalue. In some cases, it is not enough to obtain an optimal vector u. To this end, the eigenvectors which correspond to the first l smallest eigenvalue can be obtained.

B. The Relationship between 2DPCA and 2DLPP

Firstly, let us recall the 2DPCA. In general, the idea of 2DPCA is to solve the following eigenvalue problem:

$$G_t u = \lambda u$$

where $G_t = \sum_{i=1}^{M} (A_i - \overline{A})^T (A_i - \overline{A}) / M$ and $\overline{A} = \sum_{i=1}^{M} A_i / M$.

Substituting $\overline{A}$ into G_t and applying some algebra operations, we have

$$G_t = \frac{1}{M} F_1 (I_m \otimes I_M - \frac{1}{M} P \otimes I_M) F_1^T,$$

where P is an $m \times m$ matrix whose entries are 1.

The 2DPCA algorithm is to obtain the first l eigenvectors which correspond to the first l largest eigenvalues. This method can preserve the global structure. However, the 2DLPP algorithm is to obtain the first l eigenvectors which correspond to the first l smallest eigenvalues. It can preserve local information. It is interesting to note $F_1 (D \otimes I_m) F_1^T$ corresponds to weighed 2DPCA when $\overline{A} = 0$. This further verifies that effectiveness of Eq. (9.37), namely, Eq. (9.37) can preserve the local neighbor structure and simultaneously maximize the global structure.

C. A Generation of 2DLPP

In this section, we further extend 2DLPP. More specifically, one can apply two-sided projections on image matrices. By virtue of some ideas in Ye, Janardan and Li (2004), one considers the following $l_1 \times l_2$-dimensional space $L \otimes R$, where L is spanned by $\{u_1,\cdots,u_{l_1}\}$ and R is spanned by $\{v_1,\cdots,v_{l_2}\}$. Then the following matrices are defined: $L = [u_1 \cdots u_{l_1}]$ and $R = [v_1 \cdots v_{l_2}]$. It is easy to show that L should be an $m \times l_1$ matrix and R should be an $n \times l_2$ matrix. Accordingly, the image matrix A is projected on the space $L \otimes R$ by $L^T A R$ in such a case.

Similar to the discussion in Section 9.2.3, the following objective function is adopted:

$$f_2(L,R) = \frac{1}{2}\sum_{i,j}\left\|L^T A_i R - L^T A_j R\right\|_F^2 W_{ij}.$$

Applying some algebra operations, one further deals with $f_2(L,R)$.

$$f_2(L,R) = \frac{1}{2}\sum_{i,j}(\left\|L^T A_i R - L^T A_j R\right\|_F^2 W_{ij}$$

$$= \frac{1}{2}L^T\sum_{i,j}(A_i R - A_j R)W_{ij}R^T(A_i - A_j)^T L$$

$$L^T F_2 H_1 (D \otimes I_{l_2})H_1^T F_2^T L - L^T F_2 H_1 (W \otimes I_{l_2})H_1^T F_2^T L$$

$$= L^T S_1^R L,$$

where $F_2 = [A_1 ... A_s]$, $H_1 = diag(R,...,R)$, $S_1^R = F_2 H_1 (D \otimes I_{l_2} - W \otimes I_{l_2})H_1^T F_2^T$.

Similarly, one adds the following constraint:

$$D_l = L^T F_2 H_1 (D \otimes I_{l_2})H_1^T F_2^T L = L^T S_2^R L = I_{l_1}.$$

In such a case, the optimization problem can be reduced to

$$\arg\min_{L,R} f_2(L,R) \qquad\qquad (9.38)$$

subject to $L^T S_2^R L = I_{l_1}$.

It is obvious that this optimization problem involves two transformation matrices, L and R. It seems that it is very difficult to solve this optimization problem. Fortunately, we note that the optimization problem will minimize $tracef_2(L,R)$ and maximize $trace(D_l)$ for a fixed R. More specifically, under the assumption that R is the constant matrix, the optimal L can be obtained by solving the generalized eigenvalue problem $S_1^R u = \lambda S_2^R u$. The optimal L consists of the first l eigenvectors which correspond to the first l_1 smallest eigenvalues of $(S_2^R)^{-1}S_1^R$. For a fixed L, it is necessary to minimize $tracef_2(L,R)$ and simultaneously maximize $trace(D_l)$ in a similar manner. Note that $trace(AB) = trace(BA)$, for any two matrices A and B. In such a case, $tracef_2(L,R)$ and $trace(D_j)$ can be described as follows:

$$tracef_2(L,R) = \frac{1}{2}R^T \sum_{i,j}(A_i - A_j)^T LW_{ij}L^T(A_i - A_j)R$$

$$= trace(R^T F_1 H_2(D \otimes I_{l_1} - W \otimes I_{l_1})H_2^F F_1^T R),$$

where $H_2 = diag(L,...,L)$, $S_1^L = F_1 H_2(D \otimes I_{l_1} - W \otimes I_{l_1})H_2^T F_1^T$.

$$trace(D_j) = trace(R^T F_1 H_2(D \otimes I_{l_1})H_2^T F_1^T R) = trace(R^T S_2^L R).$$

Likewise, the optimal R can be obtained by solving the following eigenvaule problem $S_1^L v = \lambda S_2^L v$. Accordingly, R consists of the first l_2 eigenvectors of $(S_2^L)^{-1}S_1^L$ which corresponds to the first l_2 smallest eigenvalues.

From the above discussion, we also obtain an iterative algorithm for solving Eq. (9.38).

The iterative algorithm is briefly described as follows.

The iterative algorithm of 2DLPP

Step 1: Choose R_0 and compute S_2^R and S_1^R.
Step 2: Compute the first l_1 eigenvectors of $(S_2^R)^{-1}S_1^R$ and obtain L.
Step 3: Substitute L into S_2^L and S_1^L.
Step 4: Compute the first l_2 eigenvectors of $(S_2^L)^{-1}S_1^L$ and obtain R.
Step 5: Let $R_0 = R$, goto step 1.

It should be pointed out that the above algorithm adopts similar strategies with Ye's 2DLDA. A more detailed discussion on 2DLDA can be found in Ye, Janardan and Li (2004). The difference between 2DLDA and the iterative algorithm is that the latter can be performed in supervised or unsupervised manner while 2DLDA is supervised. Here a natural way to initialize R_0 is to use $R_0 = (I_{l2}, 0)^T$ which is discussed in Ye, Janardan and Li (2004). It is clear that the iterative algorithm is required to run several times for obtaining L and R, which results in the computational difficulty. However, it is of interest to note that the following lemma can be applied to simplify the above iterative algorithm.

Lemma 9.3 (Schott, 1997). Let A be $m \times m$ nonnegative definite matrix and B be an $m \times m$ positive definite matrix. If G is any $m \times h$ matrix with full column rank, then

$$trace((G^T BG)^{-1}G^T AG) \leq trace(B^{-1}A)_h,$$

where $trace(B^{-1}A)_h$ denotes the sum of the first h largest eigenvalues.

One can note that the minimization problem in Eq. (9.38) can be transformed into the maximization problem:

$$\max trace(L^T S_1^R L)^{-1} L^T S_2^R L).$$

Applying Lemma 9.3 , one has

$$trace(L^T S_1^R L)^{-1} L^T S_2^R L) \le trace((S_1^R)^{-1} S_2^R).$$

In order to solve $\max trace((S_1^R)^{-1} S_2^R)$, it is necessary to maximize $trace(S_2^R)$ and minimize $trace(S_1^R)$. In such a case, $trace(S_2^R)$ and $trace(S_1^R)$ can be further written

$$trace(S_2^R) = trace(R^T F_1(D \otimes I_n)F_1^T R) = trace(R^T S_2 R),$$

$$trace(S_1^R) = trace(R^T F_1(D \otimes I_n - W \otimes I_n)F_1^T R) = trace(R^T S_1 R).$$

In a similar way, we obtain R by solving the generalized eigenvalue problem $S_1 v = \lambda S_2 v$. R consists of the first l_2 eigenvectors of $(S_2)^{-1} S_1$ which corresponds to the first l_2 smallest eigenvalues. From the above discussion, we can propose the following algorithm for obtaining L and R.

Non-Iterative Algorithm of 2DLPP

Step 1: Obtain S_1 and S_2
Step 2: Compute the first l_2 eigenvector $(S_2)^{-1} S_1$ and obtain R.
Step 3: Obtain S_2^R and S_1^R.
Step 4: Compute the first l_2 eigenvectors of $(S_2^R)^{-1} S_1^R$ and obtain L.

It is clear that the above algorithm is an non-iterative method for obtaining L and R. Compared with the iterative algorithm, non-iterative algorithm has higher computational efficiency in general. As a matter of fact, non-iterative algorithm is two-level 2DLPP from our observations.

9.2.4 Multilinear LDA

Assume that $A_i \in \Re^{I_1 \times \cdots \times I_N}$, for $i = 1,...,M$, are M tensors in the dataset. These M tensors (samples) consist of c classes, with each class having n_i samples.

Let $M_i = \dfrac{1}{n_i} \sum_{j=1}^{n_i} A_j$

denote the mean tensor of the ith class, $1 \le i \le c$ and

$$\bar{M} = \frac{1}{M} \sum_{j=1}^{M} A_j$$

be the total mean tensor of all training samples. Given $U^{(1)} \in \Re^{I_1 \times R_1}$, $U^{(2)} \in \Re^{I_2 \times R_2}, \cdots, U^{(N)} \in \Re^{I_N \times R_N}$, we consider the following space $U^{(1)} \otimes \cdots \otimes U^{(N)}$., the tensor A_i is projected onto $U^{(1)} \otimes \cdots \otimes U^{(N)}$, denoted by $\hat{A}_i = A_i \times_1 ((U^{(1)})^T \times \cdots \times_N (U^{(N)})^T$

Similar to classical LDA, multilinear LDA is to find the optimal projections $U^{(1)} \in \Re^{I_1 \times R_1}$, $U^{(2)} \in \Re^{I_2 \times R_2}, \cdots, U^{(N)} \in \Re^{I_N \times R_N}$ such that the between-class scatter is maximized and the within-class scatter is minimized simultaneously. To this end, we define the following between-class distance and within-class distance in terms of the Frobenius-norm of tensors:

$$D_w = \sum_{i=1}^{c} \sum_{j=1}^{n_i} \left\| A_j - M_i \right\|_F^2 , \tag{9.39}$$

$$D_b = \sum_{i=1}^{c} n_i \left\| M_i - \bar{M} \right\|_F^2. \tag{9.40}$$

Similarly, one can define the between-class distance and within-class distance in the projection space $U^{(1)} \otimes ... \otimes U^{(N)}$ as follows:

$$\hat{D}_w = \sum_{i=1}^{c} \sum_{j=1}^{n_i} \left\| (A_j - M_i) \times_1 (U^{(1)})^T \times \cdots \times_N (U^{(N)})^T \right\|_F^2 , \tag{9.41}$$

$$\hat{D}_b = \sum_{i=1}^{c} n_i \left\| (M_i - \bar{M}) \times_1 (U^{(1)})^T \times \cdots \times_N (U^{(N)})^T \right\|_F^2. \tag{9.42}$$

It seems that it is very difficult for us to deal with Eqs. (9.41) and (9.42). However, the matrix representation of tensors provides an effective strategy for simplifying Eqs. (9.41) and (9.42). Note that two tensors satisfying the following relationship

$$S = A \times_1 (U^{(1)})^T \times_2 (U^{(2)})^T \times \cdots \times_N (U^{(N)})^T \tag{9.43}$$

can be represented in the following matrix form:

$$S_{(n)} = (U^{(n)})^T A_{(n)} (U^{(n+1)} \otimes \cdots \otimes U^{(N)} \otimes U^{(1)} \otimes \cdots \otimes U^{(n-1)}). \tag{9.44}$$

It is not difficult to verify that $\|A\|_F^2 = \|A_{(n)}\|_F^2$, for $n = 1,...,N$. In such a case, we substitute Eq. (9.44) into Eqs. (9.41) and (9.42) and obtain

$$\hat{D}_w = \sum_{i=1}^{c}\sum_{j=1}^{n_i}\left\|(U^{(n)})^T(A_j - M_i)_{(n)}(U^{(n+1)}\otimes\cdots\otimes U^{(N)})\right\|_F^2, \qquad (9.45)$$

$$\hat{D}_b = \sum_{i=1}^{c}n_i\left\|(U^{(n)})^T(M_i - \overline{M})_{(n)}(U^{(n+1)}\otimes\cdots\otimes U^{(N)})\right\|_F^2. \qquad (9.46)$$

In general, in order to obtain the optimal projections $U^{(1)}$, $U^{(2)}$,...,$U^{(N)}$, it is necessary to maximize D_b and to minimize D_w simultaneously. We note that it is very difficult to find the optimal projections simultaneously. To this end, we develop an iterative algorithm for obtaining the optimal projections $U^{(1)}$, $U^{(2)}$,...,$U^{(N)}$ like the algorithm of HOSVD or 2DLDA. Furthermore, we can see that for fixed $U^{(1)},\cdots,U^{(n-1)},U^{(n+1)}\cdots,U^{(N)}$, Eqs. (9.41) and (9.42) can be further represented as follows:

$$\hat{D}_w = \sum_{i=1}^{c}\sum_{j=1}^{n_i}\left\|(U^{(n)})^T(A_j - M_i)_{(n)}(U^{(n+1)}\otimes\cdots\otimes U^{(N)})\right\|_F^2$$

$$trace(U^{(n)T}S_b^{(n)}U^{(n)})$$

where

$$S_w^{(n)} = \sum_{i=1}^{c}\sum_{j=1}^{n_i}(A_j - M_i)_{(n)}(U^{(n+1)}\otimes\cdots\otimes U^{(N)})[(A_j - M_i)_{(n)}(U^{(n+1)}\otimes\cdots\otimes U^{(N)})]^T,$$

and $\hat{D}_b = \sum_{i=1}^{c}n_i\left\|(U^{(n)})^T(M_i - M)_{(1)}(U^{(n+1)}\otimes\cdots\otimes U^{(N)})\right\|_F^2 = trace((U^{(n)})^T S_b^{(n)}U^{(n)})$

where

$$S_w^{(n)} = \sum_{i=1}^{c}n_i[(M_i - M)_{(n)}(U^{(n+1)}\otimes\cdots\otimes U^{(N)})][(M_i - M)_{(n)}(U^{(n+1)}\otimes\cdots\otimes U^{(N)})]^T.$$

Similar to the 2DLDA algorithm, it is not difficult to obtain the optimal projection $U^{(n)}$. More specifically, for fixed $U^{(1),...,}U^{(n-1)}U^{(n+1)}U^{(N)}$, the optimal projection $U^{(n)}$ can be obtained by solving the generalized eigenvalue problem $S_b^{(n)}U^{(n)} = S_w^{(n)}U^{(n)}\Lambda$. In other words, $U^{(n)}$ consists of the first R_n eigenvectors which correspond to the first R_n largest eigenvalues of $(S_w^{(n)})^{-1}S_b^{(n)}$. In short, as a summary of the above discussion, the algorithm is shown Figure 9.1.

From the algorithm, one can note the following facts: when A_i ($i = 1,...,M$) are vectors, the algorithm is degenerated into classical LDA; when A_i ($i = 1,...,M$) are matrices, the algorithm is degenerated into 2DLDA. Therefore, in some sense, the 2DLDA method unifies current LDA and 2DLDA. It is obvious that the 2DLDA

Figure 9.1. The iterative algorithm for HDLDA

In: $A_i \in \Re^{I_1 \times \cdots \times I_N}$, for $i = 1,...,M$
Out: $U^{(n)}$, $n = 1,...,N$; $\hat{A}_i \in \Re^{R_1 \times \cdots \times R_N}$, for $i = 1,...,M$.

1. initial values: $U_0^{(n)}$ ($2 \leq n \leq N$));
2. compute the mean tensor M_i of class i and the globle mean tensor $\bar{M}$;
3. iterative until convergence

(i) compute $E_1 = (U_k^{(2)} \otimes \cdots \otimes U_k^{(N)})$,

$$(S_b)_1 = \sum_{i=1}^c n_i [(M_i - \bar{M})_{(1)} E_1][(M_i - \bar{M})_{(1)} E_1]^T$$

(ii) obtain $U_{k+1}^{(N)}$ consisting of the first R_1 eigenvectors of $[(S_w)_1]^{-1}(S_b)_1$.

(i) compute $E_N = (U_k^{(1)} \otimes \cdots \otimes U_k^{(N-1)})$,

$$(S_w)_N = \sum_{i=1}^c \sum_{j=1}^{n_i} [(A_j - M_i)_{(N)} E_N][(A_j - M_i)_{(N)} E_N]^T$$

$$(S_b)_N = \sum_{i=1}^c n_i [(M_i - \bar{M})_{(N)} E_N][(M_i - \bar{M})_{(N)} E_N]^T$$

(ii) obtain $U_{k+1}^{(N)}$ consisting of the first R_N eigenvectors of $[(S_w)_N]^{-1}(S_b)_N$.
4. Obtain converged values $U^{(1)},...,U^{(N)}$.
5. Compute $\hat{A}_i = (A_i) \times_1 (U^{(1)})^T \times \cdots \times_N (U^{(N)})^T$, for $i = 1,...,M$.

method can directly deal with multidimensional data. Since the algorithm is iterative, theoretically, the solution is local optimal. Like the HOSVD algorithm, probably it has several optimal solutions. In addition, we can see the algorithm involves setting initial values and judging the convergence. Therefore, it is necessary to discuss these two problems. By virtue of some ideas of HOSVD, we give the following strategy to obtain the initial values.

From Eqs. (9.39) and (9.40), we can obtain

$$D_w = \sum_{i=1}^c \sum_{j=1}^{n_i} \left\| A_j - M_i \right\|_F^2 \sum_{i=1}^c \sum_{j=1}^{n_i} trace[(A_j - M_i)_{(n)}][(A_j - M_i)_{(n)}]^T \, trace(\bar{S}_w)_{(n)}$$

where

$$(\overline{S}_w)_{(n)} = \sum_{i=1}^{c}\sum_{j=1}^{n_i}[(A_j - M_i)_{(n)}][(A_j - M_i)_{(n)}]^T. \tag{9.47}$$

$$D_b = \sum_{i=1}^{c} n_i \|M_i - M\|_F^2 = \sum_{i=1}^{c} trace[n_i(M_i - \overline{M})_{(n)}][(M_i - \overline{M})_{(n)}]^T = trace(\overline{S}_b)_{(n)},$$

where

$$(\overline{S}_b)_{(n)} = \sum_{i=1}^{c} n_i[(M_i - M)_{(n)}][(M_i - M)_{(n)}]^T. \tag{9.48}$$

In such a case, we obtain the initial values $U_0^{(n)}$ consisting of the first R_n eigenvectors of $[(\overline{S}_w)_{(n)}]^{-1}(\overline{S}_b)_{(n)}$. As discussed in He and Niyogi (2003), the main reason for choosing these initial values is that the optimal solution could be obtained by few iterations. In a similar way, the stop criterion used in the algorithm can take the form, for example, $\|U_{k+1}^{(n)} - U_k^{(n)}\|_F^2 \leq \varepsilon R_n$ $(1 \leq n \leq N)$, where ε is a positive number.

However, it is of interest to note that Lemma 9.3 can be applied to obtain a non iterative algorithm for HDLDA.

From Lemma 9.3, we have

$$trace(U^{(n)}S_w^{(n)}U^{(n)})^{-1}(U^{(n)})^T S_b^{(n)}U^{(n)} \leq trace(S_w^{(n)})^{-1}S_b^{(n)}. \tag{9.49}$$

From Eq. (9.49), we can see that it is necessary to minimize $trace(S_w^{(n)})$ and maximize $trace(S_b^{(n)})$ simultaneously. Note that

$$trace(S_w^{(n)}) \sum_{i=1}^{c}\sum_{j=1}^{n_i}\left\|(A_j - M_i)\times_1 (U^{(1)})^T \times_{n-1} (U^{(n-1)})^T \times_{n+1} (U^{(n+1)})^T \cdots \times_N (U^{(N)})^T\right\|_F^2 \tag{9.50}$$

$$trace(S_b^{(n)}) = \sum_{i=1}^{c} n_i\left\|(M_i - \overline{M})\times_1 (U^{(1)})^T \times_{n-1} (U^{(n-1)})^T \times_{n+1} (U^{(n+1)})^T \cdots \times_N (U^{(N)})^T\right\|_F^2 \tag{9.51}$$

Applying the matrix form of tensors from Eq. (9.50) and (9.51) and applying lemma 9.3, one can further reduce one projected matrix in Eq. (9.50) and (9.51). In a similar way, we can reduce the projected matrices until only one projected matrix is preserved. Without loss of generality, we assume that $U^{(1)}$ is preserved. In other words, there exist the following equations:

$$trace(S_w^{(n)})_{/2,\ldots,N} = \sum_{i=1}^{c}\sum_{j=1}^{n_i}\left\|(A_j - M_i)\times_1 (U^{(1)})^T\right\|_F^2 \tag{9.52}$$

$$trace(S_b^{(n)})_{/2,...,N} = \sum_{i=1}^{c} n_i \left\| (M_i - \bar{M}) \times_1 (U^{(1)})^T \right\|_F^2.$$ (9.53)

From Eq. (9.52) and (9.53), it is necessary to minimize $trace(S_w^{(n)})_{/2,...,N}$ and maximize $trace(S_b^{(n)})_{/2,...,N}$ simultaneously. In such a case, it is not difficult to verify that the optimal projected matrix $U^{(1)}$ consists of the first R_1 eigenvectors of $[(\bar{S}_w)_{(1)}]^{-1}(\bar{S}_b)_{(1)}$, where $(\bar{S}_w)_{(1)}$ and $(\bar{S}_b)_{(1)}$ are defined in Eq. (9.47) and Eq. (9.48). Furthermore, we apply lemma 9.3 to obtain other projected matrices until the last projected matrix is achieved. The corresponding algorithm is described in Figure 9.2.

From Figure 9.2, it is obvious the algorithm is non-iterative. Compared with the algorithm in Figure 9.1, the non-iterative algorithm has higher computational efficiency in general.

Figure 9.2. The non-iterative algorithm for HDLDA

In: $A_i \in \mathfrak{R}^{I_1 \times \cdots \times I_N}$, for $i = 1,...,M$
Out: $U^{(n)}$ $n = 1,...,N$; $\hat{A}_i \in \mathfrak{R}^{R_1 \times \cdots \times R_N}$, for $i = 1,...,M$.

1   compute the mean tensor M_i of class i and the global mean tensor $\bar{M}$;
2   · (i) compute $(\bar{S}_w)_1 = \sum_{i=1}^{c} \sum_{j=1}^{n_i} [(A_j - M_i)_{(1)}][(A_j - M_i)_{(1)}]^T$

   (ii) obtain $U^{(1)}$ consisting of the first R_1 eigenvectors of $[(\bar{S}_w)_1]^{-1}(\bar{S}_b)_1$.
   · (i) compute $E_1 = U^{(1)} \otimes I^{(3)} \otimes I^{(N)}$

$$(\bar{S}_w)_2 = \sum_{i=1}^{c} \sum_{j=1}^{n_i} [(A_j - M_i)_{(2)} E_1][(A_j - M_i)_{(2)} E_1]^T$$

$$(\bar{S}_b)_2 = \sum_{i=1}^{c} n_i [(M_i - \bar{M})_{(2)} E_1][(M_i - \bar{M})_{(2)} E_1]^T$$

   (ii) obtain $U^{(2)}$ consisting of the first R_2 eigenvectors of $[(\bar{S}_w)_2]^{-1}(\bar{S}_b)_2$.

   · (i) compute $E_{N-1} = U^{(1)} \otimes ... \otimes U^{(N-1)}$,

$$(\bar{S}_w)_N = \sum_{i=1}^{c} \sum_{j=1}^{n_i} [(A_j - M_i)_{(N)} E_N][(A_j - M_i)_{(N)} E_N]^T$$

$$(\bar{S}_b)_N = \sum_{i=1}^{c} n_i [(M_i - \bar{M})_{(N)} E_N][(M_i - \bar{M})_{(N)} E_N]^T$$

   (ii) obtain $U^{(N)}$ consisting of the first R_N eigenvectors of $[(S_w)_N]^{-1}(S_b)_N$.
3   Compute $\hat{A}_i = (A_i) \times_1 (U^{(1)})^T \times \cdots \times_N (U^{(N)})^T$, for $i = 1,...,M$.

9.3 APPLICATIONS TO BIOMETRIC VERIFICATION

9.3.1 The Performance of 2DLDA on Face Images

In order to verify and test the effectiveness of 2DLDA (Section 9.2.2), experiments are made on the ORL face image database (please refer to Section 3.2.3). Each face image is downsampled to 28×23 pixels to reduce the computational complexity. In all experiments, we apply the first five images of each subject for training and others are for testing. Namely, 200 samples are used for training and 200 samples are used for testing.

The first set of experiments is used for showing the effectiveness of the number of features. The parameters in 2DLDA (Section 9.2.2) are set as follows: $s_i = 1/(r + 1)$ $(i = 0,...,r)$. At the same time, 2DLDA is compared with uncorrelated image discriminant analysis (UIDA) and Liu's method (LM) (1993). In addition, the nearest neighbor classifier is adopted for classification due to the simplicity. Table 9.1 shows the classification performance of several methods when the number of feature vectors varies from 1 to 6. From Table 9.1, we can surprisedly see that the results of 2DLDA are the same as those of UIDA. One can also note that the classification performance of the 2DLDA algorithm is superior to that of Liu's method.

In the second set of experiments, similarly, the nearest neighbor classifier is used for classification and the parameters are set as follows: $s_i = 1/(r + 1)$ $(i = 0,...,r)$. In such a case, the execution time for feature extraction and classification of several methods are compared, which is shown in Table 9.2. As can be seen from Table 9.2, the methods based on image matrices including UIDA, LM and 2DLDA need less time than Eigenfaces or Fisherface. There is no remarkable difference in time for UIDA, LM and the 2DLDA method. Since both Eigenfaces and Fisherfaces need to convert image matrices into vectors in the process of recognition, the classification time of these two methods are more than that of 2D linear discriminant analysis. Moreover, 2D linear discriminant analysis is superior to classical linear discriminant analysis in terms of the computational efficiency for feature extraction.

In the third set of experiments, similar experimental conditions are set. Based on this, the classification performance of 2DLDA is compared with other methods

Table 9.1. Recognition accuracy of several methods on the ORL face database

The number of features	1	2	3	4	5	6
UIDA	0.8350	0.8900	0.8850	0.8850	0.8900	0.8900
LM	0.8350	0.8450	0.8650	0.8550	0.8550	0.8500
Ours	0.8350	0.8900	0.8850	0.8850	0.8900	0.8900

Table 9.2. the execution time for feature extraction and classification of five methods

Methods	Eigenfaces	Fisherfaces	Ours	LM	UIDA
Dimension	1×200	1×39	32×2	32×3	32×2
The time for extraction (s)	27.85	97.14	4.03	7.18	4.23
Classification time (s)	59.51	34.46	3.96	5.81	4.01
The total time (s)	87.36	131.60	7.99	12.99	8.24

including Fisherfaces , Eigenfaces, ICA , uncorrelated image discriminant analysis (UIDA), Liu's method (1993) and direct recognition method (DRM). The detailed experimental results are listed in Table 9.3. From Table 9.3, we can see that 2DLDA is better than other methods except for uncorrelated image discriminant analysis in recognition rates. To our surprise, the results of 2DLDA are the same as those of uncorrelated image discriminant analysis.

In the fourth set of experiments, we discuss the Fisher criterion values of several methods such as Liu's method (1993) and uncorrelated image discriminant analysis. Firstly, we set the parameters as follows: $s_i = 1/(r + 1)$ $(i = 0,...,r)$. In addition, we also discuss another case, namely $s_0 = 0.0001$ and $s_i = 1/r$ $(i = 1,...,r)$. In such a case, we think that the Fisher criterion plays an insignificant role and the statistical correlation between feature vectors plays an important role in feature extraction, denoted by (2). From Table 9.4, it is obvious that the Fisher criterion value of UIDA corresponding to each feature vector is the smallest in all methods. From Table 9.3, we know the classification performance of the 2DLDA algorithm is superior to that of Liu's method. This means the Fisher criterion value is not an absolute criterion for measuring the discriminatory power of discriminant vectors. We also find that the classification performance is not superior to that of uncorrelated image discriminant analysis in the second case, which also shows that statistical correlation is not an absolute criterion for measuring the discriminatory power of discriminant vectors. Therefore, in order to obtain powerful discriminant vectors, it is necessary to combine Fisher criterion values and statistical correlations among feature vectors.

Table 9.3. Recognition rates (%) of several methods

Methods	Eigenfaces	Fisherfaces	LM	UIDA	ICA	DM	Ours
Dimension	1×200	1×39	32×3	32×2	1×40	32×28	32×2
Recognition rates	88.0	86.0	86.5	89.0	84.2	83.5	89.0

Table 9.4. Fisher criterion values of several methods

$J(X_i)$	X_1	X_2	X_3	X_4	X_5	X_6
UIDA	0.8667	0.8315	0.6562	0.5804	0.5012	0.4725
LM	0.8667	0.8399	0.7479	0.6757	0.6498	0.5746
Ours (1)	0.8667	0.8315	0.6562	0.5804	0.5012	0.4725
Ours (2)	0.8667	0.8315	0.6563	0.5806	0.5014	0.4722

9.3.2 The Performance of 2DLPP on Faces Images

In order to verify and test 2DLPP described in Section 9.2.3. The experiments are made on several data sets. From iterative and non-iterative algorithms, we can see that two important parameters l_1 and l_2 are involved. For the sake of simplicity, l_1 and l_2 are set to the common value l in the following experiments. The samples belonging to the same class are considered to be closed. The weights n our experiments are set $W_{ij} = e^{-\|x_i - x_j\|/t}$. Since we focus on feature extraction by using 2DLPP, the nearest neighbor classifier is adopted.

Face images are obtained from Olivetti Research Lab. Each face image is downsampled to 28 × 23 pixels to reduce the computational complexity. Let us check the effect of the number of iterations. To this end, an experiment is carried out by using randomly chosen 5 images per class for training, the rest of image for testing. The parameter l is set to 10. Figure 9.3 denotes experimental results, where the x-axis denotes the number of iterations, and the y-axis denotes the recognition performance. As can be seen from Figure 9.3 (a), it is necessary to use several iterations to obtain good experiments results. In the meantime, we compare the performance of non-iterative algorithm (A1) with that of the iterative algorithm (A2) when the number of features changes in the interval of [1,16], where A2 is applied 10 iterations. Figure9.3 (b) denotes the experiments results. From Figure 9.3 (b), we can see that the recognition performance increases with the increase of features in general case. Non-iterative algorithm and the iterative algorithm obtain almost similar results. The smaller difference between may result from the precision of calculation. In addition, we compare our basic 2DLPP with LPP in terms of the running time for feature extraction. The running time of 2DLPP for feature extraction is 11.45s, while LPP takes 16.45s to extract features. It is obvious that 2DLPP is faster than LPP in terms of computational efficiency for feature extraction. Finally, we compare our algorithms with LPP with the change of features. In this experiment, the leave-one-out strategy is adopted. Figure 9.3 (c) lists the experimental results with the increase of *l*. As observed in Figure 9.3 (c), the recognition performance of 2DLPP is superior to that of classical LPP when the number of features is small. But

Figure 9.3. Experimental results on the ORL database (a) the effect of iterations for A1 (b) the recognition performance of A1 and A2 with the change of features.(c) the recognition performance of several methods with the change of feature by the leave-one-out strategy.

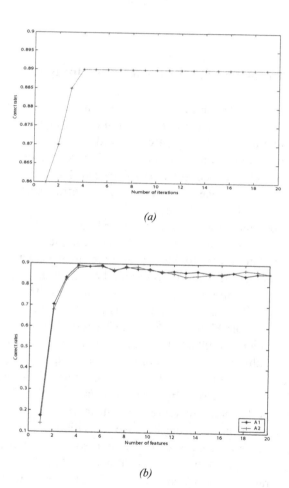

(a)

(b)

continued on following page

Figure 9.3. continued

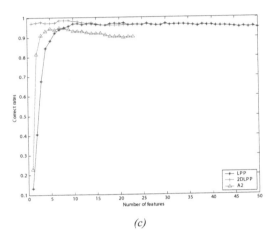

(c)

extended 2DLPP is inferior to classical LPP with respect to accuracy. The highest recognition rate of 2DLPP is 97.50%, while LPP reaches 96.75%.

9.3.3 The Performance of 2DLPP on Handwritten Character Database

The used dataset of handwritten numeral characters are from the UCI data set repository. For the description of the dataset, please refer to Section 8.3.2. Using the same procedure as shown in Section 8.3.2, we produce 256-dimensional features for each character image. We also choose only 100 samples from each class to constitute training samples and others are used for testing. As discussed in ORL experiments, the first experiment is made to show the effectiveness of iterations. In this experiment, the parameter l is set to 8. Figure 9.4 (a) shows the recognition performance with the change of iterations. From Figure 9.4 (b), it is obvious that it is not necessary to take several iterations to obtain good experimental results. However, accuracy curve is unstable with the change of iterations. In a similar way, we compare our algorithms including extended 2DLPP (non-iterative (A2) and iterative (A1)) with classical LPP in terms of the change of features. Figure 9.4 (b) denotes the recognition performance with the increase of features. As observed in Figure 9.4 (b), the performance of all the algorithms increases with the increase of features in general cases. It is noted that 2DLPP obtains almost similar experimental results with LPP, but is superior to extended 2DLPP in some cases.

Figure 9.4. Experimental results on handwritten numeral characters (a) effect of A1 in terms of the number of iterations (b) the effect of several methods in terms of the change of features.

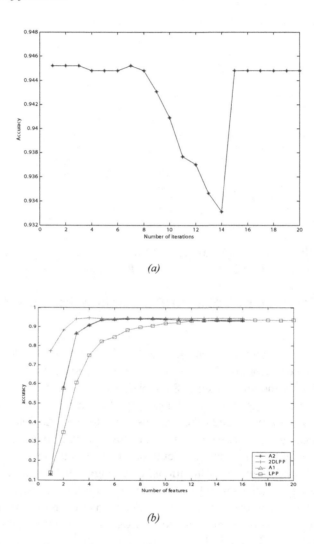

(a)

(b)

Moreover, the results of A2 are almost the same as those of A1. A2 is more efficient than A1 due to its non-iterations. We also note that Extended 2DLPP needs less coefficients that 2DLPP.

9.3.4 The Performance of Multilinear LDA

In order to test multilinear LDA, the experiments are made on color face images which can be obtained by the University of Essex (UK) face database http://cswww. essex.ac.uk/mv/ allfaces/index.html. The images in the Essex database are JPEG-compared 24-bit color images. The size of each color face image is 200 × 180. The subjects represent a wide distribution of ethnic group and both genders, but nearly all subjects are between 18 and 20 years old. It is obvious that each color face image corresponds to a three-order tensor. Hence, it is easy to apply the multilinear method to this database. In order to reduce the computational cost, we only use a subset of this face dataset. We select 40 persons with each person having 10 color images. In other words, the total number of samples is 400. Meanwhile, we subsample the original image to 50 × 45-size images. In such a case, we randomly choose 5 samples from each class to form the training samples and other samples are used for testing. In order to reduce variation, the experimental results reported in this paper are averaged over ten runs. For the sake of simplicity, we adopt the Frobenius-norm as distance measure and consider the sample with minimal distance as recognition samples. The first set of experiments is used for showing the effect of the number of iterations. Moreover, we compare the multilinear LDA method with HOSVD. Figure 9.5 shows the experimental results, where the x-axis denotes

Figure 9.5. Recognition accuracy with the change of the number of iterations

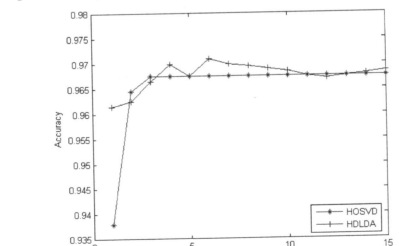

the number of iterations, and the y-axis denotes the recognition performance. In this experiment, we set $R_1 = R_2 = 10$ and $R_3 = 2$. From Figure9.5, we can see that the recognition performance is not changed violently when the number of iterations is bigger than some value. It is clear that the multilinear LDA method can obtain completive results with HOSVD. We also note that it is unnecessary for too many iterations to obtain good recognition results.

The next experiment is used to show the effect of reduced dimensions. Since the third dimension of tensors is small, we set $R_3 = 2$. Meanwhile, similar to 2DLDA, we set $R_1 = R_2 = d$. Figure 9.6 shows the recognition performance with the change of d. From Figure9.6, we note that the recognition performance firstly increases and then decreases. It is clear that the multilinear LDA method obtains slightly better results than HOSVD in terms of classification performance. Moreover, we note that the non-iterative HDLDA (NHDLDA) method obtains almost the same results with HDLDA. It shows that it may adopt the non-iterative method for solving HDLDA in order to obtain the computational efficiency in real applications.

9.4 SUMMARY AND DISCUSSION

In recent years, tensor discriminant analysis has attracted considerable interest from researchers. In this chapter, we mainly describe several variants of classical LDA including 2DLDA, 2DLPP and HOLDA after classical LDA is given.

Figure 9.6. Recognition accuracy with the change of the number features

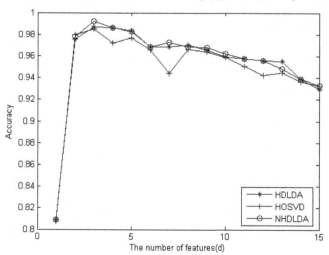

First, we describe two-dimensional linear discriminant analysis for image feature extraction. It directly utilizes image matrices to construct the Fisher criterion function, which does not need to convert image matrices into high-dimensional vectors such as classical LDA. Then discriminant vectors are obtained by maximizing Fisher criterion functions and minimizing statistical correlation between extracted features. Since the size of image matrices is much smaller that of vectors, the execution time of two-dimensional linear discriminant analysis for feature extraction is much less than that of traditional linear discriminant analysis. Moreover, we demonstrate that the Fisher criterion values of two-dimensional linear discriminant analysis are no less than the Fisher criterion values of uncorrelated discriminant vectors. In addition, the feature vectors obtained by two-dimensional linear discriminant analysis are the same as those obtained by uncorrelated discriminant vectors in some condition. It should be pointed out that the 2DLDA method requires more coefficients for feature extraction than LDA. In other words, the 2DLDA method needs more storage space than the classical LDA method, which is one of disadvantages of 2D linear discriminant analysis.

Second, two dimensional locality preserving projections are described. These algorithms are based on image matrices instead of vectors. As a result, 2DLPP is required to solve eigen-decomposition with small sizes, while LPP needs to solve eigen-decomposition with large sizes. Moreover, 2DLPP can be performed in unsupervised or supervised or semi-supervised manner. Similar to LPP, 2DLPP can preserve the local neighborhood structure as possible. However, it is worthwhile to point out that 2DLPP needs much more storage requirements since 2DLPP involutes much more coefficients than classical LPP. A feasible way to deal with this problem is to use LPP after 2DLPP is applied.

Third, a multilinear generalization of linear discriminant analysis is described. In some sense, it unifies some existing discriminant analysis methods such as LDA and 2DLDA. One of important characteristics of multilinear discriminant analysis is that it can work with the data tensor representation. In addition, it should be noted that the selection of the optimal dimension of tensors is still an open question similar to 2DLDA.

Finally, a lot of experiments are made on face images and handwritten numerical characters to demonstrate the effectiveness of these tensor subspace methods. It demonstrates that tensor subspace methods outperform classical subspace methods in some cases.

REFERENCES

Chung, F. (1997). Spectral graph theory. In *CBMS regional conference series in mathematics* (Vol. 92). RI: American Mathematical Society.

Duchene, J., & Leclercq, S. (1988). An optimal transformation for discriminant and principal component analysis. *IEEE Trans Pattern Anal. Machine Intell., 10*(6), 978-983.

Foley, D. H., & Sammon, J. W. (1975). An optimal set of discriminant vector. *IEEE Trans. Computer, C-24*(3), 281-289.

He, X. F., & Niyogi, P. (2003). Locality preserving projections. In S. Thrun, L. K. Saul, & B. Scholkopf (Eds.), *Advances in neural information processing systems,16*, 153-160. MA: The MIT Press.

Jin, Z., Yang, J-Y., Hu, Z. S., & Luo, Z. (2001). Face recognition based on the uncorrelated discriminant transformation. *Pattern Recognition, 34*(7), 1405-1416.

Jin, Z., Yang, J-Y., Tang, Z., & Hu, Z. (2001). A theorem on the uncorrelated optimal discriminant vectors. *Pattern Recognition, 34*(10), 2041-2047.

Jing, X. Y., Zhang, D., & Jin, Z. (2003). Improvements on the uncorrelated optimal discriminant vectors. *Pattern Recognition, 36*(8), 1921-1923.

Liang, Z. Z. (2006). High-dimensional discriminant analysis and its application to color face recognition. *Proceedings of the International Conference on Pattern Recognition* (pp. 917-920).

Liang, Z. Z., Shi, P. F., & Zhang, D. (2006). Two-dimensional Fisher discriminant analysis and its application to face recognition. *Proceedings of the 7th Asian Conference on Computer Vision* (pp. 130-139).

Liu, K., Cheng, Y-Q., & Yang, J-Y. (1993). Algebraic feature extraction for image recognition based on an optimal discriminant criterion. *Pattern Recognition, 26*(6), 903-911.

Schott, J. R. (1997). *Matrix analysis for statistics.* NY: Wiley-InterScience.

Xiong, H. L., Swam, M. S. S., & Ahmad, M. O. (2005). Two-dimensional FLD for face recognition. *Pattern Recognition, 38*(7), 1121-1124.

Xu, Y., Yang, J-Y., & Jin, Z. (2003). Theory analysis on FSLDA and ULDA. *Pattern Recognition, 36*(12), 3031-3033.

Xu, Y., Yang, J-Y., & Jin, Z. (2004). A novel method for Fisher discriminant analysis. *Pattern Recognition, 37*(2), 381-384.

Yan, S., Xu, D., Yang, Q., Zhang, L., Tang, X., & Zhang, H. (2005). Discriminant analysis with tensor representation. *Proceedings of the IEEE Conference on Computer Vision and Pattern Recognition* (pp. 526-532).

Yang, J., Yang, J-Y., Frangi, A. F., & Zhang, D. (2003). Uncorrelated projection discriminant analysis and its application to face image feature extraction. *Inter. J. of Pattern Recognition and Artificial Intelligence, 17*(8), 1325-1347.

Ye, J. P. (2005). Characterization of a family of algorithms for generalized discriminant analysis on undersampled problems. *Journal of Machine Learning Research, 6*(Apr), 483-502.

Ye, J. P., Janardan, R., & Li, Q. (2004). Two-dimensional linear discriminant analysis. In *Advances in neural information processing systems*. San Mateo: Morgan Kaufmann Publishers.

Ye, J. P., Janardan, R., Park, C. H., & Park, H. (2004). An optimization criterion for generalized discriminant analysis on undersampled problems. *IEEE Trans. Pattern Anal. Mach. Intell., 26*(8), 982-994.

Ye, J. P., & Li, Q. (2005). A two-stage linear discriminant analysis via QR-decomposition. *IEEE Trans. Pattern Anal. Mach. Intell., 27*(6), 929-941.

Chapter X
Tensor Independent Component Analysis and Tensor Non-Negative Factorization

ABSTRACT

In this chapter, we describe two tensor-based subspace analysis approaches (tensor ICA and tensor NMF) that can be used in many fields like face recognition and other biometric recognition. Section 10.1 gives the background and development of the two tensor-based subspace analysis approaches. Section 10.2 introduces tensor independent component analysis. Section 10.3 presents tensor nonnegative factorization. Section 10.4 discusses some potential applications of these two subspace analysis approaches in biometrics. Finally, we summarize this chapter in Section 10.5.

10.1 INTRODUCTION

Independent component analysis (ICA) (Hyvärinen & Oja, 2001) is a statistical signal processing technique. The basic idea of ICA is to represent a set of random variables using basis functions, where the components are statistically independent or as independent as possible. In general, there are two arguments for using ICA for image representation and recognition. First, the high-order relationships among images pixels may contain important information for recognition tasks. Second, ICA seeks to find the directions so that the projections of the data into those directions have maximally non-Gaussian distribution, which may be useful for classification tasks. In addition, the concept of ICA can be viewed as a generalization of PCA, since it is concerned not only with the second-order dependencies between variables but also with high-order dependencies between them.

During the past several years, the ICA algorithm has been widely used in face recognition and biomedical data. Bartlett and Sejnowski (1997) have demonstrated that the recognition accuracy using ICA basis vectors is higher than that of the PCA basis vectors with 200 face images. They found that the ICA representation of faces has the invariance to big changes in pose and small changes in illuminations. In Bartlett, Movellan and Sejnowski (2002), the authors first organized the database into a matrix X where each row vector is a different image. In this representation, the images are random variables and the pixels are trials. In this case, it makes sense to talk about independence of images or functions of images. Two images i and j are independent if when moving across pixels. In addition, they transposed the matrix X and organized the data so that images are in the columns of X. In this representation, pixels are random variables and images are trials. Here, it also makes sense to talk about independence of pixels or functions of pixels. For example, pixel and would be independent if when moving across the entire set of images. Based on these two ideas, they suggested two ICA architectures (ICA Architectures I and II) for face representation and used the Infomax algorithm (Bell & Sejnowski, 1995, 1997) to implement ICA. Both architectures were evaluated on a subset of the FERET face database and were found to be effective for face recognition. Yuen and Lai (2000, 2002) adopted the fixed-point algorithm to obtain the independent components (ICs) and used a householder transform to gain the least square solution of a face image for representations. Liu and Wechsler (1999, 2003) used an ICA algorithm to perform ICA and assessed its performance for face identification. All of these researchers claimed that ICA outperforms PCA in face recognition. Other researchers, however, reported differently. Baek, Draper, Beveridge, and She (2002) reported that PCA outperforms ICA while Moghaddam (2002), Jin and Davoine (2004) reported no significant performance difference between the two methods. Socolinsky and Selinger (2002) reported that ICA outperforms PCA on visible images but PCA outperforms ICA on infrared images.

Recently, Draper, Baek, Bartlett, and Beveridge (2003) tried to account for these apparently contradictory results. They retested ICA and PCA on the FERET face database with 1196 individuals and made a comprehensive comparison of the performances of the two methods and found that the relative performance of ICA and PCA mainly depends on the ICA architecture and the distance metric. Their experimental results showed that: (1) ICA Architecture II with the cosine distance significantly outperforms PCA with L1 (city block), L2 (Euclidean), and cosine distance metrics. This is consistent with Bartlett and Liu's results; (2) PCA with the L1 distance outperforms ICA Architecture I, which is in favour of Baek's results (2002); and (3) ICA Architecture II with L2 still significantly outperforms PCA with L2, although the degree of significance is not as great as in the ICA Architecture II with cosine over PCA. Moreover, it should be noted that this latter result is still inconsistent with Moghaddam (2002) and Jin's results (2004). Yang, Zhang, and Yang (2007) analyzed two ICA architectures and found that ICA Architecture I involves a vertically centred PCA process (PCA I), while ICA Architecture II involves a whitened horizontally centred PCA process (PCA II). Thus, it makes sense to use these two PCA versions as baselines to revaluate the performance of ICA-based face-recognition systems. Their experiments on the FERET, AR, and AT&T face-image databases showed no significant differences between ICA Architecture I (II) and PCA I (II), although ICA Architecture I (or II) may, in some cases, significantly outperform standard PCA. It is observed that the performance of ICA strongly depends on the PCA process it involves. Pure ICA projection has only a trivial effect on the performance in face recognition. More recently, motivated by multilinear algebra,some researchers proposed tensor independent component analysis.

Non-negative matrix factorization (NMF) (Lee & Seung, 1999, 2001; Li, Hou, & Zhang, 2001) is also a subspace method, which has been used for image representation and image classification. Nonnegative matrix factorization differs from other subspace methods for vector space models, for example, principal component analysis (PCA) or vector quantization (VQ), LDA, and ICA due to the use of constraints that produce nonnegative basis vectors, which make the concept of a parts-based representation possible. In the case of NMF, the basis vectors contain no negative entries. As a result, this allows only additive combinations of the vectors to reproduce the original vectors. So the perception of the whole, an image in a collection, becomes a combination of its parts represented by these basis vectors. However, some experiments show that directly using the learned feature vectors via NMF under the Euclidean distance (L2 distance) cannot improve the face recognition accuracy in contrast to traditional PCA. It is partly because that the learned bases via NMF are not orthogonal to each other. In order to improve the accuracy, Li, Hou and Zhang (2001) proposed one method called local NMF which impose additional constraints on bases. But this method has a slow speed for learning the bases. Recently Guillamet and Vitria (2003) adopted one relevant metric called earth movers distance (EMD) for parts-based representation of NMF. However the computation of EMD is too time-demanding. Liu and Zheng (2004) used two strategies to improve the accuracy of recognition. One is to adopt a Riemannian metric like distance for the learned feature vectors instead of the Euclidean distance. The other is to first orthonormalize the learned bases and then to use the projections of data based on the orthonormalized bases for further recognition. Their experiments on the USPS database demonstrate that the proposed methods can improve accuracy and even outperform PCA. Up till now, how to use the learned bases and feature vectors via NMF for further analysis such as recognition is still an open problem.

Note that in the above NMF algorithms the input data must be the vector form. However, some data are often represented as the tensor form (images). In applying traditional NMF, the 2D image matrices must be previously transformed into 1D image vectors. The resulting image vectors usually lead to a high-dimensional image vector space, where it is difficult to find good bases to approximately reconstruct original images. That is also the so-called 'curse of dimensionality' problem, which is more apparent in small-sample-size cases. To this end, some variants of NMF (Shashua & Hazan, 2005; Zhang, Chen, & Zhou, 2005) are developed in recent years. The key difference between NMF and its variants is that the latter adopts a novel representation for original images. Zhang, Chen and Zhou (2005) proposed 2-D non-negative matrix factorization. 2DNMF regards images as 2D matrices and represents them with a set of 2D bases. Their experimental results on several face databases show that 2DNMF has better image reconstruction quality than NMF under the same compression ratio. Moreover, it is also observed that the running time of 2DNMF is less that of NMF and the recognition accuracy of 2DNMF is higher than that of NMF.

10.2 TENSOR INDEPENDENT COMPONENT ANALYSIS

10.2.1 Two Architecture of ICA for Image Representations

A. ICA Architecture I

Given a set of M training samples (image column vectors), $x_1,...,x_M$ in $\mathfrak{R}^N$, the image column data matrix is written as $X = [x_1,...,x_M]$ and its transpose (image row data matrix) $Y = X^T$.

In Architecture I, the images are seen as random variables and the pixel values provide observations of these variables. This means that ICA is performed on the image row data matrix Y. Rewriting $Y = [y_1,...,y_N]$, its column vectors $y_1,...,y_N$ are used as observation vectors to estimate the unmixing matrix of the ICA model.

In Architecture I, the following steps are used to extract independent components.

1.　Centering data: Center the data Y in an observation space and obtain its mean vector $\mu_I = E\{y\} = (1/N)\sum_{j=1}^{N} y_j$. Denote $\mu_I = [\mu_1,...\mu_M]^T$. Subtracting the mean vector from each observation vector, that is, $\bar{y}_j = y_j - \mu_I$, we obtain the centered image row data matrix $Y_h = [\bar{y}_1, \cdots, \bar{y}_N]$.

2. Sphering data using PCA: Sphere the data using PCA based on the centered observation vectors $\bar{y}_1, \cdots, \bar{y}_N$. The covariance matrix Σ_I is given by

$$\Sigma_I = \frac{1}{N}\sum_{i=1}^{N} \bar{y}_i \bar{y}_i^T .$$ (10.1)

Then one can calculate the orthonormal eigenvectors $\gamma_1, \cdots, \gamma_d (d \leq M)$ of Σ_I corresponding to the d largest positive eigenvalues $\lambda_1, \dots, \lambda_d$. Letting $V = \gamma_1, \cdots, \gamma_d$ and $\Lambda = [\lambda_1, \cdots, \lambda_d]$, one can obtain the whitening matrix $P = V\Lambda^{-1/2}$ such that

$$P^T \Sigma_I P = I.$$ (10.2)

The data matrix $Y_h = [\bar{y}_1, \cdots \bar{y}_N]$ can be whitened using the transformation.

$$R = P^T Y_h.$$ (10.3)

3. ICA processing: Perform ICA on R, producing the matrix U_I with d independent basis images in its rows,

$$U_I = W_I R_h,$$ (10.4)

where W_I is the unmixing matrix generated by a given ICA algorithm based on the input data R.

Note that the unfixing matrix must be invertible, from Eq. (10.4), it follows that

$$R = (W_I)^{-1} U_I.$$ (10.5)

After vertically centering and projecting a given image x in a column vector onto the row vectors of R, one has $z = Rx$.

Therefore, in the space spanned by the row vectors of U_I, i.e., a set of d statistically independent basis images, the vector of representation coefficients of image x given by

$$s = (W_1^{-1})^T z = (W_1^{-1})^T Rx.$$ (10.6)

Overall, the transformation can be obtained by the following two steps:

$$z = Rx, \tag{10.7}$$

$$s = (W_1^{-1})^T z. \tag{10.8}$$

B. ICA Architecture II

The goal of ICA Architecture II is to find statistically independent coefficients for the input image data. In this architecture, the images are viewed as observations, and the pixel values are random variables. ICA is performed directly on the image column data matrix X. In other words, $x_1,...,x_M$ are used as observation vectors to estimate the unmixing matrix of the ICA model.

Similar to Architecture I, the following steps are used to extract independent components.

1. Centering data: centralize the data Y in an observation space and obtain its mean vector $\mu_{II} = E\{x\} = (1/M)\sum_{j=1}^{M} x_j$. When the mean vector is subtracted from every observation vector, one gets the centered image column data matrix $X_h = [\overline{x}_1, \cdots, \overline{x}_M]$.
2. Sphering data using PCA: Sphere the data using PCA based on the centered observation vectors $\overline{x}_1, \cdots, \overline{x}_M$. The covariance matrix Σ_{II} is given by

$$\Sigma_{II} = \frac{1}{M} \sum_{i=1}^{M} \overline{x}_i \overline{x}_i^T. \tag{10.9}$$

Then one can calculate the orthonormal eigenvectors $\gamma_1, \cdots, \gamma_d (d \le M)$ of Σ_{II} corresponding to the d largest positive eigenvalues $\lambda_1, \cdots, \lambda_d$. Letting $V = [\gamma_1, \cdots, \gamma_d]$ and $\Lambda = [\lambda_1, \cdots, \lambda_d]$, one can obtain the whitening matrix $P = V\Lambda^{-1/2}$ such that

$$P^T \Sigma_I P = I. \tag{10.10}$$

The data matrix $X_h = [\overline{x}_1, \ldots, \overline{x}_M]$ can be whitened using the transformation

$$R = P^T X_h. \tag{10.11}$$

3. ICA processing: Perform ICA on R, producing the matrix U_I with d independent basis images in its rows, i.e.,

$$U_I = W_I R, \tag{10.12}$$

where W_I is the unmixing matrix generated by a given ICA algorithm based on the input data R.

Note that the unfixing matrix must be invertible, from Eq. (10.12), it follows that

$$R = (W_{II})^{-1} U_I. \tag{10.13}$$

Therefore, in the space spanned by the row vectors of U_I, i.e., a set of d statistically independent basis images, the vector of representation coefficients of image x given by

$$s = (W_{II}^{-1})^T z = (W_{II}^{-1})^T P^T x. \tag{10.14}$$

Overall, the transform can be obtained by the following two steps:

$$z = P^T x, \tag{10.15}$$

$$s = (W_{II}^{-1})^T z. \tag{10.16}$$

From the above analysis, one can see that ICA Architecture I involves a vertically cantered PCA (PCA I), whereas ICA Architecture II involves a whitened horizontally cantered PCA (PCA II). Standard PCA removes the mean image of all training samples, while PCA I removes the mean of each image. PCA II is a whitened version of standard PCA. It can normalize the variances of coefficients as well as being able to make these coefficients uncorrelated. To assess the performance of two ICA architectures, it is necessary to compare them with the two different versions of PCA as well as with the standard PCA. In other words, PCA I, PCA II, and standard PCA should all be used as baseline algorithms to evaluate the ICA. Figure 10.1 illustrates two ICA-based image-representation architectures.

10.2.2 The 2DICA Algorithm

Assume that $m \times n$ matrices A_k, $k = 1,...,M$, denote original M training images. In 2DICA, one does not need to transform the 2D images into its corresponding 1D vectors. Instead one uses a more straightforward way which views an image as a 2D matrix.

One can use two successive stages to perform 2DICA. First, one aligns the M images into a $m \times nM$ matrix $X = [A_1,...,A_M]$, where each A_k denotes one of the M face images. After X is obtained, we obtain its mean vector $\mu = (1/nM)\sum_{j=1}^{nM} X_j$ and center the data X. After every vector is subtracted by the mean vector, one can get

Figure 10.1. Two ICA-based image-representation architectures

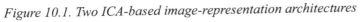
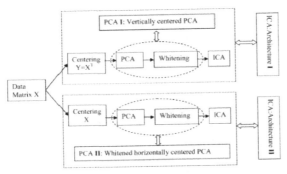

the centered image data matrix $\overline{X} = [\overline{x}_1, \cdots, \overline{x}_{nM}]$. One will sphere the data using PCA based on the centered vectors $\overline{x}_1, \cdots, \overline{x}_{nM}$. The covariance matrix Σ_I is given by

$$\Sigma_I = \frac{1}{nM} \sum_{i=1}^{nM} \overline{x}_i \overline{x}_i^T. \tag{10.17}$$

Then one can calculate the orthonormal eigenvectors $\gamma_1, \cdots, \gamma_d (d \leq nM)$ of Σ_{II} corresponding to the d largest positive eigenvalues $\lambda_1, \ldots, \lambda_d$.

Letting $V = [\gamma_1, \cdots, \gamma_d]$ and $\Lambda = [\lambda_1, \cdots, \lambda_d]$, one can obtain the whitening matrix $P = V\Lambda^{-1/2}$ such that

$$P^T \Sigma_I P = I. \tag{10.18}$$

The data matrix $\overline{X} = [\overline{x}_1, \cdots, \overline{x}_{nM}]$ can be whitened using the transformation

$$R = P^T \overline{X}. \tag{10.19}$$

Then one can perform ICA on R, producing the matrix U_I with d independent basis images in its rows, i.e.,

$$U_I = W_I R, \tag{10.20}$$

where W_I is the unmixing matrix generated by a given ICA algorithm based on the input data R.

Note that the unfixing matrix must be invertible, from Eq. (10.20), it follows that

$$R = (W_I)^{-1} U_I.$$ (10.21)

Therefore, in the space spanned by the row vectors of U_I, i.e., a set of d statistically independent basis images, the vector of representation coefficients of image x given by

$$\hat{A}_k = (W_I^{-1})^T P^T A_k = W_I P^T A_k \ k = 1, \cdots, M.$$ (10.22)

It is obvious that $\hat{A}_k(k = 1, \cdots, M)$ are $d \times n$ matrices.

Based on Eq. (10.22), we perform the second stage on $\hat{A}_k(k = 1, \dots, M)$. We first construct a matrix from submatrices $\hat{A}_k(k = 1, \dots, M)$ and define as follows $Y = [\hat{A}_1^T, \cdots, \hat{A}_M^T]$. It is obvious that Y is a $n \times dM$ matrix. After Y is obtained, we obtain its mean vector $\mu = (1/dM) \sum_{j=1}^{dM} Y_j$ and center the data Y. After the mean vector is subtracted from every vector, we get the centered image data matrix $\bar{Y} = [\bar{y}_1, \cdots, \bar{y}_{dM}]$. We will sphere the data using PCA based on the centered vectors $\bar{y}_1, \cdots, \bar{y}_{dM}$. The covariance matrix Σ_{II} is given by

$$\Sigma_{II} = \frac{1}{dM} \sum_{i=1}^{dM} \bar{y}_i \bar{y}_i^T.$$ (10.23)

Then we can calculate the orthonormal eigenvectors $\gamma_1, \dots, \gamma_d (d \leq dM)$ of Σ_{II} corresponding to the d largest positive eigenvalues $\lambda_1, \dots, \lambda_d$. Letting $V = \gamma_1, \dots, \gamma_d$ and $\Lambda = [\lambda_1, \cdots, \lambda_d]$, we obtain the whitening matrix $\tilde{P} = V \Lambda^{-1/2}$ such that

$$\tilde{P}^T \Sigma_{II} \tilde{P} = I.$$ (10.24)

The data matrix $\bar{Y} = [\bar{y}_1, \cdots, \bar{y}_{dM}]$ can be whitened using the transformation

$$R = \tilde{P}^T \bar{Y}.$$ (10.25)

Then we perform ICA on R, producing the matrix U_I with d independent basis images in its rows, i.e.,

$$U_I = W_{II} R,$$ (10.26)

where W_{II} is the unmixing matrix generated by a given ICA algorithm based on the input data R.

Note that the unfixing matrix must be invertible, from Eq. (10.26), it follows that

$$R = (W_{II})^{-1} U_I.\tag{10.27}$$

Therefore, in the space spanned by the row vectors of U_I, i.e., a set of d statistically independent basis images, the vector of representation coefficients of image x given by

$$\dddot{A}_k = (W_{II}^{-1})^T \tilde{P}^T (\hat{A}_k)^T = W_{II} \tilde{P}^T (A_k)^T P(W_I)^T, k = 1,...,M.\tag{10.28}$$

It is obvious that $\dddot{A}_k$ are $d \times d$ matrices.

From the above analysis, we know that 2DICA first performs the column ICA, then followed by row ICA operations. Figure 10.2 demonstrate how a high-dimensional image is converted into a low-dimensional image by using 2DICA.

Finally, the pseudo-code for performing 2DICA is descried as follows:

The 2DICA Algorithm

Input: $m \times n$ image matrices $\{A_k\}_{k=1}^M$ and the reduction dimension d.
Output: the matrices $W_I, W_{II}, P, \tilde{P}$.
Step 1: Align the M images into a $m \times nM$ matrix $X = [A_1, \cdots, A_M]$
Step 2: Perform classical ICA for X, and obtain matrices W_I and P.
Step 3: Construct a new matrix $Y = [\hat{A}_1^T, \cdots, \hat{A}_M^T]$
Step 4: Performing classical ICA on Y, and obtain matrices W_{II} and $\tilde{P}$,
Step 5: Obtain the approximate matrix of $\dddot{A}_k = W_{II} \tilde{P}^T (A_k)^T P(W_I)^T \ k = 1, \cdots, M$.

Figure 10.2. The dimensionality reduction by using 2DICA

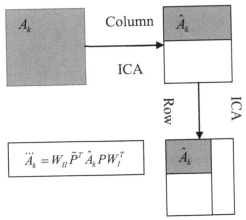

Note that in the above algorithm, we first align the M images into a $m \times nM$ matrix $X = [A_1, \cdots, A_M]$. In fact, we can also align the M images into a $m \times nM$ matrix $Y = [A_1^T, \cdots, A_M^T]$.

10.2.3 Multilinear ICA

Multilinear ICA is obtained by first representing the data tensor G as the node-n product of N mode matrices

$$G = S \times_1 U_1 \times \cdots \times_N U_N.$$

Then the N-mode ICA algorithm mainly consists of the following two steps:

1. For $n = 1, \cdots, N$, compute the mode matrix U_n.
2. obtain the core tensor as follows:

$$S = G \times_1 U_1^{-1} \times \cdots \times_N U_N^{-1}.$$

As stated in Section 10.2.1, there are also two strategies for performing multilinear independent components analysis (MICA). Architecture I forms a factorial code, where each set of coefficients that encodes people, viewpoints, illuminations, etc., is statistically independent, while Architecture II is to find a set of independent bases across people, viewpoints, illuminations, etc.

Architecture I: Transforming the flattened data tensor G into the nth mode and computing the ICA in classical mode, we can get

$$G_{(n)}^T = V_n \Sigma_n^T \bar{U}_n^T,$$

$$= (V_n \Sigma_n^T W_n^{-1})(W \bar{U}_n^T),$$

$$= K_n^T U_n^T, \tag{10.29}$$

where $G_{(n)}$ is the mode-n flattened of G. In other words, we perform the singular value decomposition on $G_{(n)}$.

The columns associated with each of the mode matrices, U_n, are statistically independent. The relationship between N-mode ICA and N-mode SVD in the context of Architecture I can be represented as follows:

$$G = Z \times_1 \bar{U}_1 \times \cdots \times_N \bar{U}_N$$

$$
\begin{aligned}
&= Z \times_1 \bar{U}_1 W_1^T W_1^{-T} \times \cdots \times_N \bar{U}_N W_N^T W_N^{-T} \\
&= Z \times_1 U_1 W_1^{-T} \times \cdots \times_N U_N W_N^{-T} \\
&= (Z \times_1 W_1^{-T} \times \cdots \times_N W_N^{-T}) \times_1 U_1 \times \cdots \times_N U_N \\
&= C \times_1 U_1 \times \cdots \times_N U_N \qquad .
\end{aligned}
\tag{10.30}
$$

Note that Z is the core tensor in N-mode SVD.

Architecture II: Flattening the data tensor G in the nth mode and computing the ICA, we obtain:

$$
\begin{aligned}
G_{(n)} &= \bar{U}_n \Sigma_n V_n^T, \\
&= (\bar{U}_n W_n^{-1})(W \Sigma_n V_n^T), \\
&= U_n K_n,
\end{aligned}
\tag{10.31}
$$

where $G_{(n)}$ is the mode-n flattened of G. In other words, one performs the singular value decomposition on $G_{(n)}$.

Architecture II results in a set of basis vectors that are statistically independent across the different modes. The relationship between N-mode ICA and N-mode SVD in the context of Architecture I is as follows:

$$
\begin{aligned}
G &= Z \times_1 \bar{U}_1 \times \cdots \times_N \bar{U}_N \\
&= Z \times_1 \bar{U}_1 W_1 W_1^{-1} \times \cdots \times_N \bar{U}_N W_N W_N^{-1} \\
&= Z \times_1 U_1 W_1^{-1} \times \cdots \times_N U_N W_N^{-1} \\
&= (Z \times_1 W_1^{-1} \times \cdots \times_N W_N^{-1}) \times_1 U_1 \times \cdots \times_N U_N \\
&= C \times_1 U_1 \times \cdots \times_N U_N \qquad .
\end{aligned}
\tag{10.32}
$$

Note that Z is the core tensor in N-mode SVD.

10.3 TENSOR NON-NEGATIVE FACTORIZATION (NF)

10.3.1 Classical NMF

The key characteristic of NMF is the non-negativity constraints imposed on the two factors, and the non-negativity constraints are compatible with the intuitive notion of combining parts to form a whole. NMF can also be interpreted as a parts-based representation of the data due to the fact that only additive, not subtractive, combinations are allowed. Assume that the image database is represented as an $N \times M$ matrix V, each column containing N non-negative pixel values corresponding to one of the M face images. In order to compress data or reduce the dimensionality, NMF finds two nonnegative matrix factors W and H such that

$$(V)_{i\mu} \approx (WH)_{iu} = \sum_{a=1}^{d} W_{ia} H_{q\mu} \tag{10.33}$$

Here the d columns of W are called NMF bases, and the columns of H are its combining coefficients. The dimensions of W and H are $N \times d$ and $d \times m$ respectively. The rank (d) of the factorization is usually chosen such that $(N+M)r < NM$, and hence the compression or dimensionality reduction is achieved. The compression ratio of NMF is easily gotten as $(Nd+Md)$.

To obtain an approximate factorization $V \approx W H$, a cost function is needed to quantify the quality of the approximation. NMF uses the following divergence measure as the objective function:

$$D(V,WH) = \sum_{i=1}^{N} \sum_{j=1}^{M} (V_{ij} \ln \frac{V_{ij}}{(WH)_{ij}} - V_{ij} + (WH)_{ij}), \tag{10.34}$$

After some simplification and elimination of pure data terms, one can obtain

$$D(V,WH) = \sum_{i=1}^{N} \sum_{j=1}^{M} (\sum_{k=1}^{d} W_{ik} H_{kj} - V_{ij} \ln \sum_{k=1}^{d} W_{ik} H_{kj}). \tag{10.35}$$

Taking the derivative with respect to H gives

$$\frac{\partial}{\partial H_{ab}} D(V,WH) = \sum_{i=1}^{N} W_{ia} - \sum_{i=1}^{N} \frac{V_{ib} W_{ia}}{\sum_{k=1}^{d} W_{ik} H_{kb}}. \tag{10.36}$$

Then the gradient algorithms can be described as follows:

$$H_{ab} \leftarrow H_{ab} - \eta_{ab} \frac{\partial}{\partial H_{ab}} D(V,WH), \tag{10.37}$$

$$H_{ab} \leftarrow H_{ab} - \eta_{ab} (\sum_{i=1}^{N} W_{ia} - \sum_{i=1}^{N} \frac{V_{ib} W_{ia}}{\sum_{k=1}^{d} W_{ik} H_{kb}}), \tag{10.38}$$

where η_{ab} is a step size.

Let $\eta_{ab} = . \dfrac{H_{ab}}{\sum\limits_{i=1}^{N} W_{ia}}$ Then the multiplicative rule is:

$$H_{ab} \leftarrow H_{ab} \dfrac{\sum\limits_{i=1}^{N} W_{ia} V_{ib} / \sum\limits_{k=1}^{d} W_{ik} H_{kb}}{\sum\limits_{i=1}^{N} W_{ia}}. \qquad (10.39)$$

Similarly, taking the derivative with respect to W gives

$$\dfrac{\partial}{\partial H_{cd}} D(V, WH) = \sum\limits_{j=1}^{M} H_{dj} - \sum\limits_{j=1}^{M} \dfrac{V_{cj} W_{dj}}{\sum\limits_{k=1}^{d} W_{ck} H_{kj}}. \qquad (10.40)$$

Then the gradient algorithms can be described as follows:

$$H_{cd} \leftarrow H_{cd} - \nu_{cd} \dfrac{\partial}{\partial H_{cd}} D(V, WH), \qquad (10.41)$$

$$H_{cd} \leftarrow H_{cd} - \nu_{cd} (\sum\limits_{i=1}^{M} H_{dj} - \sum\limits_{j=1}^{N} \dfrac{V_{cj} W_{dj}}{\sum\limits_{k=1}^{d} W_{ck} H_{k}}), \qquad (10.42)$$

where ν_{cd} is a step size.

Let $\nu_{cd} = \dfrac{W_{cd}}{\sum\limits_{j=1}^{M} H_{dj}}$. Then the multiplicative rule is :

$$W_{cd} \leftarrow W_{cd} \dfrac{\sum\limits_{i=1}^{M} H_{di} V_{ci} / \sum\limits_{k=1}^{d} W_{ck} H_{ki}}{\sum\limits_{i=1}^{M} H_{di}}. \qquad (10.43)$$

Overall, the pseudo-code for computing the matrices W and H is described as follows:

The Algorithm of NMF

Input: the $N \times M$ matrix V, and reduction dimension d.
Output: Matrices W and H
Step 1: initialize the matrices W and H and set $k \leftarrow 1$.

Step 2: while not convergent
    (a) update the bases W using Eq. (10.43)
    (b) update the coefficients H using Eq. (10.42)
Step 3: end while

10.3.2 The 2DNMF Algorithm

Assume that $m \times n$ matrices A_k, $k = 1,...,M$, denote original M training images. In 2DNMF, one does not need to transform the 2D images into its corresponding 1D vectors. Instead, one can use a more straightforward way which views an image as a 2D matrix.

In (Zhang, Chen, & Zhou, 2005), The authors used two successive stages to perform 2DNMF. First, they align the M images into a $m \times nM$ matrix $X = [A_1,...,A_M]$, where each A_k denotes one of the M face images. After X is obtained, one can perform classical NMF on the matrix X. That is, one needs to find a $m \times d$ non-negative matrix L and a $d \times nM$ non-negative matrix H such that

$$X \approx LH, \tag{10.44}$$

Note that L and H are the bases and combining coefficients respectively. Partitioning the matrix H into M submatrices, denoted as $H = [H_1,\cdots,H_M]$, one can write Eq. (10.44) as follows

$$[A_1,\cdots,A_M] \approx L[H_1,\cdots,H_M]. \tag{10.45}$$

Furthermore, one can obtain

$$A_k = LH_k \ (k = 1,...,M). \tag{10.46}$$

From Eq. (10.46), one can note that the image A_k is a weighted sum of the column bases L. Since H_k is an $d \times n$ matrix, there are dn coefficients for the image A_k. In order to further reduce the number of coefficients, Zhang, Chen, and Zhou (2005) performed the second stage to find row bases. They constructed a matrix from submatrices $[H_1,\cdots,H_M]$ and defined as follows $\hat{H} = [H_1^T,\cdots,H_M^T]$. It is obvious that $\hat{H}$ is a $nd \times M$ matrix. Based on $\hat{H}$, they seeked a $n \times d$ non-negative matrix R and a $d \times dM$ non-negative matrix C such that

$$\hat{H} \approx RC. \tag{10.47}$$

Here R and C are the bases and combing coefficients respectively. It is obvious that R and C can be obtained by performing classical NMF on the matrix $\hat{H}$. Partitioning the matrix C into M submatrices, denoted as $C = [C_1, \cdots, C_M]$, one can write Eq. (10.47) as follows

$$[H_1^T, \cdots, C_1^T] \approx R[C_1, \cdots, C_M].\tag{10.48}$$

Furthermore, one can obtain

$$H_k^T \approx RC_k \ (k = 1, \cdots, M).\tag{10.49}$$

From Eq. (10.49), one can note that the image H_k^T is a weighted sum of the rows bases.

Substituting Eq. (10.49) into Eq. (10.46), one can obtain

$$A_k \approx LC_k^T R^T \ (k = 1, \cdots, M).\tag{10.50}$$

From Eq. (10.50), one can find that each image is decomposed into three matrices. Note that C_k is a coefficient matrix and its dimension is $d \times d$.

Let $L = [l_1, \cdots, l_d]$ and $R = [r_1, \cdots, r_d]$. Define the outer product between the column base l_i and the row base r_j as follows.

$$E_{ij} = l_i \circ r_j \ 1 \le i \le d, 1 \le j \le d,\tag{10.51}$$

According to Eq. (10.51), one can write Eq. (10.50) into

$$A_k \approx LC_k^T R^T = \sum_{i=1}^{d} \sum_{j=1}^{d} (D_k)_{ij} E_{ij}.\tag{10.52}$$

From Eq. (10.52), the image A_k is a linear combination of 2D bases. Note that 2D bases E_{ij} have the following properties.

(a)   the dimension of E_{ij} is equal to the size of the original images.
(b)   The intrinsic dimensionality of E_{ij} is 1.

From the above analysis, one can know that 2DNMF first performs the column NMF, then followed by row NMF operations. Figure 10.3 shows how a high-dimensional image is transformed into a low-dimensional image by using 2DNMF.

Finally, the pseudo-code for performing 2DNMF is descried as follows.

The 2DNMF Algorithm

Input: $m \times n$ image matrices $\{A_k\}_{k=1}^{M}$ and the reduction dimension d.
Output: the matrices L, R, and D_k ($k = 1, \cdots, d$).
Step 1: Align the M images into a $m \times nM$ matrix $X = [A_1, ..., A_M]$
Step 2: Perform classical NMF on $X = LH$, and obtain matrices L and H.
Step 3: Partition H into $H = [H_1, ..., H_M]$, construct a new matrix from H, denoted as $\hat{H} = [H_1^T \cdots H_M^T]$
Step 4: Performing classical NMF on $\hat{H} = RC$, and obtain matrices R and C,
Step 5: Obtain the approximate matrix of $A_k \approx LC_k^T R^T$ ($k = 1, ...M$).

Note that in the above algorithm, one first aligns the M images into a $m \times nM$ matrix $X = [A_1, ..., A_M]$. In fact, one can also align the M images into a $n \times mM$ matrix $Y = [A_1^T, \cdots, A_M^T]$. The dimension d in two stages may be different. It can be bigger than or smaller than the dimension of images.

10.3.3 Multilinear Non-Negative Factorization

A tensor G of dimensions $[d_1] \times \cdots [d_n]$ is indexed by n indices $i_1, \cdots, i_n$ with $1 \le i_j \le d_j$. It is of rank at most k if it can be expressed as a sum of k rank-1 tensors, i.e. a sum of n-fold outer-product: $G = \sum_{i=1}^{k} u_1^j \otimes u_2^j \otimes \cdots \otimes u_n^j$. Although the rank of a matrix can be found in the polynomial time using the SVD algorithm, the rank of a tensor is an NP-hard problem.

Given an n-way array G, we expect to find a non-negative rank-k tensor $\sum_{i=1}^{k} u_1^j \otimes u_2^j \otimes \cdots \otimes u_n^j$ described by nk vectors u_i^j. The following optimization problem is constructed:

Figure 10.3. An illustration of dimensionality reduction by using 2DNMF

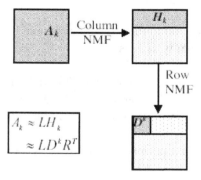

$$\min f(u_i^j) = \min \frac{1}{2} \left\| G - \sum_{i=1}^{k} \otimes u_i^j \right\|_F^2, \tag{10.53}$$

subject to, $u_i^j \geq 0$,

where $\| \ \|_F$ is the square Frobenious norm, i.e., the sum of squares of all entries of the tensor elements. The direct approach is to form a positive preserving gradient descent scheme.

Let $\langle A, B \rangle$ denote the inner-product operation, i.e. $\sum_{i_1, \cdots, i_n} A_{i_1 \cdots i_n} B_{i_1 \cdots i_n}$. Since the differential commutes with inner-products, i.e., $d\langle A, A \rangle = 2\langle A, dA \rangle$, we have

$$\frac{1}{2} d \left\langle G - \sum_{j=1}^{k} \otimes_{i=1}^{n} u_i^j, G - \sum_{j=1}^{k} \otimes_{i=1}^{n} u_i^j \right\rangle,$$

$$\left\langle G - \sum_{j=1}^{k} \otimes_{i=1}^{n} u_i^j, d[G - \sum_{j=1}^{k} \otimes_{i=1}^{n} u_i^j] \right\rangle. \tag{10.54}$$

Taking the differential with respect to u_r^s and noting that

$$d[G - \sum_{j=1}^{k} \otimes_{i=1}^{n} u_i^j] = - \otimes_{i=1}^{r-1} u_i^s \otimes d(u_r^s) \otimes_{i=r+1}^{n} u_i^s,$$

The differential becomes

$$df(u_r^s) = \left\langle \sum_{j=1}^{k} \otimes_{i=1}^{n} u_i^j, \otimes_{i=1}^{r-1} u_i^s \otimes d(u_r^s) \otimes_{i=r+1}^{n} u_i^s \right\rangle - \left\langle G, \otimes_{i=1}^{r-1} u_i^s \otimes d(u_r^s) \otimes_{i=r+1}^{n} u_i^s \right\rangle.$$

The differential with respect to the lth coordinate u_{rl}^s is

$$df(u_{rl}^s) = \left\langle \sum_{j=1}^{k} \otimes_{i=1}^{n} u_i^j, \otimes_{i=1}^{r-1} u_i^s \otimes e_l \otimes_{i=r+1}^{n} u_i^s \right\rangle - \left\langle G, \otimes_{i=1}^{r-1} u_i^s \otimes e_l \otimes_{i=r+1}^{n} u_i^s \right\rangle,$$

where e_l is the lth column of the $d_r \times d_r$ identity matrix. Let $S \in [d_1] \times \cdots [d_n]$ denote an n-tuple index $\{i_1, \cdots, i_n\}$. Let S / i_r denote the set $\{i_1, \cdots, i_{r-1}, i_{r+1}, \cdots, i_n\}$ and $S_{i_r \leftarrow l}$ denote the set of indices S where the index i_r is replaced by the constant l. Then, using the identity $\langle x_1 \otimes y_1, x_2 \otimes y_2 \rangle$, one can obtain the partial derivative

$$\frac{\partial f}{\partial u_{rl}^s} = \sum_{j=1}^{k} u_{rl}^j \prod_{i \neq r} (u_i^j)^T u_i^s - \sum_{S/i_r} (G_{S_{i_r \leftarrow l}} \prod_{m \neq r} u_{m,i_m}^s). \tag{10.55}$$

Using the multiplicative update rule by setting the constant μ_{rl}^s of the gradient descent formula

$$u_{rl}^s \leftarrow u_{rl}^s - \mu_{rl}^s \frac{\partial f}{\partial u_{rl}^s} \text{ to be,}$$

$$\mu_{rl}^s = \frac{u_{rl}^s}{\sum_{j=1}^k u_{rl}^j \prod_{i \neq r} (u_i^j)^T u_i^s}, \tag{10.56}$$

one can obtain

$$u_{rl}^s \leftarrow \frac{u_{rl}^s \sum_{S/i_r} G_{S_{i_r} \leftarrow l} \prod_{m \neq r} u_{m,i_m}^s}{\sum_{j=1}^k u_{rl}^j \prod_{i \neq r} (u_i^j)^T u_i^s}. \tag{10.57}$$

It is shown that this update rule can make the value of the optimization function become small. The following proposition will provide the theoretical foundation for the update rule.

Proposition 10.1: Let $f(x_1,...,x_n)$ be a real quadratic function with Hessian of the form $H = cI$ with $c > 0$. Given a point $x^t = (x_1^t, \cdots, x_n^t)$ and a point $x^{t+1} = x^t - \mu(\nabla f(x^t)$ with $0 < \mu < \frac{1}{c}$, then $f(x^{t+1}) < f(x^t)$.

10.4 APPLICATIONS TO BIOMETRIC VERIFICATION

In this section, the performances of 2DICA, ICA, 2DNMF, NMF and tensor NF are demonstrated. Zhang, Chen, and Zhou (2005) computed the bases of NMF and 2DNMF from the training set. They also computed the bases of PCA and 2DPCA [26]. They did the experiment on the FERET face databases as shown in Section 3.4.4, and 200 face images are used as the training set. Figure 10.4 plots parts of the bases gotten from the four methods respectively. The bases in Figure 10.4 (a) and (b) are obtained by using the method (Zhang, Chen, & Liu, 2005). For NMF the first 16 columns of W are transformed into the representation in matrix form, whereas for 2DNMF the 16 bases ($1 \le i \le 4$, $1 \le j \le 4$) are directly described as the images. From Figure 10.4, one can see that both the bases of PCA and 2DPCA are global. It is also observed that 2DPCA possess some strips or blocks like structures. A possible explanation is that 2DPCA is essentially a kind of line-based PCA. As a result, the bases of 2DPCA cannot yet reflect any local or part-based features. On the other hand, Figure 10.4 (c) indicates that although NMF is a part-based algorithm, its bases still take on some holistic properties similar to PCA. In contrast, one can notice from Figure 10.4 (d) that the bases of 2DNMF are much sparser than those of NMF. It is worth noting that although the bases of 2DNMF are sparse, they have no parts-based (like eye, mouth, etc. in face image) features any more due to the essence of 2D methods. That is, 2DNMF is essentially a kind of line-based NMF. Consequently, what 2DNMF really learns is some parts of 'lines'. Moreover, because each base of 2DNMF can be generated using a d-dimensional column base and a *d*-dimensional row base, its storing coefficients (*d+d*) are much fewer than that of the NMF base (which is *d*d*). Thus one can use much more sparse-distributed 2D bases to represent the original image. As a result, in some sense, 2DNMF has higher compression ratio than NMF.

The 1th row of Figure 10.5 shows some of the NMF factors generated from a set of 2429, 19×19, images from the MIT CBCL database. One can clearly see that ghost structures and the part decomposition is complicated .The NTF factors (rank-1 matrices), shown in the 2nd row, have a sharper decomposition into sparse components. The 2nd row shows an overlap of rank-1 factors whose energy is localized in the same image region. One can clearly see that the parts (which now correspond to higher rank matrices) corresponding to eyes, cheeks, and shoulders are shown.

Figure 10.4. (Zhang, Chen, & Zhou, 2005). Bases obtained from PCA (a), 2DPCA (b), NMF (c) and 2DNMF (d) respectively. For NMF the first 16 columns of matrix W are retransformed to matrix for plotting, while for 2DNMF the 16 bases Eij (1≤i≤4, 1≤j≤4) are directly plotted as images.

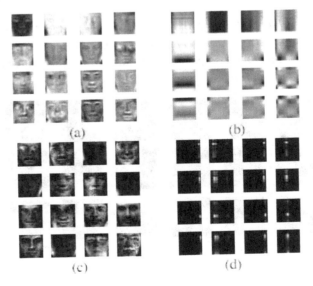

In the following, we compare the performances of NMF, 2DNMF, ICA and 2DICA when they are used for the classification tasks. The recognition accuracy, which is defined as the percentage of correctly recognized images in test images, is used as the performance measure. The experiment is first made to classify test images on two face databases: UMIST and Yale Face images. The UMIST Face Database consists of 564 images of 20 people. Each covers a range of poses from profile to frontal views. Subjects cover a range of race/sex/appearance. Each subject exists in their own directory and images are numbered consecutively as they were taken. Each image is resized to 112 × 92 pixels. As for the description of the Yale face database, please refer to Section 3.3.3. In this database, the facial portion of each original image was automatically cropped based on the location of eyes and the cropped image was resized to 80×80 pixels. In both face databases, we randomly choose five images from each person as training samples and others are used as testing samples. In addition, the experiments are made to test the classification accuracy of the fourth methods under partial occlusions (10%). In order to reduce variations, the final results are averaged over ten runs. Table 10.1 demonstrate the experimental results. Note that the dimensions are chosen based on the Fisher criterion. The 3rd and 4th rows denote performance under partial occlusions. From Table 1, one can observe that the 2D Methods (including 2DICA and 2DNMF) outperform classical 1D methods. Moreover, NMF is not superior to ICA in terms of the classification performance. In the case of occlusions, the performances of two methods become worse. These experiments show that it is reasonable to adopt the 2D methods for feature extraction in real-world applications.

Figure 10.5. (Shashua & Hazan, 2005). The first row: leading NMF factors of CBCL face dataset, compared to leading NTF factors in the 2nd row. The 3rd row: summed factors of NTF located in the same region (resulting in higher rank factors) — see texts for further explanation.

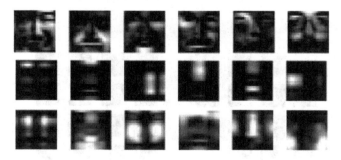

Table 10.1. Performance comparisons of four methods on two face databases (%)

	ICA	2DICA	NMF	2DNMF
UMIST	73.45(5.31)	75.68(6.30)	71.22(7.22)	72.34(4.33)
Yale	70.13(8.37)	72.37(7.25)	66.90(7.39)	68.76(9.12)
UMIST(10%)	68.39(6.34)	69.68(8.15)	60.05(8.99)	62.33(9.44)
Yale(10%)	61.22(7.15)	69.23(10.12)	59.22(8.34)	64.67(9.56)

10.5 SUMMARY

In this chapter, two tensor subspace methods: tensor ICA and tensor NMF, are introduced. Although independent components analysis (ICA) maximizes the statistical independence of the representational components of a training image ensemble, it cannot distinguish between the different factors, or modes, inherent to image formation including scene structure, illumination, and imaging. Fortunately, the multifactor models for ICA can deal with these problems. Specifically, the multilinear ICA (MICA) model of image ensembles can learn the statistically independent components of multiple factors. In addition, one can notice that ICA employs linear (matrix) algebra, whereas MICA exploits multilinear (tensor) algebra. Different from ICA, NMF is an effective method for finding parts-based representation of non-negative data such as face images. Although it has been successfully applied in real world, directly using NMF for face recognition often leads to low classification performance. Moreover, when performing on large databases, NMF needs considerable computational costs. To overcome the disadvantages of classical NMF, tensor NMF is developed. The key difference between classical NMF and tensor NF and is that the latter adopts a novel representation for original images. Specifically, NMF is a special case of tensor NF based on multilinear algebra.

REFERENCES

Baek, K., Draper, B. A., Beveridge, J. R., & She, K. (2002). PCA vs. ICA: A comparison on the FERET data set. *Proc. Joint Conf. Inf. Sci.* (pp. 824-827).

Bartlett, M. S., Movellan, J. R., & Sejnowski, T. J. (2002). Face recognition by independent component analysis. *IEEE Trans. Neural Netw.*, *13*(6), 1450-1464.

Bartlett, M. S., & Sejnowski, T. J. (1997). Independent of face images: a representation for face recognition. *Proceedings of the Fourth Annual Joint Symposium on Neural computation*, *3299*, 528-539.

Bell, A. J., & Sejnowski, T. J. (1995). An information-maximization approach to blind separation and blind deconvolution. *Neural Comput.*, *7*(6), 1129-1159.

Bell, A. J., & Sejnowski, T. J. (1997). The 'independent components' of natural scenes are edge filters, *Vis. Res.*, *37*(23), 3327-3338.

Draper, B. A., Baek, K., Bartlett, M. S., & Beveridge, J. R. (2003). Recognizing faces with PCA and ICA. *Comput. Vis. Image Underst.*, *91*(1-2), 115-137.

Guillamet, D., & Vitria, J. (2003). Evaluation of distance metrics for recognition based on non-negative matrix factorization. *Pattern Recognition Letters*, *24*(9-10), 1599-1605.

Hyvärinen, A., & Oja, E. (2001). Independent component analysis: algorithms and applications. *Neural Netw.*, *13*(4-5), 411-430.

Jin, Z., & Davoine, F. (2004). Orthogonal ICA representation of images. *Proc. 8th Int. Conf. Control, Autom., Robot. and Vis.* (pp. 369-374).

Lee, D. D., & Seung, H. S. (1999). Learning the parts of objects by non-negative matrix factorization. *Nature*, *401*, 788-791.

Lee, D. D., & Seung, H. S. (2001). Algorithms for non-negative matrix factorization. *Adv. Neural Inform. Process. Syst.*, *13*, 556-562.

Li, S. Z., Hou, X. W., & Zhang, H. J. (2001). Learning spatially localized parts-based representation. *Proceedings of IEEE International Conference on Computer Vision and Pattern Recognition* (pp. 207-212).

Liu, C., & Wechsler, H. (1999). Comparative assessment of independent component analysis for face recognition. *Proc. 2nd Int. Conf. Audio and Video-Based Biometric Person Authentication* (pp. 211-216).

Liu, C., & Wechsler, H. (2003). Independent component analysis of Gabor features for face recognition. *IEEE Trans. Neural Netw.*, *14*(4), 919-928.

Liu, W. X., & Zheng, N. N. (2004). Non-negative matrix factorization based methods for object recognition. *Pattern Recognition Letters*, *25*(8), 893-897.

Moghaddam, B. (2002). Principal manifolds and probabilistic subspaces for visual recognition.*IEEE Trans. Pattern Anal. Mach. Intell.*, *24*(6), 780-788.

Shashua, A., & Hazan, T. (2005). Non-negative tensor factorization with application to statistics and computer vision. *Proceedings of the Int'l Conference on Machine Learning* (pp. 792-799).

Socolinsky, D., & Selinger, A. (2002). A comparative analysis of face recognition performance with visible and thermal infrared imagery. *Proc. Int. Conf. Pattern Recog.* (pp. 217-222).

Yang, J., Zhang, D., & Yang, J-Y. (2007). Constructing PCA baseline algorithms to reevaluate ICA-based face-recognition performance. *IEEE Trans. Systems, Man, and Cybernetics—Part B: Cybernetics, 37*(4), 1015-1021.

Yuen, P. C., & Lai, J. H. (2000). Independent component analysis of face images. *Proc. IEEE Int. Conf. Biological Motivated Comput. Vis.*, 545-553.

Yuen, P. C., & Lai, J. H. (2002). Face representation using independent component analysis. *Pattern Recognit., 35*(6), 1247-1257.

Zhang, D. Q., Chen, S. C., & Liu, J. (2005). Representing image matrices: Eigen-images vs. Eigenvectors. *Proceedings of the International Symposium on Neural Networks (ISNN'05), vol. 2, Chongqing, China* (pp. 659-664).

Zhang, D. Q., Chen, S. C., & Zhou, Z. H. (2005). Two-dimensional non-negative matrix factorization for face representation and recognition. *Proceedings of the International Conference on Computer Vision* Workshop on Analysis and Modeling of Faces and Gestures (pp. 35.-363)

Chapter XI
Other Tensor Analysis and Further Direction

ABSTRACT

In this chapter, we describe tensor-based classifiers, tensor canonical correlation analysis and tensor partial least squares, which can be used in biometrics. Section 11.1 gives background and devolvement of these tensor methods. Section 11.2 introduces tensor-based classifiers. Section 11.3 gives tensor canonical correlation analysis and tensor partial least squares. We summarize this chapter in Section 11.4.

11.1 INTRODUCTION

In general, a biometric system consists of data acquisition phase, feature extraction phase and the classification phase. In the data acquisition phase, the data obtained are often represented by multidimensional arrays, that is, tensors, such as the grey face image, the colour faces in image classification and the gene expression data. In the feature extraction phase, multilinear subspace methods mentioned in Chapters VIII, IX, and X can be used for data representation and feature extraction. In the classification phase, the classifiers (Bousquet, Boucheron, & Lugosi, 2004; Duda, Hart, & Stock, 2001; Muller, Mika, Ratsch, Tsuda, & Scholkopf, 2001; Highleyman, 1962) play an important role in the biometric system and how to design a good classifier is of interest for researchers. Traditionally, the classifier design is almost based on vector pattern, that is, before using them, any non-vector pattern such as an image should be first vectorized into the vector pattern by the techniques such as concatenation. However, the Ugly Duckling Theorem (Chen, Wang, & Tian, 2007) indicates that it cannot be said that one pattern representation is always better than another. As a result, it is not always reasonable to design classifiers based on traditional vector patterns.

Motivated by the tensor ideas in feature extraction, some researchers have designed some classifiers based on tensor ideas in recent years. For example, Chen, Wang and Tian (2007) designed the classifiers using a set of given matrix patterns. They first represented a pattern in matrix form and extended existing vector-based classifiers to their corresponding matrixized versions. Specifically, considering a similar principle to the support vector machine which maximizes the separation margin and has superior generalization performance, the modified HK algorithm (MHKS) (Leski, 2003) is chosen and then a matrix-based MHKS (MatMHKS) classifier is developed. Their experimental results on ORL, Letters and UCI data sets show that MatMHKS is more powerful in generalization than MHKS. Further, Wang and Chen (2007) proposed a new classifier based on matrix patterns and LS-SVM. This method is referred to as MatLSSVM. The MatLSSVM method can not only directly operate on original matrix patterns, but also efficiently reduce memory for the weight vector in LS-SVM. However, one of disadvantages of MatLSSVM is that there exist unclassifiable regions when it is extended to the multi-class problems. To avoid this point, a corresponding fuzzy version of MatLSSVM (MatFLSSVM) is further proposed to remove unclassifiable regions for multi-class problems. Experimental results on some benchmark datasets show that their proposed method is competitive in classification performance compared to LS-SVM and fuzzy LS-SVM (FLS-SVM). In Tao, Li, Hu, Maybank and Wu (2005; Tao, Li, Wu, Hu, & Maybank, 2006) a supervised tensor learning (STL) framework is established for convex optimization techniques such as support vector machines (SVM) and minimax probability machines (MPM). Within the STL framework, many conventional learning machines can be generalized to take nth-order tensors as inputs. These generalized algorithms have several advantages: (1) reduce the problem of "the curse of dimensionality" in machine learning and data mining; (2) avoid the failure to converge; and (3) achieve better separation between the different categories of samples. Further, they generalized MPM to the STL version, which is called tensor MPM (TMPM). The TMPM method can obtain a series of tensor projection vector by an iterative algorithm. The experiments on a binary classification problem show that TMPM significantly outperforms the original MPM.

In addition to introducing tensor-based classifiers, we also demonstrate more examples of tensor analysis including tensor canonical correlation analysis and tensor partial least squares. Canonical Correlation Analysis (CCA), firstly developed by Hotelling (1936) in 1930s, is a powerful statistical technique to measure the linear relationship between two multidimensional variables. It finds two linear combinations, one for each multidimensional variable, which are optimal with respect to correlations. In other words, the goal of CCA is to find the directions of maximum data correlation. Up till now, the CCA method has been widely used in several fields such as signal processing, medical studies, and pattern recognition (Melzer, Reiter, & Bischof, 2003; Sun, Zeng, Liu, Heng, & Xia, 2005; Zheng, Zhou, Zou, & Zhao, 2006). However, this method always suffers from the small sample size (SSS) problem in the applications. To this end, two-dimensional CCA based on classical CCA is developed. Sample images in 2DCCA are represented as 2D matrices instead of vectors, and discriminative features are extraction from the image covariance matrix. In addition, partial least squares (PLS) (Wold, 1982, 1985; Helland, 1988; Oskuldsson, 1988; Lewi, 1995) are developed for the regression problem and have proven to be popular and effective approaches to the problems in biometrics such as predicting the bioactivity of molecules. The PLS method can be used for multivariate as well as univariate regressions. Moreover, the PLS algorithms can reduce the variance by introducing a small bias. Since Wold (1982, 1985) proposed PLS in the field of econometrics, the PLS methods had found a variety of applications in the areas such as bioinformatics, face recognition and character recognition. For example, in (Tan, Shi, Tong, Hwang, & Wang, 2004), the authors used discriminant partial least squares (DPLS) to classify different types of human tumors and showed good prediction performance of DPLS on four microarray datasets. In Baek and Kim (2004) the PLS algorithm is used to extract facial features and the experimental results show the PLS algorithm can obtain lower recognition error rate than PCA. However, classical PLS often suffers from the small sample size problem. To this end, 2DPLS and multilinear PLS are developed in this chapter.

11.2 TENSOR-BASED CLASSIFIERS

11.2.1 Tensor Ho-Kashyap (HK) Classifier

11.2.1.1 Classical Ho-Kashyap and MHKS Algorithm

For a two-class (ω_1, ω_2) problem, assume that $S = \{(x_i, y_i) | i = 1, \cdots, M\} \subset \Re^N \times \{+1, -1\}$ is a set of M samples. Let $\hat{x}_i = [x_i^T, 1]^T$. In general, a linear discriminant function for two-class problems can be defined as

$$g(\hat{x}_i) = u^T \hat{x}_i, \tag{11.1}$$

where u is the weight vector or a projection vector. If $g(\hat{x}_i)$ is bigger than zero, the corresponding sample $\hat{x}_i$ is considered as ω_1 class. Otherwise, it belongs to ω_2 class.

Further, applying the class label, one can obtain

$$y_i g(\hat{x}_i) = y_i u^T \hat{x}_i > 0, \ (i = 1, \cdots, M). \tag{11.2}$$

Eq. (11.2) shows that the samples can be correctly classified by the linear discriminant function $g(\hat{x}_i)$.

Let $Y = [y_1 \hat{x}_1, \cdots, y_M \hat{x}_M]^T$. We denote Eq. (11.2) in matrix form

$$Yu > 0. \tag{11.3}$$

In (Leski, 2003), the optimization function of the Ho-Kashyap (HK) algorithm is defined as the following quadratic loss function:

$$J(u,b) = \|Yu - b\|^2, \tag{11.4}$$

where b is the margin vector and $b > 0$.

Taking the derivative of Eq.(11.4) with respect to u and b gives

$$\frac{\partial J}{\partial u} = 2Y^T (Yu - b), \tag{11.5}$$

$$\frac{\partial J}{\partial b} = -2(Yu - b). \tag{11.6}$$

In addition, for any value of b, one has

$$u = Y^+ b, \tag{11.7}$$

where Y^+ denotes the pseudo-inverse.

Note that $b > 0$ and b should avoid converging to zero in the gradient descent procedure. Consequently, the following update rule for b is adopted.

$$\begin{cases} b(1) > 0 \\ b(k+1) = b(k) + \rho(e(k) + |e(k)|), \end{cases} \tag{11.8}$$

where $e(k) = Yu(k) - b(k)$, k is the index of iterations and ρ is the learning rate. To avoid the HK algorithm being sensitive to outliers, Leski (2003) modified the HK algorithm and defined the canonical hyperplane as

$$Yu \geq 1_{M \times 1}. \tag{11.9}$$

Based on Eq.(11.9), Leski (2003) developed the following optimization function to obtain the projection vector u and the margin vector b,

$$\min I(u,b) = \min(\|Yu - 1_{N \times 1} - b\|^2 + Cu^T u), \tag{11.10}$$

where C is the regularization parameter. The optimal parameters u and b are obtained by alternately optimizing

$$u = (Y^T Y + CI)^{-1} Y^T (b + 1_{M \times 1}), \tag{11.11}$$

$$b = Yu - 1_{M \times 1}, \tag{11.12}$$

where I is a matrix by setting the last element of an identity matrix to zero and $1_{M \times 1}$ denotes a column vector whose elements are 1.

11.2.1.2 Matrix-Pattern-Oriented HK Classifier

Assume that m × n matrices A_k, $k = 1,\cdots,M$, denote M images and y_k, $k = 1,\cdots,M$, are the corresponding M labels.

Chen et al. (2007) developed a matrix-pattern-oriented, two-sided linear classifier based on the HK algorithm with the regularization learning, as an extension to the HK algorithm.

Based on the matrix notation, they defined the following decision function

$$f(A) = u^T Av + b_0, \tag{11.13}$$

where $u \in \Re^m$, $v \in \Re^n$, and b_0 is a bias.

From Eq. (11.13), one can design a classifier based on the matrix pattern. In such a case, the two-sided linear function for two-class (ω_1, ω_2) problems can be given

$$g(A_i) = u^T A_i v + b_0 \begin{cases} > 0 & A_i \in \omega_1 \\ < 0 & A_i \in \omega_2 \end{cases}. \tag{11.14}$$

Further, from Eq. (11.14), one has

$$y_i g(A_i) = y_i (u^T A_i v + b_0) > 0, \ (i = 1, \cdots, M). \tag{11.15}$$

Similar to classical HK algorithm, a canonical hyperplane is defined as

$$y_i g(A_i) = y_i (u^T A_i v + b_0) > 1, \ (i = 1, \cdots, M). \tag{11.16}$$

Based on Eq. (11.16), Chen et al. (2007) defined the following optimization problem

$$\min I (u, v, b_0, b) = \min[\sum_{i=1}^{M} y_i (u^T A_i v + b_0) - 1 - b_i)^2 + C(u^T S_1 u + v^T S_2 v)], \tag{11.17}$$

where $b = [b_1, \ldots, b_M]^T$, $S_1 = mI$ and $S_2 = nI$ are two regularization matrices, the regularization parameter C controls the generalization ability of the classifier.

Let $Y = [\hat{y}_1, \cdots, \hat{y}_M]^T$, $\hat{y}_i = y_i [u^T A_i, 1]^T$, and $\hat{v} = [v^T, b_0]^T$. We transform Eq. (11.17) into the following matrix form

$$\min I(u, \hat{v}, b) = \min(\| Y\hat{v} - 1_{N \times 1} - b \|^2 + C(u^T S_1 u + \hat{v}^T \hat{S}_2 \hat{v})), \tag{11.18}$$

where $\hat{S}_2$ is a matrix with dimension of $(n + 1) \times (n + 1)$ and $\hat{S}_2 = \begin{bmatrix} S_2 & 0 \\ 0 & 0 \end{bmatrix}$.

Taking the derivative of the function with respect to $u, \hat{v}$ and b gives

$$\frac{\partial I}{\partial u} = 2\sum_{i=1}^{M} y_i A_i v [y_i (u^T A_i v + b_0) - 1_{N \times 1} - b_i] + 2CS_1 u, \tag{11.19}$$

$$\frac{\partial I}{\partial b} = -2(Y\hat{v} - 1_{M \times 1} - b), \tag{11.20}$$

$$\frac{\partial I}{\partial \hat{v}} = -2(Y\hat{v} - 1_{M \times 1} - b). \tag{11.21}$$

By setting $\dfrac{\partial I}{\partial u} = 0$ and $\dfrac{\partial I}{\partial \hat{v}} = 0$, one can get

$$\hat{v} = (Y^T Y + C\hat{S}_2)^{-1} Y^T (1_{M \times 1} + b), \tag{11.22}$$

$$u = (\sum_{i=1}^{M} A_i vv^T A_i^T + CS_1)^{-1} (\sum_{i=1}^{M} y_i (1 + b_i - y_i b_0) A_i v). \tag{11.23}$$

From Eqs. (11.22) and (11.23), one can notice that the weight vectors u and $\hat{v}$ are all determined by the margin vector b whose components determine the distance of the corresponding sample to the separation hyperplane. Moreover, because u and $\hat{v}$ are mutually dependent, it is necessary to use the iterative procedure to obtain them.

Based on the above discussion, Chen et al. (2007) summarized MatMHKS as follows.

The algorithm for matrix-pattern-oriented HK classifiers

Step 1: Fix $C \geq 0, 0 < \rho < 1$, initialize $b(1) \geq 0$ and $u(1)$, set $k = 1$
Step 2: $\hat{v} = (Y^T Y + C\hat{S}_2)^{-1} Y^T (1_{M \times 1} + b(k))$
Step 3: $e = Y\hat{v} - 1_{M \times 1} - b$
Step 4: $b(k+1) = b(k) + \rho(e(k) + |e(k)|)$,
Step 5: if $\| b(k+1) - b(k) \| > \varepsilon$, then $k = k + 1$, goto Step (6); else stop

Step 6: $u(k+1) = (\sum_{i=1}^{M} A_i v(k) v(k)^T A_i^T + CS_1)^{-1} (\sum_{i=1}^{M} y_i (1 + b_i(k) - y_i b_0) A_i v(k))$, go to step 2

where k denotes the index of iterations, and ε is a preset parameter.

Note that this algorithm is degenerated into MHKS when $m=1$, $u=1$ and step 6 is omitted. When C is set to 0, the algorithm is degenerated into the original Ho-Kashyap algorithm. As a result, Ho-Kashyap and MHKS algorithms are two special cases of MatMHKS. In addition, Chen et al. (2007) pointed out that there exists the relationship between MatMHKS and MHKS by the Kronecker product. That is, MatMHKS is equivalent to MHKS with the Kronecker product decomposability constraint. In some sense, MatMHKS is guided by some prior information such as the structural or local contextual information which is reflected in the representation of the Kronecker product. Moreover, the advantages of MatMHKS are that it can avoid overtraining and reduction in dimensionality for weights.

11.2.2 Tensor LS-SVM

11.2.2.1 Classical LS-SVM

Let $S = \{(x_i, y_i) | i = 1, \cdots, M\} \subset \Re^N \times \{+1, -1\}$ be a set of examples. In LS-SVM (Suykens & Vandewalle, 1999), the decision function is written as

$$f(x) = \sum_{i=1}^{M} \alpha_i y_i K(x, x_i) + b, \tag{11.24}$$

where α_i are a real constant, b is a bias, and $K(x, x_i)$ is a kernel function. The output of $f(x)$ is 1 if its value is greater than 0, -1 otherwise. In general, parameters b and α_i can be obtained by solving the following primal optimization problem

$$\min \frac{1}{2} w^T w + \frac{C}{2} \sum_{i=1}^{M} \zeta_i^2, \tag{11.25}$$

subject to $y_i(w^T \phi(x_i) + b) = 1 - \zeta_i, i = 1, \ldots, M.$
where $\phi()$ is a linear or nonlinear function which maps the input space into a higher dimensional feature space, w is a weight vector to be determined, C is a regularization constant and ζ_i is a slack variable.

From Eq. (11.25), one can construct the following Lagrangian function

$$L(w, b, \zeta_i, \alpha_i) = \frac{1}{2} w^T w + \frac{C}{2} \sum_{i=1}^{M} \zeta_i^2 - \sum_{i=1}^{M} \alpha_i [y_i(w^T \phi(x_i) + b) - 1 + \zeta_i]$$

$$\tag{11.26}$$

Taking the derivative with respect to w, b, ζ_i, α_i gives

$$\frac{\partial L}{\partial w} = 0 \Rightarrow w = \sum_{i=1}^{M} \alpha_i y_i \phi(x_i), \tag{11.27}$$

$$\frac{\partial L}{\partial b} = 0 \Rightarrow 0 = \sum_{i=1}^{M} \alpha_i y_i, \tag{11.28}$$

$$\frac{\partial L}{\partial \zeta_i} = 0 \Rightarrow \alpha_i = C\zeta_i, \tag{11.29}$$

$$\frac{\partial L}{\partial \alpha_i} = 0 \Rightarrow 0 = y_i(w^T \phi(x_i) + b) - 1 + \zeta_i = 0. \tag{11.30}$$

From Eqs. (11.27), (11.28), (11.29) and (11.30), one can obtain

$$\begin{bmatrix} 0 & -Y^T \\ Y & \Omega + C^{-1}I \end{bmatrix} \begin{bmatrix} b \\ a \end{bmatrix} = \begin{bmatrix} 0 \\ 1 \end{bmatrix}$$ (11.31)

where $Y = [y_1,...,y_M]^T$, $(\Omega)_{ij} = y_i y_j K(x_i, x_j)$ and $a = [\alpha_1, \cdots, \alpha_M]$.

From Eq. (11.31), one can obtain a and b. Thus, a decision function in Eq.(11.24) is obtained.

11.2.2.2 Matrix LS-SVM

Assume that $m \times n$ matrices A_k, $k = 1, \cdots, M$ denote M images and y_k, $k = 1, \cdots, M$ are the corresponding label $k = 1, \cdots, M$.

Based on LS-SVM, Wang and Chen (2007) proposed a variant of LS-SVM, called MatLSSVM, for two-class problems. This method can directly deal with the data in the form of matrices. In their method, the decision function is defined as the following form:

$$f(A) = u^T A v + b,$$ (11.32)

where $u \in \mathfrak{R}^m$ and $v \in \mathfrak{R}^n$.

It is obvious that the MatLS-SVMs method needs to store $m + n$ coefficients for u and v, while the classical LSSVMs method needs to store mn coefficients. As a result, the higher dimension the pattern has, the less memory the MatLSSVMs method needs to store weight vectors.

In MatLSSVMs, the following optimization problem is constructed:

$$\min \frac{1}{2}u^T u + \frac{C}{2}\sum_{i=1}^{M}\zeta_i^2 + \frac{1}{2}v^T v.$$ (11.33)

subject to $y_i(u^T A_i v + b) = 1 - \zeta_i$, $i = 1, \cdots, M$.

From the above optimization problem, one can see that it is difficult to find the optimal u and v simultaneously. However, when one fixes one of variables (u,v), it is easy to solve Eq. (11.33). In other words, the variable u can be obtained by a similar procedure of LS-SVMs in the case of the fixed v and the variable v can be obtained by a similar procedure of LS-SVMs in the case of the fixed u.

Wang and Chen (2007) do not use this alternating optimization procedure to obtain u and v. They obtain u and v by the following equations:

$$u = \sum_{i=1}^{M}\alpha_i y_i A_i v,$$ (11.34)

$$v_{t+1} = v_t - \eta(-\sum_{i=1}^{M} \alpha_i y_i A_i^T u_t), \tag{11.35}$$

where η is the learning rate and t is the iterative index.

Overall, the algorithm of MatLSSVMs proposed by Wang and Chen (2007) is summarized as follows.

The Algorithm of MatLSSVMs

Step 1: initialize v_0, η, MaxIter, ε, and C.
Step 2: For $t = 1$: MaxIter
   (a)   obtain α_i by solving classical LSSVM in the fixed v_{t-1} and obtain

$$u_t = \sum_{i=1}^{M} \alpha_i y_i A_i v_{t-1} \text{ by}$$

update v by Eq.(11.35),
   (b)   if $\|v_{t+1} - v_t\| > \varepsilon$ and $t < MatIter$, then step 2, else go to step 3.
Step 3: stop

From the algorithm of MatLSSVMs, one can see that the MatLSSVMs method consists of two phases. First, the solution to v can be gotten by an iterative algorithm. Second, for every fixed v, an analytical solution to u similar to LS-SVM can be obtained. Here, for a fixed v, the solution to u is free of local minima due to the fact that it is a convex optimization problem. However, in solving v, its optimality may not be guaranteed due to non-convexity of the criterion for v. In addition, it is worth noting that if we want the problem to be convex, we may alternatively take only u instead of both u and v as unknown and view the vector v as a hyperparameter in such a case.

11.2.3. Classification Learning Based on Convex Optimization Programming

11.2.3.1 Convex Programming

In general, learning models can be formulated as optimization problems. In this subsection, we first introduce convex optimization and then give a general formulation for convex optimization-based learning.

The convex optimization problem has the following expression

$$\min f_0(u) \tag{11.36}$$
$$\text{subject to } f_i(u) \le 0 (1 \le i \le m),$$
$$f_i(u) = 0 (m+1 \le i \le p),$$

where $f_i(u)$ $(0 \le i \le m)$ are convex functions and $f_i(u)(m+1 \le i \le p)$ are affine functions.

The convex optimization problem defined in Eq.(11.36) consists of a large number of popular special cases, such as the linear programming (LP) (Vanderbei, 2001), the linear fractional programming (LFP) (Boyd & Vandenberghe, 2004), the quadratic programming (QP), the quadratically constrained quadratic programming (QCQP), the second-order cone programming (SOCP) (Lobo, Vandenberghe, Boyd, & Lebret, 1998), the semidefinite programming (SDP) (Vandenberghe & Boyd, 1996), and the geometric programming (GP) (Boyd, Kim, Vandenberghe, & Hassibi, 2006). All of these special cases have been widely applied in different areas, such as computer networks, machine learning, computer vision, psychology, the health research, the automation research, and economics.

The significance of a convex optimization problem is that the solution is unique (i.e., the locally optimal solution is also the globally optimal solution). Consequently, the convex optimization theory has been widely applied to pattern classification for many years, such as LP in the linear programming machine (LPM) (Hardoon, Szedmak, & Taylor, 2004) QP in the support vector machines (SVM), SDP in the distance metric learning (DML).

In the following, we give a general formula for convex optimization-based learning

$$\min f(u, b, \zeta_i) \tag{11.37}$$

subject to $y_i c_i (u^T x_i + b) \ge \zeta_i$ $(i = 1, \cdots, M)$, where $c_i: \mathfrak{R}^{N+M+1} \to R, f: \mathfrak{R}^{N+M+1} \to R$ a criterion (convex function) for classification0, $c_i: \mathfrak{R}^{N+M+1} \to R$ for all $1 \le i \le M$ are convex constraint functions, $x_i \in$ $1 \le i \le M$ are training samples and their class labels are given by $y_i \in \mathfrak{R}^N \{1, -1\}$, $\zeta_1, \cdots, \zeta_M$ are slack variables, and $u \in \mathfrak{R}^N$ and $b \in \mathfrak{R}$ determine the classification hyperplane, that is, $sign(u^T x + b)$. By defining different classification criteria f and convex constraint functions c_i, we can obtain a large number of learning machines, such as SVM, MPM, and DML.

11.2.3.2 Supervised Tensor Learning: A Framework

Supervised tensor learning (STL) (Tao et al., 2005) generalizes the vector-based learning algorithms to accept general tensors as input. In STL, assume that there are M training samples $A_i \in \mathfrak{R}^{I_1 \times \cdots I_N}$ $(i = 1, \cdots, M)$ represented by tensors associated with class label information $y_i \in \{1, -1\}$. One wants to separate the positive sample ($y_i = 1$) from the negative samples ($y_i = -1$) based on a criterion. This extension is obtained by using $A_i \in \Re^{I_1 \times \cdots I_N}$. Therefore, STL is defined by

$$\min f(\{u_k\}_{k=1}^N, b, \{\zeta_i\}_{i=1}^M), \qquad (11.38)$$

$$\text{subject to } y_i c_i (A_i \prod_{k=1}^N \times_k u_k + b) \geq \zeta_i, \ 1 \leq i \leq M.$$

There are two different points between the vector-based learning and the tensor-based learning: (1) the training samples are represented by vectors in vector-based learning, whereas they are represented by tensors in tensor-based learning; and (2) the classification decision function which is defined by $u \in \Re^N$ and $b \in \Re$ in vector-based learning is $sign(u^T x + b)$, whereas the classification decision function which is defined by $u_i \in \Re^N$ and $b \in \Re$ in tensor-based learning is $sign(A \times_k u_k|_{k=1}^N + b)$. In the vector-based learning, one has the classification hyperplane, $(u^T x + b) = 0$, whereas in the tensor-based learning, one defines the classification tensorplane, that is, $(A \times_k u_k|_{k=1}^N + b) = 0$.

From Eq.(11.38), one can obtain the following Lagrangian function

$$L(\{u_k\}_{k=1}^N, b, \{\zeta_i\}_{i=1}^M, \alpha) = f(\{u_k\}_{k=1}^N, b, \{\zeta\}_{i=1}^M) - \sum_{i=1}^M \alpha_i (y_i c_i (A_i \prod_{k=1}^N \times_k u_k + b) - \zeta_i)$$

$$= f(\{u_k\}_{k=1}^N, b, \{\zeta_i\}_{i=1}^M) - \sum_{i=1}^M \alpha_i y_i c_i (A_i \prod_{k=1}^N \times_k u_k + b) + \sum_{i=1}^M \alpha_i \zeta_i$$

$$(11.39)$$

where $\alpha_1, \cdots, \alpha_N$ are Lagrangian multiplies.

Further, the solution of Eq. (11.39) can be obtained by solving the following saddle point of the optimization function.

$$L(\{u_k\}_{k=1}^N, b, \{\zeta_i\}_{i=1}^M, \alpha). \qquad (11.40)$$

The derivative of $L(\{u_k\}_{k=1}^N, b, \{\zeta_i\}_{i=1}^M, \alpha)$ with respect to u_j is

$$\frac{\partial L}{\partial u_j} = \frac{\partial f}{\partial u_j} - \sum_{i=1}^M \alpha_i y_i \frac{\partial}{\partial u_j} (c_i (A_i \prod_{k=1}^N \times_k u_k + b))$$

$$= \frac{\partial f}{\partial u_j} - \sum_{i=1}^M \alpha_i y_i \frac{dc_i}{dz} \frac{\partial}{\partial u_j} (A_i \prod_{k=1}^N \times_k u_k + b) \qquad (11.41)$$

$$= \frac{\partial f}{\partial u_j} - \sum_{i=1}^M \alpha_i y_i \frac{dc_i}{dz} \frac{\partial}{\partial u_j} (A_i \bar{\times}_j u_j) ,$$

where $z = A_i \prod_{k=1}^{N} \times_k u_k + b$.

The derivative of $L(\{u_k\}_{k=1}^{N}, b, \{\zeta_i\}_{i=1}^{M}, \alpha)$ with respect to b is

$$\frac{\partial L}{\partial b} = \frac{\partial f}{\partial b} - \sum_{i=1}^{M} \alpha_i y_i \frac{\partial}{\partial b}(c_i(A_i \prod_{k=1}^{N} \times_k u_k + b))$$

$$= \frac{\partial f}{\partial b} - \sum_{i=1}^{M} \alpha_i y_i \frac{dc_i}{dz} \frac{\partial}{\partial b}(A_i \prod_{k=1}^{N} \times_k u_k + b)$$

$$= \frac{\partial f}{\partial b} - \sum_{i=1}^{M} \alpha_i y_i \frac{dc_i}{dz}, \tag{11.42}$$

where $z = A_i \prod_{k=1}^{N} \times_k u_k + b$.

To obtain a solution of STL, one needs to set $\frac{\partial L}{\partial b} = 0$ and $\frac{\partial f}{\partial u_j} = 0$. Further, one has

$$\frac{\partial f}{\partial u_j} = \sum_{i=1}^{M} \alpha_i y_i \frac{dc_i}{dz} \frac{\partial}{\partial u_j}(A_i \bar{\times}_j u_j), \tag{11.43}$$

$$\frac{\partial f}{\partial b} = \sum_{i=1}^{M} \alpha_i y_i \frac{dc_i}{dz}, \tag{11.44}$$

Based on Eq. (11.43), one can notice that the solution u_j depends on u_k ($1 \le k \le N$, $k \ne j$). That is, directly obtaining the solution of STL is intractable. Fortunately, the alternating projection scheme can provide a strategy for obtaining the solution of STL. The key idea in the alternating projection optimization for STL is to obtain u_j with the fixed u_k ($1 \le k \le N$, $k \ne j$) in an iterative way.

Finally, Tao et al. (2005) proposed the following algorithm for the supervised tensor learning.

The Algorithm for the Supervised Tensor Learning

Input: The training samples $A_i \in \Re^{I_1 \times \cdots \times I_N}$ and class label information $y_i \in \{1, -1\}$ $i = 1, \cdots, M$.
Output: The parameters in classification tensor plane $\{u_k\}_{k=1}^{N}$ and b, such that the STL objective function $f(\{u_k\}_{k=1}^{N}, b, \{\zeta_i\}_{i=1}^{M})$ defined in Eq. (11.38) is minimized.
Step 1: Set $\{u_k\}_{k=1}^{N}$ equal to random unit vectors,

Step 2: Carry out steps 3–5 iteratively until convergence;

Step 3: For k = 1 to N:

Step 4: Obtain $\{u_k\}_{k=1}^{N}$ by optimizing

Step 5: end

Step 6: convergence checking. if the calculated $\{u_k\}_{k=1}^{N}$ have been converged. Here $u_{i,t}$ is the current projection vector and $u_{i,t-1}$ is the previous projection vector.

11.3 OTHER TENSOR SUBSPACE ANALYSIS

11.3.1 Tensor Canonical Correlation Analysis

11.3.1.1 Classical CCA

Given a set of samples $S = (x_1, y_1),...,(x_M, y_M)$ of (x, y), where $x_i, y_i \in \mathfrak{R}^N$. Let $X = [x_1,\cdots, x_M]$ and $Y = [y_1,\cdots, y_M]$. Choosing a direction $u \in \mathfrak{R}^N$ and projecting X onto the direction u, we have

$$\hat{X} = X^T u. \tag{11.45}$$

Choosing a direction $v \in \mathfrak{R}^N$ and projecting Y onto the direction v, one has

$$\hat{Y} = Y^T v. \tag{11.46}$$

The first stage of canonical correlation is to choose u and v such that the correlation between two vectors is maximized. In other words, the following objective function needs to be maximized

$$\rho = \max corr(\hat{X}, \hat{Y})$$

$$= \max \frac{<\hat{X}, \hat{Y}>}{\|\hat{X}\|\|\hat{Y}\|} = \max \frac{<X^T u, Y^T v>}{\|X^T u\|\|Y^T v\|}, \tag{11.47}$$

where $< \cdot, \cdot >$ denotes the Euclidean inner product of the vector and $\| \|$ is the norm of a vector. If we use $Ef(x,y)$ to denote the empirical expectation of the function $f(x,y)$, then

$$Ef(x, y) = \frac{1}{M} \sum_{i=1}^{M} f(x_i, y_i). \tag{11.48}$$

Based on Eq. (11,48), we can rewrite Eq. (11.47) as

$$\rho = \max \frac{E(u^T xy^T v)}{\left\| E(x^T u) \right\| \left\| E(y^T v) \right\|} = \max \frac{u^T E(xy^T)v}{\left\| E(x^T u) \right\| \left\| E(y^T v) \right\|}. \tag{11.49}$$

Note that the covariance matrix of (x,y) is

$$C(x,y) = E\left[\begin{pmatrix} x \\ y \end{pmatrix} \begin{pmatrix} x \\ y \end{pmatrix}^T \right] = \begin{bmatrix} C_{xx} & C_{xy} \\ C_{yx} & C_{yy} \end{bmatrix}. \tag{11.50}$$

The total covariance matrix $C(x,y)$ is a block matrix where the within-set covariance matrices are C_{xx} and C_{yy}, and the between-set covariance matrices are C_{xy} and C_{yx}. Using Eq. (11.50), we can rewrite the function ρ as

$$\rho = \max \frac{u^T C_{xy} v}{\sqrt{u^T C_{xx} u} \sqrt{v^T C_{yy} v}}. \tag{11.51}$$

Note that the solution of Eq. (11.51) is not affected by scaling u and v either together or independently. In other words, replacing u by αu gives the same results for ρ. Based on this point, the following conditions must be imposed in order to maximize the function ρ.

$$u^T C_{xx} u = 1, \tag{11.52}$$

$$v^T C_{yy} v = 1. \tag{11.53}$$

From Eqs. (11.51), (11.52) and (11.53), one can obtain the corresponding Lagrangian

$$L(\lambda, u, v) = u^T C_{xy} v - \lambda_x (u^T C_{xx} u - 1)/2 - \lambda_y (v^T C_{yy} v - 1)/2. \tag{11.54}$$

Taking derivatives with respect to u and v, one can obtain

$$\frac{\partial L}{\partial u} = C_{xy} v - \lambda_x C_{xx} u = 0, \tag{11.55}$$

$$\frac{\partial L}{\partial v} = C_{yx} u - \lambda_y C_{yy} v = 0. \tag{11.56}$$

From Eqs. (11.55) and (11.56), one further has

$$0 = \lambda_y v^T C_{yy} v -, \lambda_x u^T C_{xx} u \tag{11.57}$$

which together with the constraints implies that $\lambda_y = \lambda_x$. Let $\lambda_y = \lambda_x = \lambda$. Assume that C_{yy} is invertible, one has

$$v = C_{yy}^{-1} C_{yx} u / \lambda. \tag{11.58}$$

Substituting Eq. (11.58) into (11.55) gives

$$C_{xy} C_{yy}^{-1} C_{yx} u = \lambda^2 C_{xx} u. \tag{11.59}$$

It is obvious that Eq. (11.59) is a generalized eigenproblem. Hence, we can obtain projection vectors by solving this generalized eigenproblem. In some real applications, some regularization parameters are used to avoid the singularity problem in the covariance matrices.

11.3.1.2 2DCCA

Assume that $m \times n$ matrices A_k, $k = 1, \cdots, M$, denote M images and $m \times n$ matrices B_k, $k = 1, \cdots, M$, denote another M images. In 2DCCA, one does not need to transform the 2D images into its corresponding 1D vectors. Instead one uses a more straightforward way which views an image as a matrix.

We use two successive stages to perform 2DCCA. First, we align the M images (A_k) into a $m \times nM$ matrix $X = [A_1, \cdots, A_M]$ and align the M images (B_k) into a $m \times nM$ matrix $Y = [B_1, \cdots, B_M]$. After X and Y is obtained, one can perform classical CCA on the matrices X and Y. That is, one needs to find two directions $u, v \in \mathfrak{R}^m$ such that the following objective function is maximized:

$$\rho = \max \frac{< X^T u, Y^T v >}{\left\| X^T u \right\| \left\| Y^T v \right\|} \tag{11.60}$$

In such a case, we obtain u and v by performing classical CCA on Eq.(11.60). After obtaining u and v, one can easily compute

$$\hat{X} = X^T u, \tag{11.61}$$

$$\hat{Y} = Y^T v. \tag{11.62}$$

It is straightforward to verify that $\hat{X}$ and $\hat{Y}$ are $nM \times 1$ vectors. Further, we partition vectors $\hat{X}$ and $\hat{Y}$ into M blocks respectively, each block having dimensions of n, denoted by $(\hat{X})^T = [(\hat{X}_1)^T, \cdots, (\hat{X}_M)^T]$ and $(\hat{Y})^T = [(\hat{Y}_1)^T, \cdots, (\hat{Y}_M)^T]$. Let $\bar{X} = [\hat{X}_1, \cdots, \hat{X}_M]$

and $\bar{Y} = [\hat{Y}_1, \cdots, \hat{Y}_M]$. Note that $\bar{X}$ and $\bar{Y}$ are $n \times M$ matrices. In the second phage, we continue to perform classical CCA on the matrices $\bar{X}$ and $\bar{Y}$. That is, one needs to find two directions $\hat{u}, \hat{v} \in \mathfrak{R}^n$ such that the following objective function is maximized:

$$\rho = \max \frac{< \bar{X}^T \hat{u}, \bar{Y}^T \hat{v} >}{\left\| \bar{X}^T \hat{u} \right\| \left\| \bar{Y}^T \hat{v} \right\|} \tag{11.63}$$

Likewise, it is not difficult to obtain $\hat{u}$ and $\hat{v}$ by solving Eq.(11.63).

From the above analysis, we briefly summary the 2DCCA algorithm as follows.

The 2DCCA Algorithm

Input: $m \times n$ image matrices $\{A_k\}_{k=1}^M$ and $\{B_k\}_{k=1}^M$.

Output: the vectors u and v, $\hat{u}$ and $\hat{v}$

Step 1: Align the M images $\{A_k\}_{k=1}^M$ into a $m \times nM$ matrix $X = [A_1, \cdots, A_M]$ and Align the M images $\{B_k\}_{k=1}^M$ into a $m \times nM$ matrix $Y = [B_1, \cdots, B_M]$,

Step 2: Perform classical CCA on X and Y, and obtain vectors u and v,

Step 3: Compute $\hat{X} = X^T u$ and $\hat{Y} = Y^T v$ and partition $\hat{X}$ and $\hat{Y}$ into $(\hat{X})^T = [(\hat{X}_1)^T, \cdots, (\hat{X}_M)^T]$ and $(\hat{Y})^T = [(\hat{Y}_1)^T, \cdots, (\hat{Y}_M)^T]$. Let $\bar{X} = [\hat{X}_1, \cdots, \hat{X}_M]$ and $\bar{Y} = [\hat{Y}_1, \cdots, \hat{Y}_M]$.

Step 4: Performing classical CCA on $\bar{X}$ and $\bar{Y}$, and obtain vectors $\hat{u}$ and $\hat{v}$,

Step 5: Compute $\hat{A}_k \approx u^T A_k \hat{u}$ $\hat{B}_k \approx v^T B_k \hat{v}$ $k = 1, \cdots, M$).

Note that in the above algorithm, we first align the M images into a $m \times nM$ matrix $X = [A_1, \cdots, A_M]$. In fact, we can also align the M images into a $n \times mM$ matrix $\bar{Y} = [\hat{Y}_1, \cdots, \hat{Y}_M]$. In addition, we only obtain two pairs of vectors (u, v) and $(\hat{u}, \hat{v})$. In real applications, it is often needs multiple pairs of vectors. The methods for obtaining multiple pairs of vectors in 2DCCA are similar to those in classical CCA.

11.3.1.3 Multilinear CCA

Assume that $A_k \in \mathfrak{R}^{I_1 \times \cdots \times I_N}$ and $B_k \in \mathfrak{R}^{I_1 \times \cdots \times I_N}$, $k = 1, \ldots, M$, are two groups of tensors. Given $U^{(1)} \in \mathfrak{R}^{I_1 \times R_1}, U^{(2)} \in \mathfrak{R}^{I_2 \times R_2}, \cdots, U^{(N)} \in \mathfrak{R}^{I_N \times R_N}$, and $V^{(1)} \in \mathfrak{R}^{I_1 \times R_1}, V^{(2)} \in \mathfrak{R}^{I_2 \times R_2}, \cdots,$ $V^{(N)} \in \mathfrak{R}^{I_N \times R_N}$, we consider the following spaces $U^{(1)} \otimes \cdots \otimes U^{(N)}$ and $V^{(1)} \otimes \cdots \otimes V^{(N)}$. The tensors , A_k, $k = 1, \cdots, M$, are projected onto $U^{(1)} \otimes \cdots \otimes U^{(N)}$, denoted by $\hat{A}_k = A_k \times_1 ((U^{(1)})^T \times \cdots \times_N (U^{(N)})^T$ and the tensors B_k, $k = 1, \cdots, M$, are projected onto $V^{(1)} \otimes \cdots \otimes V^{(N)}$, denoted by $\hat{B}_k = B_k \times_1 ((V^{(1)})^T \times \cdots \times_N (V^{(N)})^T$.

Similar to classical CCA, multilinear CCA is to find the optimal projection matrices $U^{(1)} \in \mathfrak{R}^{I_1 \times R_1}, U^{(2)} \in \mathfrak{R}^{I_2 \times R_2}, \cdots, U^{(N)} \in \mathfrak{R}^{I_N \times R_N}$ such that the following objective function is maximized.

$$\rho = \max \frac{E < \hat{A}, \hat{B} >}{\left\| E(\hat{A}) \right\| \left\| E(\hat{B}) \right\|}, \tag{11.64}$$

where $E(\hat{A}, \hat{B}) = \frac{1}{M} \sum\limits_{i=1}^{M} < \hat{A}_i, \hat{B}_i >$, $E(\hat{A}) = \| \frac{1}{M} \sum\limits_{i=1}^{M} \hat{A}_i \|$ and $E(\hat{B}) = \| \frac{1}{M} \sum\limits_{i=1}^{M} \hat{B}_i \|$.

It seems that it is very difficult for us to deal with Eq. (11.64). However, the matrix representation of tensors provides an effective strategy for simplifying Eq. (11.64). Note that two tensors satisfying the following relationship

$$S = A \times_1 (U^{(1)})^T \times_2 (U^{(2)})^T \times \cdots \times_N (U^{(N)})^T. \tag{11.65}$$

can be represented in the following matrix form:

$$S_{(n)} = (U^{(n)})^T A_{(n)} (U^{(n+1)} \otimes \cdots \otimes U^{(N)} \otimes U^{(1)} \otimes \cdots \otimes U^{(n-1)}). \tag{11.66}$$

It is not difficult to verify that $\|A\|_F^2 = \|A_{(n)}\|_F^2$, for $n = 1, \ldots, N$. For the sake of notational simplicity, let $(U^{(n+1)} \otimes \cdots \otimes U^{(N)} \otimes U^{(1)} \otimes \cdots \otimes U^{(n-1)}) = U^{(\backslash n)}$ and $(V^{(n+1)} \otimes \cdots \otimes V^{(N)} \otimes V^{(1)} \otimes \cdots \otimes V^{(n-1)}) = V^{(\backslash n)}$. In such a case, we have

$$< (\hat{A}_i)_{(n)}, (\hat{B}_i)_{(n)} > = < \hat{A}_i, \hat{B}_i > = < (U^{(n)})^T (A_i)_{(n)} U^{(\backslash n)}, (V^{(n)})^T (B_i)_{(n)} V^{(\backslash n)} >$$

$$= \text{trace} \left[(U^{(n)})^T (A_i)_{(n)} U^{(\backslash n)} (V^{(\backslash n)})^T (B_i)_{(n)}^T (V^{(n)}) \right] \tag{11.67}$$

$$\left\| \sum_{i=1}^{M} \hat{A}_i \right\|^2 = < \sum_{i=1}^{M} (\hat{A}_i)_{(n)}, \sum_{i=1}^{M} (\hat{A}_i)_{(n)} >$$

$$= < (U^{(n)})^T \sum_{i=1}^{M} (A_i)_{(n)} U^{(\backslash n)}, (U^{(n)})^T \sum_{i=1}^{M} (A_i)_{(n)} U^{(\backslash n)} >$$

$$= trace[(U^{(n)})^T \sum_{i=1}^{M} (A_i)_{(n)} U^{(\backslash n)} (\sum_{i=1}^{M} (A_i)_{(n)} U^{(\backslash n)})^T U^{(n)}]. \tag{11.68}$$

In a similar way, we have

$$\left\| \sum_{i=1}^{M} \hat{B}_i \right\|^2 = \text{trace} \left[(V^{(n)})^T \sum_{i=1}^{M} (B_i)_{(n)} V^{(\backslash n)} (\sum_{i=1}^{M} (B_i)_{(n)} V^{(\backslash n)})^T V^{(n)} \right]. \tag{11.69}$$

In general, in order to obtain the optimal projections $U^{(1)}$, $U^{(2)}$,···,$U^{(N)}$, it is necessary to maximize Eq.(11.64). We note that it is very difficult to find the optimal projections simultaneously. To this end, an iterative algorithm is developed for obtaining the optimal projections $U^{(1)}$, $U^{(2)}$,···,$U^{(N)}$, like the algorithm of HOSVD. Further, we can see that for fixed $U^{(1)}$,···, $U^{(n-1)}$,···,$U^{(n+1)}$,···, $U^{(N)}$ it is not difficult to obtain the optimal projection $U^{(n)}$ similar to the CCA algorithm.

Let $C_{AA}^{(n)} = [\sum_{i=1}^{M} (A_i)_{(n)} U^{(\backslash n)} (\sum_{i=1}^{M} (A_i)_{(n)} U^{(\backslash n)})^T]$, $C_{BB}^{(n)} = [\sum_{i=1}^{M} (B_i)_{(n)} V^{(\backslash n)} (\sum_{i=1}^{M} (B_i)_{(n)} V^{(\backslash n)})^T]$,

and $C_{AB}^{(n)} = [\sum_{i=1}^{M} (A_i)_{(n)} U^{(\backslash n)} (\sum_{i=1}^{M} (B_i)_{(n)} V^{(\backslash n)})^T]$.

Assume that $C_{BB}^{(n)}$ is invertible. Then the optimal projection $U^{(n)}$ can be obtained by solving the generalized eigenvalue problem

$$C_{AB}^{(n)} (C_{BB}^{(n)})^{-1} C_{BA}^{(n)} U^{(n)} = C_{AA}^{(n)} U^{(n)} \Lambda. \qquad (11.70)$$

and $V^{(n)}$ can be obtained by

$$V^{(n)} = (C_{BB}^{(n)})^{-1} C_{BA}^{(n)} U^{(n)} \Lambda^{-\frac{1}{2}}. \qquad (11.71)$$

As a summary of the above discussion, the algorithm is shown as follows. The iterative algorithm of Multilinear CCA

In: $A_i \in \Re^{I_1 \times \cdots \times I_N}$, $B_i \in \Re^{I_1 \times \cdots \times I_N}$ for $i = 1,\cdots, M$
Out: $U^{(n)}$, $V^{(n)}$ $n = 1,\cdots, N$.
Step 1: Initial values: $U_0^{(n)}$ and $V_0^{(n)}$ $(2 \leq n \leq N)$;
Step 2: Compute the mean tensor M_i of class i and the globle mean tensor $\bar{M}$;
Step 3: iterative until convergence

(a) (i) compute $E_1 = (U_k^{(2)} \otimes \cdots \otimes U_k^{(N)})$, $F_1 = (V_k^{(2)} \otimes \cdots \otimes V_k^{(N)})$

$(S_b)_1 = \sum_{i=1}^{c} n_i [(M_i - \bar{M})_{(1)} E_1][(M_i - \bar{M})_{(1)} E_1]^T$,

(ii) obtain $U_{k+1}^{(1)}$ by solving Eq.(11.70) and $V_{k+1}^{(1)}$ by Eq.(11.71)

(N) (i) compute $E_N = (U_k^{(1)} \otimes \cdots \otimes U_k^{(N-1)})$, $F_1 = (V_k^{(1)} \otimes \cdots \otimes V_k^{(N-1)})$,

(ii) obtain $U_{k+1}^{(1)}$ by solving Eq.(11.70) and $V_{k+1}^{(1)}$ by Eq.(11.71)

Obtain converged values $U^{(1)}, \ldots, U^{(N)}, V^{(1)}, \ldots, V^{(N)}$.

Step 4: Compute $\hat{A}_i = (A_i) \times_1 (U^{(1)})^T \times \cdots \times_N (U^{(N)})^T$,

$$\hat{B}_i = (B_i) \times_1 (V^{(1)})^T \times \cdots \times_N (V^{(N)})^T \text{ for } i = 1, \cdots, M.$$

From the above algorithm, we note the following facts: when A_i $(i = 1, \cdots, M)$ are vectors, the algorithm is degenerated into classical CCA. Therefore, in some sense, the proposed method unifies current CCA and 2DCCA. It is obvious that multilinear CCA can directly deal with multidimensional data. Since the algorithm is iterative, the solution is theoretically local optimal. Like the HOSVD algorithm, probably the algorithm has several optimal solutions. In addition, we can see the algorithm involves setting initial values and judging the convergence. Therefore, it is necessary to further discuss these two problems in the future.

11.3.2 Tensor Partial Least Squares

11.3.2.1 Classical Partial Least Squares

Let $X = [x1, \cdots, xM]^T$ be the $(M \times N)$ matrix of M input and Y be $M \times L$ matrix of the corresponding L-dimensional response, where x_i $(i = 1, \cdots, n) \in \Re^N$. Without loss of generality, we assume that the matrix X and Y should be centralized in the PLS regression. They are easily obtained by a translation of data. In general, PLS is to approximate X and Y by some variables and to model the relationship between X and Y. Specifically, the PLS method decomposes X and Y matrices into the following form:

$$X = TP^T + E \tag{11.72}$$

$$Y = UQ^T + F \tag{11.73}$$

where T and U are $M \times k$ matrices of the extracted k score vectors , P and Q are matrices of loadings, and E and F are matrices of resides.

In addition, the PLS regression model can also be represented with the regression coefficient matrix B and the residual matrix R as follows:

$$Y = XB + R \tag{11.74}$$

$$B = W(P^T W)^{-1} C^T, \tag{11.75}$$

where P is the $N \times k$ matrix containing loading vectors. The matrix $P^T W$ is upper triangular and invertible. Note that Rannar, Lindgram, Geladi, and World (1994) obtained the following equalities:

$$P = X^T T (T^T T)^{-1}, \qquad\qquad (11.76)$$

$$C = Y^T T (T^T T)^{-1}, \qquad\qquad (11.77)$$

$$W = X^T U, \qquad\qquad (11.78)$$

$$T = XW (P^T W)^{-1}, \qquad\qquad (11.79)$$

Substituting Eqs. (11.76), (11.77) and (11.78) into Eq. (11.75) and using the orthogonality of the matrix T, we obtain B in the following form:

$$B = X^T U (T^T X X^T U)^{-1} T^T Y. \qquad\qquad (11.80)$$

Further, substituting into Eqs. (11.78) and (11.79) into Eq. (11.80), one can obtain

$$B = W (W^T X^T X W)^{-1} W^T X^T Y. \qquad\qquad (11.81)$$

It is obvious that Eq.(11.81) only contains an unknown matrix W.

Assume that Y can be constructed by XB when enough dimensions are adopted. In other words, R is a zero matrix. In such a case, we obtain

$$Y = XW (W^T X^T X W)^{-1} W^T X^T Y. \qquad\qquad (11.82)$$

We multiple $Y^T = XW$ in right-side in Eq. (11.82) and multiple X^T in the left-side in Eq. (11.82). Then we obtain

$$X^T Y Y^T X W = X^T X W (W^T X^T X W)^{-1} W^T X^T Y Y^T X W. \qquad\qquad (11.83)$$

Let $\Gamma = (W^T X^T X W)^{-1} W^T X^T Y Y^T X W$. Then we obtain

$$X^T Y Y^T X W = X^T X W \, \Gamma. \qquad\qquad (11.84)$$

It is not difficult to verify that Γ is a diagonal matrix when W consists of the eigenvector matrix of Eq. (11.84) in Fukunaga (1990).

Note that the solutions of Eq. (11.84) are conjugate orthogonal with respect to $X^T X$. However, in some PLS regression problems, it is required the W should be a column orthogonal matrix. In such a case, we can obtain the orthogonal matrix $\bar{W}$ by Gram- Schmidt orthogonalization. In addition, we can see that $X^T X$ is singular when the number of samples is smaller than the dimension of samples. Fortunately, some effective algorithms (Howland & Park, 2004; Ye, Janardan, Park, & Park, 2004) for overcoming the singular problem in generalized eigenvalue problems have been developed recently.

11.3.2.2 2D Partial Least Squares (2DPLS)

Assume that $m \times n$ matrices A_k, $k = 1,..., M$, denote M images and $\hat{Y}$ is an $M \times c$ matrix of the corresponding c-dimensional response. In 2DPLS, one does not need to transform the 2D images into its corresponding 1D vectors.

First, we align the M images (A_k) into a $mM \times n$ matrix $X = [A_1^T, \cdots, A_M^T]^T$.

Let $Y = [\underbrace{\hat{Y}_1, \cdots, \hat{Y}_1}_{m}, \cdots, \underbrace{\hat{Y}_M, \cdots, \hat{Y}_M}_{m}]$,

where $\hat{Y}_i$ is the transpose of the ith row of matrix $\hat{Y}_i$. After X and Y is obtained, one can perform classical PLS on the matrices X and Y. That is, one needs to find projection matrices $W_1 \in \mathfrak{R}^{n \times d}$ such that

$$X^T YY^T XW_1 = X^T X \, W_1 \Gamma. \tag{11.85}$$

It is obvious that Eq. (11.85) is a generalized eigenvalue problem. It is not difficult to verify that Γ is a diagonal matrix when

W_1 consists of the eigenvector matrix of Eq. (11.85).
Further, we obtain the following matrix:

$$B = W_1 (W_1^T X^T X W_1)^{-1} W_1^T X^T Y. \tag{11.86}$$

Second, we align the M images (A_k) into a $nM \times m$ matrix $U = [A_1,...,A_M]^T$. Let

$$T = [\underbrace{\hat{Y}_1, \cdots, \hat{Y}_1}_{n}, \cdots, \underbrace{\hat{Y}_M, \cdots, \hat{Y}_M}_{n}],$$

where $\hat{Y}_i$ is the ith column of matrix $\hat{Y}^T$. After U and T are obtained, one can perform classical PLS on the matrices U and T. That is, one needs to find the projection matrices $W_2 \in \mathfrak{R}^{m \times d}$ such that

$$U^T T T^T U W_2 = U^T U \, W_2. \tag{11.87}$$

It is obvious that Eq. (11.87) is a generalized eigenvalue problem. It is not difficult to verify that Γ is a diagonal matrix when W_2 consists of the eigenvector matrix of Eq. (11.87).

Further, we obtain the following matrix:

$$C = W_2 (W_2^T U^T U W_2)^{-1} W_2^T U^T T. \tag{11.88}$$

From Eqs. (11.86) and (11.88), one can notice that B *is* an $n \times c$ matrix and C is an $m \times c$ matrix. After a test sample A is put, we have

$$\bar{Y} = C^T A B \tag{11.89}$$

From $\hat{Y}$, one can see that the response of each sample is a vector. However, from Eq. (11.89), we can know $\bar{Y}$ is a $c \times c$ matrix. To be consistent with the original form, one can obtain the response of a test sample by using $\bar{Y}$, denoted by

$$Y_{final} = mean(\bar{Y}), \text{ or } \max(\bar{Y}), \text{ or } \min(\bar{Y}). \tag{11.90}$$

From the above analysis, we briefly summary the 2DPLS algorithm as follows.

The 2DPLS Algorithm

Input: $m \times n$ image matrices $\{A_k\}_{k=1}^{M}$ and the responses $\{Y_k\}_{k=1}^{M}$.

Output: the vectors B and C

Step 1: Align the M images (A_k) into a $nM \times m$ matrix $X = [A_1^T, \cdots, A_M^T]^T$ and Let $Y = [\underbrace{\hat{Y}_1, \cdots, \hat{Y}_1}_{m}, \cdots, \underbrace{\hat{Y}_M, \cdots, \hat{Y}_M}_{m}]$, where $\hat{Y}_i$ is the transpose of the ith row of matrix $\hat{Y}$.

Step 2: Perform classical PLS B on X and Y, obtain W_1 by Eq. (11.85) and B by Eq.(11.86)

Step 3: align the M images (A_k) into a $nM \times m$ matrix $U = [A_1, ... A_M]^T$. Let

$$T = [\underbrace{\hat{Y}_1, \cdots, \hat{Y}_1}_{n}, \cdots, \underbrace{\hat{Y}_M, \cdots, \hat{Y}_M}_{n}],$$

where $\hat{Y}_i$ is the ith column of matrix $\hat{Y}^T$.

Step 4: Performing classical PLS on U and T, and obtain W_2 by Eq. (11.87) and C by Eq. (11.88),

Step 5: compute the final response by Eq. (11.90).

11.3.2.3 Multilinear Partial Least Squares

Assume that $A_k \in \mathfrak{R}^{I_1 \times \cdots \times I_N}$, $k = 1, \cdots, M$, are M tensors and $\hat{Y}$ is a $M \times c$ matrix of the corresponding c-dimensional response. The matrix representation of tensors provides an effective strategy for dealing with multilinear PLS.

Let B be an $I_1 \times \cdots \times I_N \times M$ tensor which consists of a group of tensors $A_k \in \mathfrak{R}^{I_1 \times \cdots \times I_N}$ and $B_{(n)}$ be an $(I_1 \cdots I_{n-1} I_{n+1} \cdots I_N M) \times I_n$ matrix by unfolding the matrix B. Let

$$Y_{(n)} = [\ \underbrace{\hat{Y}_1, \cdots, \hat{Y}_1}_{I_1 \cdots I_{n-1} I_{n+1} \cdots I_N}, \cdots, \underbrace{\hat{Y}_M, \cdots, \hat{Y}_M}_{I_1 \cdots I_{n-1} I_{n+1} \cdots I_N}],$$

where $\hat{Y}_i$ is the ith column of matrix $\hat{Y}^T$.

After $B_{(n)}$ and $Y_{(n)}$ are obtained, one can perform classical PLS on the matrices $B_{(n)}$ and $Y_{(n)}$. That is, one needs to find the projection matrices $W^{(n)} \in \mathfrak{R}^{I_n \times R_d}$ such that

$$B_{(n)}^T Y_{(n)} Y_{(n)}^T B_{(n)} W^{(n)} = B_{(n)}^T B_{(n)} W^{(n)}. \tag{11.91}$$

Further, we obtain the following matrix:

$$C^{(n)} = W^{(n)} ((W^{(n)})^T B_{(n)}^T B_{(n)} W^{(n)})^{-1} (W^{(n)})^T B_{(n)}^T Y_{(n)}. \tag{11.92}$$

After a test sample A is put, we have

$$\bar{Y} = A \times_1 (C^{(1)})^T \times_2 (C^{(2)})^T \times \cdots \times_N (C^{(N)})^T, \tag{11.93}$$

In general, one can see that the response of each sample is a vector. However, from Eq. (11.93), we can know $\bar{Y}$ is a tensor. To be consistent with the original form, we can obtain the response of a test sample by using $\bar{Y}$, denoted by

$$Y_{final} = mean(\bar{Y}_{(n)}), \text{ or } \max(\bar{Y}_{(n)}), \text{ or } \min(\bar{Y}_{(n)}), \tag{11.94}$$

where $\bar{Y}_{(n)}$ is the unfolding matrix of tensor $\bar{Y}$ in Eq. (11.93).

11.4 SUMMARY

In this chapter, we introduce tensor-based classifiers and tensor canonical correlation analysis and tensor partial least squares. First, the vector-based classifiers are extended to accept tensors as input, which is the multilinear extension of classifiers.

The results provide a unified framework for classifier design. Among these classifiers, we mainly introduce tensor Ho-Kashyap HK classifiers, Tensor LS-SVM and classification learning based on convex optimization programming. To obtain the solutions of these learning algorithms, the alternating optimization is adopted. Second, we also demonstrate tensor canonical correlation analysis and tensor partial least squares. Tensor CCA and tensor PLS give a reformative framework of classical CCA and classical PLS. In this framework, these two tensor subspaces can directly use the image matrix to extract the features instead of matrix-to-vector transformation, which can effectively avoid the singularity of matrices occurring in classical subspace analysis. Overall, these two tensor subspace analysis can efficiently solve the small sample size problem. Although we describe more examples of tensor analysis in this chapter, some tensor analysis such as tensor cluster analysis is not involved because the ideas in this chapter are easily extended to tensor cluster analysis and other classical statistical learning methods.

REFERENCES

Baek, J., & Kim, M. (2004). Face recognition using partial least squares components. *Pattern Recognition, 37*(6), 1303-1306.

Bousquet, O., Boucheron, S., & Lugosi, G. (2004). Introduction to statistical learning theory, *Advanced Lectures on Machine Learning, LNCS 3176*, 169-207.

Boyd, S., Kim, S. J., Vandenberghe, L., & Hassibi, A. (2006). A tutorial on geometric programming. *Optim Eng., 8*(1), 67-127.

Boyd, S., & Vandenberghe, L. (2004). *Convex optimization*. Cambridge, UK: Cambridge University Press.

Chen, S. C., Wang, Z., & Tian, Y. J. (2007). Matrix-pattern-oriented Ho-Kashyap classifier with regularization learning. *Pattern Recognition, 40*(5), 1533-1543.

Duda, R. O., Hart, P. E., & Stock, D. G. (2001). *Pattern classification* (2nd ed.). New York: Wiley.

Fukunaga, K. (1990). *Introduction to statistical pattern recognition* (2nd ed.). New York, Academic Press.

Hardoon, D. R., Szedmak, S., & Taylor, J. S. (2004). Canonical correlation analysis: An overview with application to learning methods. *Neural computation, 16*(12), 2639-2664.

Helland, I. S. (1988). On structure of partial least squares regression. *Communications in Statistics of Simulation and Computation, 17*(2), 581-607.

Highleyman, W. H. (1962). Linear decision functions with application to pattern recognition. *Proceedings of the IRE*, (Vol. 50, No. 1, pp. 1501-1514).

Hotelling, H. (1936). Relations between two sets of vitiates. *Biometrika, 28*, 321-377.

Howland, P., & Park, H. (2004). Generalized discriminant analysis using the generalized singular value decomposition. *IEEE Trans. on Pattern Analysis and Machine Intelligence, 26*(8), 995-1006.

Leski, J. (2003). Ho–Kashyap classifier with generalization control. *Pattern Recognition Lett., 24*(14), 2281-2290.

Lewi, P. J. (1995). Pattern recognition, reflections from a chemometric point of view. *Chemometrics and Intelligent Laboratory Systems, 28*(1), 23-33.

Lobo, M. S., Vandenberghe, L., Boyd, S., & Lebret, H. (1998). Applications of second-order cone programming. *Linear Algebr. Appl., 284*(1-3), 193-228.

Melzer, T., Reiter, M., & Bischof, H. (2003). Appearance models based on kernel canonical correlation analysis. *Pattern Recognition, 36*(9), 1961-1971.

Muller, K.-R., Mika, S., Ratsch, G., Tsuda, K., & Scholkopf, B. (2001). An introduction to kernel-based learning algorithms. *IEEE Trans. Neural Networks, 12*(2), 181-202.

Oskuldsson, A. H. (1988). PLS regression methods. *Journal of Chemometrics, 2*(3), 211-228.

Rannar, S., Lindgren, F., Geladi, P., & World, S. (1994). A PLS kernel algorithm for data sets with many variables and fewer objects, Part I: Theory and algorithm. *Chemometrics and Intelligent laboratory System, 8*(2), 111-125.

Sun, Q., Zeng, S., Liu, Y., Heng, P., & Xia, D. (2005). A new method of feature fusion and its application in image recognition. *Pattern Recognition, 38*(12), 2437-2448.

Suykens, J. A. K., & Vandewalle, J. (1999). Least squares support vector machine classifiers. *Neural Processing Letters, 9*(3), 293-300.

Tan, Y., Shi, L., Tong, W., Hwang, G., & Wang, C. (2004). Multi-class tumour classification by discriminant partial least squares using microarray gene expression data and assessment of classification models. *Computational Biology and Chemistry, 28*(3), 235-244.

Tao, D., Li, X., Hu, W., Maybank, S. J., & Wu, X. (2005). Supervised tensor learning. *Proceedings of the IEEE international conference on data mining* (pp. 450-457).

Tao, D., Li, X., Wu, X., Hu, W., & Maybank, S. J. (2006). Supervised tensor learning. *Knowledge and Information Systems, 13*(1), 1-42.

Vandenberghe, L., & Boyd, S. (1996). Semidefinite programming. *SIAM Rev., 38*(1), 49-95.

Vanderbei, R. (2001). *Linear programming: foundations and extensions* (2nd ed.). Berlin: Springer.

Wang, Z., & Chen, S. C. (2007). New least squares support vector machines based on matrix patterns. *Neural Processing Letters, 26*(1), 41-56.

Wold, H. (1982). Soft modelling: the basic design and some extensions. *Systems Under Indirect Observation: Causality and Prediction*, Amsterdam, North Holland, 1-54.

Wold, H. (1985). Partial least squares. In N. L. Johnson & S. Kotz (Eds.), *Encyclopaedia of statistical sciences* (pp. 581-591). New York: Wiley.

Ye, J., Janardan, R., Park, C. H., & Park, H. (2004). An optimization criterion for generalized discriminant analysis on undersampled problems. *IEEE Trans. on Pattern Analysis and Machine Intelligence, 26*(8), 982-994.

Zheng, W., Zhou, X., Zou, C., & Zhao, L. (2006). Facial expression recognition using kernel canonical correlation analysis (KCCA). *IEEE Trans. Neural Networks, 17*(1), 233-238.

Section III
Biometric Fusion

Chapter XII
From Single Biometrics to Multi–Biometrics

ABSTRACT

In the past decades while biometrics attracts increasing attention of researchers, people also have found that the biometric system using a single biometric trait may not satisfy the demand of some real-world applications. Diversity of biometric traits also means that they may have different performance such as accuracy and reliability. Multi-biometric applications emerging in recent years are a big progress of biometrics. They can overcome some shortcomings of the single biometric system and can perform well in improving the system performance. In this chapter we describe a number of definitions on biometrics, categories and fusion strategies of multi-biometrics as well as the performance evaluation on the biometric system. The first section of this chapter describes some concepts, motivation and justification of multi-biometrics. Section 12.2 provides some definitions and notations of biometric and multi-biometric technologies. Section 12.3 is mainly related to performance evaluation of various types of biometric systems. Section 12.4 briefly presents research and development of multi-biometrics.

12. 1 INTRODUCTION

As mentioned in previous chapters, biometric technologies play an important role in access control and other systems that depend on secure personal authentication.

The fact that biometrics may possess excellent properties such as universality (every person has biometric traits), uniqueness (generally, no two people have identical biometric traits), permanence (most biometric traits do not vary over time), collectability (biometric traits can be measured quantitatively) and good performance (biometric technologies can achieve accurate results under varied environmental circumstances) (Ross & Jain, 2004; Jain, Ross, & Prabhakar, 2004) provides a solid base for these systems. Indeed, biometric technology is a methodology to achieve fast, user-friendly authentication with high accuracy. As mentioned in Chapter I, compared with biometric systems, traditional security systems, such as passwords or tokens-based methods, have some serious disadvantages.

Biometric technologies have many applications (Jain, Bolle, & Pankanti, 1999; Zhang & Jain (Eds.), 2006; Wayman, 2001; Bolle, Connell, Pankanti, Ratha, & Senior, 2004; Herzog & Reithiger, 2006; Jain & Ross, 2004; Jain, 2003). Biometrics can be incorporated in solutions to provide for Homeland Security including applications for improving airport security, strengthening border management control, in visas and in preventing ID theft. Biometrics can be also applied to secure electronic banking, investing and other financial transactions, enterprise-wide network security infrastructures, retail sales, law enforcement, and health and social services. Biometrics can also be integrated with other technologies such as encryption keys or smart cards to produce a hybrid security system. This way of exploiting biometrics is also called two-factor authentication, please refer to web site (http://www.answers.com/topic/two-factor-authentication). As shown in Chapter I, biometric applications can be categorized into several categories.

Varieties of biometric traits can be individually applied for personal authentication (Zhang, Jing, & Yang, 2005; Zhang & Jain (Eds.), 2004; Zhang, 2004); however, the biometric system using a single biometric trait usually suffers from some problems such as unsatisfactory accuracy, spoof attacks, and restricted degrees of freedom (Bubeck, 2003). For example, manual workers with damaged or dirty hands may not be able to provide high-quality fingerprint images. In this case, fingerprint authentication seems not to be a good means for authenticating personal identity. For an iris identification system, the existing registration failure risk would reduce the reliability of the system. For a biometric system using speech, some factors, such as ambient noise, changes in behavioral attributes of the voice, and voice change due to aging, will affect the system's performance. For a biometric system using face images, some challenges, such as variations in facial expression, pose and lighting, will limit the system's performance. One's keystroke trait and signature trait may vary to some extent and also bring side effects into the single biometric system using keystrokes or signature traits. All these examples imply that the single biometric system may not be guaranteed to provide a high accuracy.

In the past some means to improve biometric systems' reliability have been investigated. It has been proven that the simultaneous use of two or more biometric traits of the same identity is an effective way to enhance the performance of the biometric system (Jain, Prabhakar, & Chen, 1999; Ross & Jain, 2003; Prabhakar & Jain, 2002; Zhang & Jain (Eds.), 2006). Biometric systems that integrate multiple biometric traits are called multi-biometric systems or multimodal biometric system. Biometric systems that use only one biometric trait are called single biometric systems. It is well recognized that the combination of typical physiological or behavioral traits make biometric systems more accurate. Moreover, it is reported that non-conventional traits, i.e. the so-called soft traits such as color of skin, color of iris and height of the subject might also be integrated with conventional biometric traits to enhance the overall performance of the system. Different from "soft traits", the term "hard traits" is used to denote conventional biometric traits such as iris, face and palm print. By far, many multi-biometric techniques have been proposed and evaluated (Jain, Bolle, & Pankanti, 1999; Ross & Jain, 2003; Jain, Pankanti, & Chen, 1999; Hong & Jain, 1998; Kresimir & Mislav, 2004; Snelick, Uludag, & Mink, 2005). The promising results of multi-biometric systems encourage engineers and practitioners to devote themselves to the development of biometric systems. The significance of multi-biometrics is also partially reflected by the following statement: "Multi modal technology makes biometric work" ("Aurora Defense", 2002).

One of the methodological rationales of multi-biometrics is as follows: since different biometric traits such as the iris and the fingerprint can be considered independent of each other, the combination of them means that more information is used, which is theoretically helpful to improve the performance of biometric systems. Indeed, higher accuracy, which may be considered one of the essential goals of biometric technology, is also the primal reason of the appeal of multi-biometric systems.

The multi-biometric system will also provide strong feasibility and reliability, which can be explained in twofold: First, multi-biometric technology is able to improve the anti-spoofing performance of the system because it is much more difficult for an intruder to simultaneously spoof multiple biometric traits. Second, in the case where one biometric trait of an individual is not accessible (due to illness or injury), a multi-biometric system may still work, as long as the other traits are accessible. However, a single biometric system cannot work in the case where the user does not possess the required particular biometric trait. Varieties of studies and experiments have shown that multi-biometrics does perform better than single biometrics. For example, biometrics using face and fingerprint (Snelick et al., 2005; Hong & Jain, 1998), iris and face (Wang, Tan, & Jain, 2003), ear and face (Chang, Bowyer & Sarkar, 2003), palm print and hand geometry (Kumar, Wong, Shen, &

Jain, 2003), or face and speech data (Ben-Yacoub, Abdeljaoued, & Mayoraz, 1999) all are capable to obtain a higher accuracy than the corresponding single biometric technologies.

12.2 BIOMETRIC AND MULTI-BIOMETRIC FUSION: DEFINITION AND NOTATION

12.2.1 Definitions

Total Risk

Let R be the set that consists of similarity values representing genuine users. The total risk of a biometric system using a single trait can be defined as $E(R) = C_{FAR}$ * $FAR(R) + C_{FRR}$ * $FRR(R)$, where C_{FAR} and C_{FRR} are respectively the costs of falsely accepting an imposter and of falsely rejecting an genuine user. It is clear that if $C_{FAR} = C_{FRR}$, then the total risk $E(R)$ is the same as the total error, $FAR(R) = FRR(R)$. We can define the minimum total risk as follows (Hong, Jain, & Pankanti, 2000):

$$E_{min}(R) = \min_t (C_{FAR} * FAR(R) + C_{FRR} * FRR(R)), \qquad (12.1)$$

where t denotes the threshold. It has been theoretically demonstrated that a multi-biometric system which fuses multiple biometric traits at the matching score level or decision level can obtain lower total risk than the corresponding single biometric system using a single biometric trait (Hong, Jain, & Pankanti, 2000).

Verification

A verification process can be described formally as follows: given an input feature vector X_G of the single biometrics and the claimed identity of the user, determine if X_G belongs to class ω_1 or ω_2, where ω_1 means that the claim is true (a genuine user) and ω_2 means that the claim is false (an impostor). Generally, we should match X_G against the registered biometric template of the claimed identity, to determine whether the user is a genuine user. If the similarity between feature vector X_G and the registered biometric template of the claimed identity is greater than a predefined threshold, we can consider that the user is a genuine user; otherwise the user is considered to be an impostor.

Identification

Identification can be described as follows: given an input feature vector X_G of the single biometric trait of a user, determine the identity of the user. Generally, we can compute the similarities between X_G and the registered biometric templates of different identities and select the identity having the maximum similarity as the identity of the user.

FAR, FRR

False reject rate (*FRR*) of a genuine user *n* is defined as

$$FRR(n) = \frac{\text{Number of rejected verification attempts for a genuine user n}}{\text{Number of all verification attempts for the same genuine user n}}.$$

The overall *FRR* for *N* genuine users is defined as follows:

$$FRR = \frac{1}{N} \sum_{n=1}^{N} FRR(n).$$

False accept rate (*FAR*) of an imposter *n* is defined as

$$FAR(n) = \frac{\text{Number of accepted verification attempts for an imposter } n}{\text{Number of all verification attempts for the same imposter } n}.$$

The overall *FAR* for *N* imposters is defined as follows:

$$FAR = \frac{1}{N} \sum_{n=1}^{N} FAR(n).$$

FMR

In the case of identification, False Match Rate (FMR) is defined as the rate that the biometric system incorrectly declares a successful match between the input pattern and a nonmatching pattern in the database. In the case of verification, FMR refers to the rate of the impostor whose (similarity) score is greater than the decision threshold.

FNMR

In the case of identification, False Non-match Rate (FNMR) is defined as the rate that the biometric system incorrectly declares failure of match between the input pattern and a matching pattern in the database. In the case of verification, FNMR refers to the rate of the genuine user whose (similarity) score is smaller than the decision threshold.

FTAR

FTAR refers to failure to acquire rate (FTAR). FTARs of practical biometric systems are affected by the nature of the capture device and the biometric traits as well as the cooperation of the user.

FTER

FTER refers to failure to enroll rate (FTER) in the system register (enroll) stage. Usually failure to enroll happens when the obtained enroll data are considered invalid or of poor quality.

Receiver Operating Characteristic (ROC)

ROC represents a graphic means for assessing the ability to discriminate between genuine users and imposters. The ROC plot can be obtained by graphing the values of FAR and FRR, changing the threshold implicitly. Note that both the theoretical and the experimental studies show that in a biometric system in a practical situation attempts for achieving a low FAR by adjusting the predefined threshold for verification usually should at the cost of a high FRR (Golfarelli, Maio, & Maltoni, 1997). In other words, it is almost impossible for a certain system to simultaneously reduce the FAR and FRR of the system only by adjusting the predefined threshold for verification. For real-world applications, it is an important issue to select an appropriate threshold and to obtain the best trade-off between FAR and FRR.

EER

Equal error rate (EER) refers to the rate at which both accept and reject errors are equal. The EER is obtained from the ROC plot by taking the point where FAR and FRR have the same value. The ERR is usually used to compare performances of two systems. The lower the EER is, the more accurate the system is considered to be.

12.2.2 Categories of Multi-Biometrics

Though the formal definition and categories of types of biometric fusion systems is still an active topic, INCITS (InterNational Committee for Information Technology

Standards) Secretariat, Information Technology Industry Council (ITI) classifies them into three primary categories, defined as follows:

A. Multi-Modal. Multi-modal biometrics means the use of two or more fundamentally different types of raw biometric samples, such as face image and fingerprint image data. This includes cases where the same body part is sampled in two fundamentally different ways. Examples include a hand that can be sampled as a palm print or an outline (hand geometry).
B. Multi-Instance. Multi-instance biometrics means the use of the same type of raw biometric sample and processing on multiple instances of similar body parts, such as two fingers, or two irises.
C. Multi-Algorithmic. Multi-algorithmic biometrics means the use of multiple algorithms of processing on the same raw biometric samples, such as minutia and ridge pattern algorithms applied to the same finger image data.

Raw sample means the data captured by a biometric capture system before any processing by biometric algorithms that perform either registration (determination of landmarks or features) or template creation.

Multi-biometrics can also be categorized in other ways. For example, as presented in Section 12.2.3, multi-biometrics can also be categorized depending on the stage in which of the authentication process the information of different biometric traits is combined. In addition, two terms bimodal-biometrics and multi-modal biometrics are also used to categorize biometrics in some cases where people care how many biometric traits are used in the multi-biometric system. While bimodal-biometrics is usually referred to as the biometric system that uses simultaneously two biometric traits, multi-modal biometrics can be referred to as the biometric system that uses simultaneously not less than three biometric traits. Indeed, bimodal biometrics can be regarded as the simplest case of generalized multi-modal biometrics.

A single biometric system can be presented by the flowchart as shown in Figure 12.1, while a multi-biometric system can be presented by the flowchart as shown in Figure 12.2. The "fusion process" as shown in Figure 12.2 implements the information fusion of multi-modal biometrics. The meanings of the terms in the flowchart are explained as follows:

The **Stored Bio Record** is the template or image data enrolled for each user.

The **Demographic Record** is the user specific information deemed advantageous for decision making in the case where the biometric trait of the subject is not accessible.

The **Decision Record** is the information created and transmitted after the decision process.

Figure 12.1. Flowchart of a single biometric system

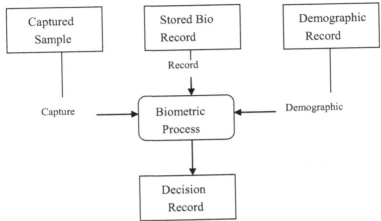

Figure 12.2. Flowchart of a multi-modal biometric system

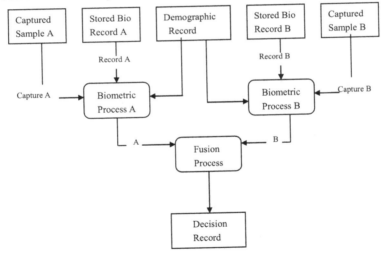

12.2.3 Fuse Information of Multi-Biometrics at Different Levels

If the systems are categorized according to the stage in which of the authentication process the information from the different sensors is combined, there are three categories of fusion strategies: fusion at the feature level, fusion at the matching

Figure 12.3. Fusion at the feature level

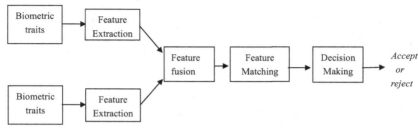

Figure 12.4. Fusion at the matching score level

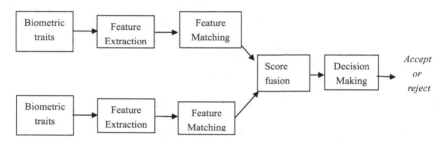

score level, and fusion at the decision level. Fusion at the feature level means immediate data integration at the beginning of the authentication process whereas fusion at the decision level represents data integration at the end of the process.

Fusion at the feature level can be described as follows. The data obtained from each sensor is used to compute a feature vector. As the feature extracted from one biometric trait is independent of that extracted from the other, it is reasonable to concatenate the two vectors into a single new vector for performing multi-biometrics based personal authentication. Note that the new feature vector now has a higher dimensionality than the original feature vector generated from each sensor. Feature reduction techniques may be employed to extract useful features from the new feature vector. This class of fusion is illustrated in Figure 12.3.

Fusion at the matching score level can be depicted as follows. Each subsystem using one biometric trait of the multi-biometric system provides a matching score indicating the proximity of the feature vector with the template vector. These scores can be combined to assert the veracity of the claimed identity. Fusion at the matching score level is illustrated in Figure 12.4.

Fusion at the decision level for verification can be implemented using the following procedures. First, each sensor captures one of multiple biometric traits

Figure 12.5. Fusion at the decision level

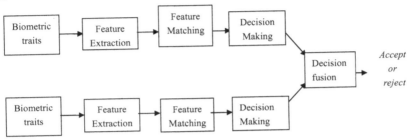

and the resulting feature vectors are individually classified into the two decisions – accept or reject the claimed identity. Then a scheme that exploits the known decisions to make the final decision is used. Fusion at the decision level is illustrated in Figure 12.5.

In the field of multi-biometrics, a number of studies of feature level fusion (Chang, Bowyer, Sarkar, & Victor, 2003; Ross & Govindarajan, 2005; Kong, Zhang, & Kamel, 2006; Kober, Harz, & Schiffers, 1997; Gunes & Piccardi, 2005; Jing, Yao, Zhang, Yang, & Li, 2007), matching score level fusion (Dass, Nandakumar, & Jain, 2005; Schmid, Ketkar, Singh, & Cukic, 2006) and decision level fusion (Verlinde & Cholet, 1999; Chatzis, Bors, & Pitas, 1999; Osadciw, Varshney, & Veeramachaneni, 2003; Gökberk & Akarun, 2006) have been made. Although fusion of multi-biometrics are generally recognized as three classes as described above, in real-world applications of multi-modal biometrics it is possible that the "fusion process" is simultaneously involved in different levels such as in both the matching score level and the decision level (Jain, Chen, & Demirkus, 2007).

12.3 PERFORMANCE EVALUATION OF BIOMETRIC TECHNIQUES

While various types of biometric techniques have been developed, people find that biometric traits have different natures and these techniques also have different performance. As shown in Table 12.1, biometric techniques can be scored in terms of the nature of the biometric trait such as universality (1), distinctiveness (2), permanence (3), collectability (4), performance (5), and acceptability (6).

From Table 12.1, we can see that almost no one biometric trait simultaneously have high "distinctiveness", "permanence", "collectability", "performance" and "acceptability". Table 12.2 shows accuracies of state of art of biometric recognition

Table 12.1. Performance scores of different biometric techniques

	universality	distinctiveness	permanence	collectability	performance	acceptability
Face	H	L	M	H	L	H
Hand geometry	M	M	M	H	M	M
Fingerprint	M	H	H	M	H	M
Iris	H	H	H	M	H	L
Retina	H	H	M	L	H	L
Signature	L	L	L	H	L	H
Voice	M	L	L	M	L	H

"H", "M" and "L" represent "high", "medium" and "low", respectively

Table 12.2. State of art of biometric recognition systems

	EER	FAR	FRR	Number of Subjects	Comment	Reference
Face	n.a.	1%	10%	37437	Varied lighting, indoor/outdoor	FRVT
Fingerprint	n.a.	1%	0.1%	25000	US Government operational data	FpVTE
Fingerprint	2%	2%	2%	100	Rotation and exaggerated skin distortion	FVC
Hand geometry	1%	2%	0.1%	129	With rings and improper placement	(2005)
Iris	< 1%	0.94%	0.99%	1224	Indoor environment	ITIRT
Iris	0.01%	0.0001%	0.2%	132	Best conditions	NIST
Voice	6%	2%	10%	310	Text independent, multilingual	NIST

systems. We should point out aside the nature of the biometric trait, the accuracy of the biometric system is also directly related to the sensor, scalability of the user, and the algorithm. As a result, Table 12.2 does not mean that when we use a biometric trait shown in this table we can obtain the same accuracy. Indeed, we can consider that the accuracy shown in Table 12.2 was obtained under the condition of zero FTAR and FTER. It is probably that real-world application of the biometric trait usually produces a lower accuracy than that shown in Table 12.2 because of nonzero

FTAR and FTER and other uncertain factors such as lack of accessibility to the biometric trait due to illness or injury. Jain, Pankanti, Prabhakar, Hong, and Ross (2004) indicated that a large gap exists between the current biometric technology and the performance requirement.

12.4 RESEARCH AND DEVELOPMENT OF MULTI-BIOMETRICS

12.4.1 Basis and Potential of Multi-Biometrics

The basis and potential of multi-biometrics can be shown from theory or practical perspective. We first briefly present some significant theory research on the basis and potential of multi-biometrics as follows. Kittler, Hatef, Duin, and Matas (1998) studied the problem of combining classifiers that used different representations of the patterns to be classified and developed a common theoretical framework for classifier combination. They also showed that under different assumptions and using different approximations they could derive the commonly used classifier combination schemes such as the product rule, sum rule, min rule, max rule, median rule, and majority voting. Golfarelli Maio and Maltoni (1997) studied the problem of performance evaluation in biometric verification systems. They derived two statistical expressions for theoretically calculating FRR and FAR. They also demonstrated the fundamental relation between FRR and FAR. Hong, Jain and Pankanti (2000) theoretically proved that it was possible to improve performance of the biometric system by integrating multiple biometric traits. Kuncheva, Whitaker, Shipp, and Duin (2000) studied the limits on the major voting accuracy produced by the combination of dependent classifiers. Jain, Nandakumar, and Ross (2005) analyzed and compared the performance of different normalization techniques and fusion rules. Dass, Nandakumar and Jain (2005) proposed an optimal framework for combining the matching scores from multiple modalities using the likelihood ratio statistic computed using the generalized densities estimated from the genuine and impostor matching scores. A theoretical analysis of a novel approach was proposed based on the "dynamic selection" of matching scores (Tronci, Giacinto, & Fabio, 2007). Such a selector aims at choosing, for each user to be authenticated, just one of the scores produced by the different biometric systems available. Dass, Zhu,and Jain (2006) analyzed and discussed the problem of constructing confidence regions based on the ROC curve for validating the claimed performance levels and the problem of determining the required number of biometric samples needed to establish confidence regions of pre-specified width for the ROC curve. Osadciw, Varshney and Veeramachaneni (2003) explored optimum fusion rules for multimodal biometrics. Sim, Zhang, Janakiraman, and Kumar (2007) presented the theory, architecture and implementation of the multimodal biometric verification system that continuously verifies the presence of a logged-in user. They also argued that the usual performance metrics of false accept and false reject rates were insufficient yardsticks for continuous verification and proposed new metrics. Oermann, Scheidat, and Vielhauer (2006) presented a theoretical concept of a methodology to improve those fusions and strategies independently of their application levels. They showed that the fusion could be potentially improved by extracting and merging certain semantic information and integrating it as additional knowledge (e.g. metadata) into the fusion process. Zhang and Zuo (2007) and Xiao (2007) summarized intelligent computation technologies in the fields of biometrics from different view of points.

There is also a variety of practical research on multi-biometrics. Chang, Bowyer, Sarkar, and Victor (2003) combined the ear and face image to perform identity recognition and could obtain the accuracy of 90.9%, whereas the accuracies of the ear-based and face-based identity recognition are 71.6% and 70.5%, respectively. Other examples for illustrating that the use of multi-modal biometrics brings performance improvement include the combination of, fingerprint and face (Hong & Jain, 1998), iris and face (Wang, Tan, & Jain, 2003), speech and face (Ben-Yacoub et al., 1999; Teoh, Samad, & Hussain, 2002), visual and acoustic signals for command-word recognition (Kober, Harz , & Schiffers, 1997). etc. In addition, studies on the multi-instance biometrics such as personal authentication using two irises (Wu, Wang, Zhang, & Qi, 2007), two palm prints (Wu, Wang, & Zhang, 2007), hand geometry and texture (Kumar & Zhang, 2006; Kumar, Wong, Shen, & Jain, 2003), the combination of shape contexts and local features of signature (Li, Zhang, & Wang, 2006) also suggested clear performance improvement. Jain, Chen and Demirkus (2007) recently made a significant progress in fingerprint verification. They proposed to verify fingerprint using level 3 features (ridge flow and pattern type, minutia points and pores as well as ridge contours) and achieved a relative performance gain of 20 percent in terms of EER over the Level 2 matcher.

Besides the integration of different types of biometric technologies and the combination of multi-instances can improve the performance of the biometric system; the advancement in the sensor and algorithm design also allows the biometric system to produce a higher accuracy. Take face recognition as an example, while the 2002 Face Recognition Vendor Test (FRVT 2002) reported that "the best 2002 face recognition probability of verification using a single face image with controlled illumination was 90 percent" (Philips, Grother, Micheals, Blackburn, Tabassi, & Bone, 2002), 2006 Face Recognition Vendor Test (FRVT 2006) obtained a FRR of 0.01 at a FAR of 0.001 by using very high-resolution still images and Viisage (V-3Dn algorithm) on the 3D images. Development of palm print verification is another example. Zhang, Kong, You and Wong (2003) developed a CCD-based plamprint device and collected a palm print image database, 7,752 images from 386 different palms. Using this database, they obtained a 98 percent genuine acceptance rate and a 0.04 percent false acceptance rate with the threshold 0.3425. Wu, Zhang and Wang (2006) extracted the palm line feature, one of the most important feature of the palm print image. Palm print verification using the obtained palm lines obtained the EER of 0.0084. In addition fusion of phase and orientation information of the palm print image also can obtain a satisfactory accuracy (Wu, Zhang, & Wang, 2006; Kong, Zhang, & Kamel, 2006).

12.4.2 Use and Application of Multi-Biometrics

In recent years many governments have increasing concerns about the multi-biometric technology. In May 2005 the German Upper House of Parliament approved the implementation of the ePass, which enables the passport issued to all German citizens to contain biometric traits (please refer to: http://www.itsmig.de/best_practices/eP-ass_en.php). The issued ePass contains a chip that holds a digital photograph and one fingerprint from each hand, usually of the index fingers, though others may be used if these fingers are missing or have extremely distorted prints. In Germany, the new work visas will also include fingerprinting, iris scanning, and digital photos" (please refer to: http://www.filipinoexpress.com/19/19_news.html). In Israel the biometric technology has been used for several years. For example, at the border crossing points from Israel to the Gaza Strip and West Bank, authorized Palestinians can pass through the turnstiles through the authorization check based on their biometric traits and the held smartcard with stored information of fingerprints, facial geometry and hand geometry. At peak periods more than 15,000 people an hour pass through the gates. In Israel another example of biometric application is in the Tel Aviv Ben Gurion Airport. This airport has a frequent flyer's fast check-in system based on the use of a smartcard that holds information of the hand geometry and fingerprints of the holders. In Iraq, biometric technologies are also being used extensively (please refer to: http://www.csc.com/solutions/security/casestudies/2829.shtml). For example, during account creation, the collected biometric information can be inputted into a central database. Also, additional information such as individual personal history can be added to each account record. Besides the governments mentioned above, the United States government has also become a strong advocate of biometrics in recent years.

REFERENCES

Aurora Defense LLC. (2002). PRWeb Press Release. From http://www.prweb.com/releases/2002/2/prweb33800.php.

Ben-Yacoub, S., Abdeljaoued, Y., & Mayoraz, E. (1999). Fusion of face and speech data for identity verification. *IEEE Trans. Neural Networks, 10*(5), 1065-1075.

Bubeck, U. M. (2003). *Multibiometric authentication- an overview of recent developments.* San Diego: San Diego State University.

Chang, K., Bowyer, K. W., Sarkar, S., & Victor, B. (2003). Comparison and combination of ear and face images in appearance-based biometrics. *IEEE Trans. Pattern Anal. Machine Intell., 25*(9), 1600-1165.

Chatzis, V., Bors, A. G., & Pitas, I. (1999). Multimodal decision-level fusion for person authentication. *IEEE Trans. on SMC-A, 29* (6), 674-680.

Dass, S. C., Nandakumar, K., & Jain, A. K. (2005). A principled approach to score level fusion in multimodal biometric systems. *Proc. of Audio- and Video-based Biometric Person Authentication (AVBPA)* (pp. 1049-1058).

Dass, S., Zhu, Y., & Jain, A. (2006). Validating a biometric authentication system: sample size requirements. *IEEE Trans. Pattern Anal. Machine Intell., 28*(12), 1902-1913.

Golfarelli, M., Maio, D., & Maltoni, D. (1997). On the error-reject tradeoff in biometric verification systems. *IEEE Trans. Pattern Anal. Machine Intell., 19*(7), 786-796.

Gökberk, B., & Akarun, L. (2006). Comparative analysis of decision-level fusion algorithms for 3D face recognition. *Proc. of International Conference on Pattern Recognition (ICPR)* (pp. 1018-1021).

Gunes, H., & Piccardi, M. (2005). Affect recognition from face and body: early fusion vs. late fusion. *Proc. of 2005 IEEE International Conference on , Systems, Man and Cybernetics* (pp. 3437-3443).

Herzog, G., & Reithiger, N. (2006). *The SmartKom: foundations of multimodal dialogue systems* (pp. 43-58). New York: Springer-Verlag New York Inc.

Hong, L., & Jain, A. (1998). Integrating faces and fingerprints for personal identification. *IEEE Trans. Pattern Anal. Machine Intell., 20*(12), 1295-1307.

Hong, L., Jain, A., & Pankanti, S. (2000). Can multibiometrics improve performance?. *Proceedings AutoID* (pp. 59-64).

Jain, A. (2003, November). Multimodal user interfaces: Who's the user? *Invited talk in Fifth International Conference on Multimodal Interfaces*. Vancouver, British Columbia, Canada.

Jain, A., Bolle, R., & Pankanti, S. (1999). *Biometrics: personal identification in networked society*. Boston Hardbound: Kluwer Academic Publishers.

Jain, A. K., Chen, Y., & Demirkus, M. (2007). Pores and ridges: high-resolution fingerprint matching using level 3 features. *IEEE Trans. Pattern Anal. Machine Intell.*, *29*(1), 15-27.

Jain, A. K., Jain, K., & Ross, A. (2005). Score normalization in multimodal biometric systems. *Pattern Recognition*, 38, 2270 – 2285.

Jain, A. K., Prabhakar, S., & Chen, S. (1999). Combining multiple matchers for a high security fingerprint verification system. *Pattern Recognition Letters*, *20*(11-13), 1371-1379.

Jain, A. K., Pankanti, S., Prabhakar, S., Hong., L., & Ross, A. (2004). Biometrics: a grand challenge. *Proc. of the 17th International Conference on Pattern Recognition*, *2*, 935–942.

Jain, A., & Ross, A. (2004). Multibiometric systems. *Communications of the ACM, Special Issue on Multimodal Interfaces*, *47*(1), 34-40.

Jain, A. K., Ross, A., & Prabhakar, S. (2004). An introduction to biometric recognition. *IEEE Trans. on Circuits and Systems for Video Technology, Special Issue on Image- and Video-Based Biometrics*, *14*(1), 4-20.

Jing, X. Y., Jing, Y. F., Zhang, D., Yang, J. Y., & Li, M. (2007). Face and palmprint pixel level fusion and Kernel DCV-RBF classifier for small sample biometric recognition. *Pattern Recognition*, *40*(11), 3209-3224.

Kittler, J. Hatef, M., Duin, R. P. W., & Matas, J. (1998). On combining classifiers. *IEEE Trans. Pattern Anal. Machine Intell.*, *20*(3), 226-239.

Kober R., Harz U., & Schiffers J. (1997). Fusion of visual and acoustic signals for command-word recognition, *Proc. of International Conference on Acoustics, Speech and Signal Processing* (pp. 1495-1497).

Kong, A., Zhang, D., & Kamel, M. (2006). Palmprint identification using feature-level fusion. *Pattern Recognition*, *39*(3), 478-487.

Kresimir, D., & Mislav, G. (2004). A survey of biometric recognition methods. *Proceedings of the 46th International Symposium Electronics in Marine(ELMAR-2004)* (pp.16-18).

Kumar, A., Wong, D. C. M., Shen, H. C., & Jain, A. K. (2003). Personal verification using palmprint and hand geometry biometric. *Proceedings of the fourth International Conference on Audio-and Video-Based Biometric Person Authentication (AVBPA)* (pp. 668-678).

Kumar, A., & Zhang, D. (2006). Personal recognition using hand shape and texture. *IEEE Trans. Image Processing, 15*(8), 2454-2461, 2006.

Kuncheva, L. I., Whitaker, C. J., Shipp, C. A., & Duin, R. P. W. (2000). Is independence good for combining classifiers? *Proc. International Conference on Pattern Recognition (ICPR)* (pp. 168-171).

Li, B., Zhang, D., & Wang, K. (2006). Online signature verification by combining shape contexts and local features. *Pattern Recognition, 39*(11), 2244-2247.

Oermann, A., Scheidat, T., Vielhauer, C., & Dittmann, J. (2006). Semantic fusion for biometric user authentication as multimodal signal processing. *Proceedings of international workshop Multimedia content representation, classification and security (MRCS)* (pp. 546-553).

Osadciw, L. A., Varshney, P. K., & Veeramachaneni, K. (2003). *Multisensor surveillance systems: a fusion perspective*. Boston: Kluwer Academic Publishers.

Prabhakar, S., & Jain, A. K. (2002). Decision-level fusion in fingerprint verification. *Pattern Recognition, 35*(4), 861-874.

Ross, A., & Govindarajan, R. (2005). Feature level fusion using hand and face biometrics. *Proc. of SPIE Conference on Biometric Technology for Human Identification II* (pp. 196-204).

Ross, A., & Jain, A. (2003). Information fusion in biometrics. *Pattern Recognition Letters, 24*(13), 2115-2125.

Ross, A., & Jain, A. K. (2004). Multimodal biometrics: An overview. *Proc. of the 12th European Signal Processing Conference* (pp. 1221-1224).

Schmid, N. A., Ketkar, M., Singh, H., & Cukic, B. (2006). Performance analysis of iris-based identification system at the matching score level. *IEEE Trans. on Information Forensics and Security, 1*(2), 154-168.

Sim, T., Zhang, S., Janakiraman, R., & Kumar, S. (2007). Continuous verification using multimodal biometrics. *IEEE Trans. Pattern Analysis and Machine Intelligence, 29*(4), 687-700.

Snelick, R., Uludag, U., Mink, A., Indovina, M., & Jain, A. (2005). Large-scale evaluation of multimodal biometric authentication using state-of-the-art systems. *IEEE Trans. Pattern Anal. Machine Intell.*, *27*(3), 450-455.

Teoh, A. B. J., Samad, S. A., & Hussain, A. (2002). Decision fusion comparison for a biometric verification system using face and speech. *Malaysian Journal of Computer Science*, *15*(2), 17-27.

Tronci, R., Giacinto, G., & Roli, F.(2007). Dynamic score selection for fusion of multiple biometric matchers. *14th International Conference on Image Analysis and Processing (ICIAP 2007)* (pp. 15-22).

Verlinde, P., & Cholet, G. (1999). Comparing decision fusion paradigms using k-NN based classifiers, decision trees and logistic regression in a multi-modal identity verification application. *Proceedings of International Conference on Audio and Video-Based Biometric Person Authentication (AVBPA)* (pp. 188-193).

Wang, Y., Tan, T., & Jain, A. K. (2003). Combining face and iris biometrics for identity verification. *Proc.of International Conference on Audio and Video-Based Biometric Person Authentication (AVBPA)* (pp. 805-813).

Wayman, J. L. (2001). Fundamentals of biometric authentication technologies. *International Journal of Image and Graphics*, *1*(1), 93-113.

Wu, X., Wang, K., & Zhang, D. (2007). Automated personal authentication using both palmprints. *Proceedings of the International Conference on Entertainment Computing* (pp. 450-453).

Wu, X., Wang, K., Zhang, D., & Qi, N. (2007). Combining left and right irises for personal authentication. *Proceedings of the 6th International Conference Energy Minimization Methods in Computer Vision and Pattern Recognition* (pp. 145-152).

Wu, X., Zhang, D., & Wang, K. (2006). Fusion of phase and orientation information for palmprint authentication. *Pattern Anal. Appl.*, *9*(2-3), 103-111.

Wu, X., Zhang, D., & Wang, K. (2006). Palm-line extraction and matching for personal authentication. *IEEE Trans. SMC-A*, *36*(5), 978-987.

Xiao, Qinghan (2007). Biometrics—technology, application, challenge, and computational intelligence solutions. *IEEE Computational Intelligence Magazine*, *2*(2), 5-25.

Zhang, D. (2004). *Palmprint Authentication*. Boston: Kluwer Academic Publishers.

Zhang, D., & Jain, A. K. (Eds.) (2004). *Biometric authentication.* New York: Springer-Verlag New York, Inc.

Zhang, D., & Jain, A. (Eds.) (2006). *Advances in biometrics.* New York: Springer-Verlag New York, Inc.

Zhang, D., Jing, X., & Yang, J. (2005). *Biometric Images Discrimination (BID) Technologies.* Hershey: Idea Group Publishing.

Zhang, D., Kong, W., You, J., & Wong, M. (2003). Online palmprint identification. *IEEE Trans. Pattern Anal. Machine Intell., 25*(9), 1041-1050.

Zhang, D., & Zuo, W. (2007). Computational intelligence-based biometric technologies. *IEEE Computational Intelligence Magzine,* 26-36.

Chapter XIII
Feature Level Fusion

ABSTRACT

This chapter introduces the basis of feature level fusion and presents two feature level fusion examples. As the beginning, Section 13.1 provides an introduction to feature level fusion. Section 13.2 describes two classes of feature level fusion schemes. Section 13.3 gives a feature level fusion example that fuses face and palm print. Section 13.4 presents a feature level fusion example that fuses multiple feature presentations of a single palm print trait. Finally, Section 13.5 offers brief comments.

13.1 INTRODUCTION

Fusion at the feature level means that the combination of different biometric traits occurs at an early stage of the multi-biometric system (Chang, Bowyer, & Sarkar, 2003; Gunatilaka & Baertlein, 2001; Gunes & Piccardi, 2005; Jain, Ross, & Prabhakar, 2004; Kober, Harz, & Schiffers, 1997; Kong, Zhang, & Kamel, 2006; Ross & Govindarajan, 2005; Ross & Jain, 2003). The traits fused at the feature level will be used in the matching and decision-making modules of the multi-biometric system to obtain authentication results. As pointed out by Jain, Ross and Prabhakar (2004) and other researchers (Choi, Choi, & Kim, 2005; Ratha, Connell, & Bolle, 1998; Singh, Vatsa, Ross, & Noore, 2005), it is likely that the integration at the feature level is able to produce a higher accuracy than fusion at the matching score level and fusion at the decision level. This is because the feature representation conveys richer information than the matching score or the verification decision (i.e. accept or reject) of a biometric trait. In contrast, the decision level is so coarse that much information loss will be caused (Sim, Zhang, Janakiraman, & Kumar, 2007). Following are some examples of fusion at the feature level in the field of biometrics. Chang, Bowyer and Sarkar (2003) fused appearance traits of the face and ear at the feature level. They concatenated the traits of the face and ear and exploited the resultant new one-dimensional data to perform personal authentication. To reduce the dimensionality of the new data, they extracted features from the new data. Ross and Govindarajan (2005) discussed fusion at the feature level in the following different scenarios such as fusion of PCA and LDA coefficients of face images and fusion of face and hand modalities. Kong, Zhang and Kamel (2006) fused the phase information of different Gabor filtering results at the feature level to perform palm print identification. Gunatilaka and Baertlein (2001) proposed a feature-level fusion approach for fusing data generated from non-coincidently sampled sensors. Other feature level fusion examples include fusion of visual and acoustic signals (Kober, Harz, & Schiffers, 1997), the fusion of face and body information (Gunes & Piccardi, 2005), fusion of face and fingerprint (Rattani, Kisku, Bicego, & Tistarelli, 2006,2007), fusion of side face and gait (Zhou & Bhanu, 2008), fusion of iris and face and (Son & Lee, 2005), fusion of palm print and palm vein (Wang, Yau, Suwandy, & Sung, 2008), fusion of lip and audio (Chetty & Wagner, 2008), etc. Feature level fusion is also implemented for other fields such as medical image fusion (Kor & Tiwary, 2004; Patnaik, 2006) object classification (Wender & Dietmayer, 2007), machinery fault diagnosis (Liu, Ma, & Mathew, 2006) and content-based image retrieval (Rahman, Desai, & Bhattacharya, 2006).

A number of techniques or approaches may be incorporated with feature level fusion. For example, when feature level fusion is implemented, linear feature extraction methods are usually employed to reduce the dimension of the resultant data of the fusion process (Son & Lee, 2005). This is also helpful for reducing the risk of curse of dimensionality (Rattani, KisKu, Bicego, & Tistarelli, 2006). When the fused data are in the form of color images, the approach of respectively fusing data at different channels (Liu & Liu, 2007; Ross & Govindarajan, 2005) is a good way. In addition, some approaches were used to overcome the problem that multiple modalities have incompatible feature sets. For example, in order to address the issue that the minutiae feature point sets of fingerprint are not compatible with the appearance-based image feature, Rattani, KisKu, Bicego and Tistarelli (2007) proposed to make the minutiae feature point rotation and translation invariant and introduced the keypoint descriptor (Ross & Govindarajan, 2005). Feature selection technique may be involved in feature level fusion (Kumar & Zhang, 2006; Liu, Meng, Hong, Wang, & Song, 2007).

13.2 SCHEMES TO FUSE FEATURES AT THE FEATURE LEVEL

Fusion at the feature level can be broadly grouped into two classes. The first class covers the direct combination of different trait features obtained by the feature extraction procedures of different subsystems of the multi-biometric system. The combined features are then used to perform identification or verification (as shown in Figure 13.1). The second class covers feature fusion which involves first combining different original biometric traits and then carrying out a certain feature extraction or feature selection process on the combined biometric traits to obtain the final features for personal authentication (as shown in Figure 13.2). Note that previous definitions of fusion at the feature level primarily focus on the first class of fusion. However, as shown later in Section 13.3, the second class of fusion is also feasible and can be adopted by a multi-biometric system. In Section 13.3, the feature fusion procedure can be viewed as the second class of fusion. This is because after the face and palm print traits are combined to form x_{norm}, the KDCV Algorithm is then

Figure 13.1. Flow chart of the first class of feature level fusion

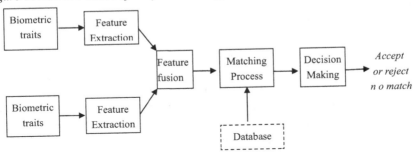

Figure 13.2. Flow chart of the second class of feature level fusion

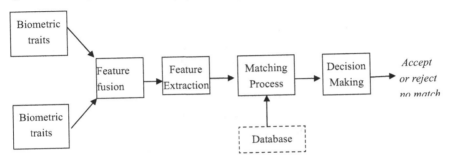

used to extract features from x_{norm}. The feature fusion scheme in Chang, Bowyer and Sarkar (2003) also belongs to the second class of fusion.

The following sections of this chapter will present two examples of feature level fusion. The first example is typical for multi-modal biometrics and clearly shows the typical fusion process of the first class of feature level fusion. It first extracts features of two biometric traits using the same feature extraction algorithm and then combines these features to perform personal authentication. The second example uses multiple presentations of a biometric trait to identify personal identities. This can be regarded as a typical instance of multi-algorithmic biometrics. Indeed, the multiple presentations are obtained by applying different algorithms to the same biometric trait.

13.3 FACE AND PALM PRINT FUSION AT THE FEATURE LEVEL

In this section, we present a novel fusion approach to multi-biometrics at the feature level. We first combine two kinds of biometrics: the face feature, which is a representative contactless biometric trait, and the palm print feature, which is a typical contacting biometric trait. We perform the Gabor transform on face and palm print images and combine them at the feature level. The correlation analysis shows that there is very small correlation between their normalized Gabor-transformed images. This section also presents a novel classifier, KDCV-RBF, to classify the fused biometric images. It extracts the image discriminative features using a kernel discriminative common vectors (KDCV) approach and classifies the features by using the radial basis function (RBF) network. Two large public face databases (AR and FERET) and a large palm print database are used to test the fusion approach. Experimental results demonstrate that the proposed biometric fusion recognition approach is an effective solution to the small sample size problem.

13.3.1 Gabor Transform of Face and Palm Print Images

2D Gabor filters are used mostly in image presentation. Gabor filters are also applied to texture segmentation, target detection, document analysis, edge detection, etc. A Gabor filter is basically a Gaussian function modulated by a complex sinusoid. At the same time, a Gabor filter can be also viewed as a sinusoidal plane of particular frequency and orientation, modulated by a Gaussian envelope. This can be written as $h(x,y) = s(x,y)g(x,y)$, where $s(x,y)$ is a complex sinusoid, and $g(x,y)$ is a 2-D Gaussian shaped function, known as an envelope. The complex sinusoid is defined as $s(x,y) = e^{-j2\pi(ux\cos\theta + uy\sin\theta)}$.

The 2-D Gaussian function is defined as follows: $g(x, y) = \dfrac{1}{\sqrt{2\pi}\sigma} e^{-\frac{x^2 + y^2}{2\sigma^2}}$.

Thus, the Gabor filter is generally defined as follows:

$$G(x, y, \theta, u, \sigma) = \frac{1}{\sqrt{2\pi}\sigma} e^{-\frac{x^2 + y^2}{2\sigma^2}} e^{-j2\pi(ux\cos\theta + uy\sin\theta)}. \tag{13.1}$$

where u is the frequency of the sinusoidal wave, θ is the orientation of this filter, and σ is the standard deviation of the Gaussian envelop. Note that the filtering result is a complex number.

The images in the first row are the resultant images of the Gabor transform under the conditions of $\sigma = 2$. The images in the second, third and forth rows are the resultant images of the Gabor transform under the condition of $\sigma = 4, \sigma = 8$, and $\sigma = 16$, respectively. For resultant images shown in each row, the orientation of the Gabor function increases rightwards. That is, the first image shown in each row is associated with $\theta = 0$ while the last image shown in each row is associated with

$$\theta = \frac{7\pi}{8}.$$

The Gabor function as defined in (13.1) is used as the filter operator. The size of the face image is 60×60. For the filter parameters, σ is set as 2, 4, 8, 16, respectively, $u = \dfrac{1}{\sigma}$,

and θ is respectively set as

$$0, \frac{\pi}{8}, \frac{2\pi}{8}, \frac{3\pi}{8}, \frac{4\pi}{8}, \frac{5\pi}{8}, \frac{6\pi}{8} \text{ and } \frac{7\pi}{8}.$$

Thus the Gabor transform used in this section contains four scales and eight orientations. Using the above Gabor function with different parameter values, we can transform an original image into 32 resultant images. Figure 13.3 shows an original face image. Figure 13.4 shows the results of Gabor filtering (expressed by magnitude values). The size of the original palm print image is also 60×60.

Figure 13.3. An original face image

Figure 13.4. Resultant images of Gabor transform on the face image shown in Figure 13.3

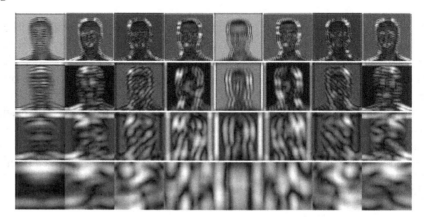

13.3.2 Fusion Procedure

The feature level fusion is implemented using the following procedure (Jing, Yao, Zhang, Yang, & Li, 2007):

(i) Let X_{face} and X_{palm} respectively denote sample sets of the face and palm print images. x_{face} is used to denote a sample of X_{face} with the size 60×60. Performing the Gabor transform on X_{face}, we obtain 32 resultant images (such as the ones shown in Figure 13.4). Combining them, we get a Gaborface image sample $x_{Gaborface}$, the initial size of which is 240×480. To reduce the computational cost, we downsample each Gaborface image by a ratio equal to 4. Hence the size of $x_{Gaborface}$ is reduced to 60×120. Similarly, for a sample x_{palm} from X_{palm}, we obtain its Gaborpalm image $x_{Gaborpalm}$.

(ii) We combine $x_{Gaborface}$ and its corresponding $x_{Gaborpalm}$ vertically to obtain a fusion image sample x_{fuse} with the size of 120 × 120. We thus get a fusion image sample set X_{fuse}. Note that the imaging conditions such as lighting conditions and camera focus settings for the face and palm print images are different. Thus, it is necessary to perform pixel normalization for fusion images. x_{fuse} can be normalized as follows:

$$x_{norm} = \frac{x_{fuse} - \mu_{fuse}}{\sigma_{fuse}},$$

where μ_{fuse} and σ_{fuse} are the mean and variance of x_{fuse}, respectively. We denote the normalized sample set consisting of x_{norm} by X_{norm}.

To show the dependency of $x_{Gaborpalm}$ on $x_{Gaborpalm}$, we analyze the correlation between $x_{Gaborface}$ and $x_{Gaborpalm}$ as follows. Let a and b respectively represent the face and palm print image parts of x_{norm}. We use the following expression to evaluate their correlation coefficient

$$cor(a,b) = \frac{\sum_{i=1}^{60} \sum_{j=1}^{120} |(a_{ij} - \overline{a})(b_{ij} - \overline{b})|}{\sqrt{(\sum_{i=1}^{60} \sum_{j=1}^{120} (a_{ij} - \overline{a})^2) \cdot (\sum_{i=1}^{60} \sum_{j=1}^{120} (b_{ij} - \overline{b})^2)}},$$

where $|\quad|$ means the absolute value, and $\overline{a}, \overline{b}$ are the mean values of a and b, respectively. We calculate the correlation coefficients for all samples in X_{norm}, and then obtain the average correlation coefficient $cor(X_{norm})$. Table 13.1 shows the correlation analysis of the face and palm print images. For the original image sets X_{palm} and X_{face}, we calculate their correlation coefficients using the same method presented above. Table 13.1 shows that the correlation of the face and palm print images is quite small, especially for normalized Gabor-transformed images. This means that the Gabor transform is helpful in reducing the correlation between different biometric images.

Table 13.1. Correlation coefficients between original face and palm print images and correlation coefficients between resultant images of Gabor transforms of face and palm print images

The set of samples	Combined Face and palm print images	Average correlation coefficient
X_{norm}	AR and palm print	0.0344
	Feret and palm print	0.0395
X_{face} and X_{palm}	AR and palm print	0.1351
	Feret and palm print	0.1185

13.3.3 KDCV-Based Feature Extraction and RBF Classification

13.3.3.1 Kernel-Based Nonlinear Discrimination Analysis (Jing, Yao, Zhang, Yang, & Li, 2007)

For a given nonlinear mapping function ϕ, the input data space R^n can be mapped into a feature space F. Suppose that the sample set X contains c known pattern classes, l_i is the training sample number of the *ith* class, and there are a total of $l = \sum_{i=1}^{c} l_i$ training samples. Then S_b^ϕ, S_w^ϕ defined as in (13.1) respectively denote the between-class scatter matrix and within-class scatter matrix of the feature space.

$$S_b^\phi = \frac{1}{l}\sum_{i=1}^{c}\left(m_i^\phi - m^\phi\right)\left(m_i^\phi - m^\phi\right)^T, S_w^\phi = \sum_{i=1}^{c}\sum_{j=1}^{l_i}\left(\phi\left(x_j^i\right) - m_i^\phi\right)\left(\phi\left(x_j^i\right) - m_i^\phi\right)^T,$$

(13.1)

where $\phi(x_j^i), j = 1,2,...,l_i$ means the *jth* sample of the *ith* class, m_i^ϕ is the mean value of the *ith* class, and m^ϕ denotes the mean value of all the training samples. Then the Fisher criterion in the feature space is as follows:

$$J_1(\varphi) = \frac{\varphi^T S_b^\phi \varphi}{\varphi^T S_w^\phi \varphi},$$

(13.3)

For the feature space, the optimal discriminant vector φ should make $J_1(\varphi)$ reach its maximum value, which implies that if we transform the feature space into a new space by taking φ as the transforming axis, the new space will have the maximal linear seperability (Xu, Yang, Lu, & Yu, 2004; Xu, Yang, & Jin, 2003). It has been proven that a transforming axis φ can be expressed in terms of

$$w = \sum_{i=1}^{l}\alpha_i \phi(x_i).$$

(13.4)

We define a kernel function

$$k\left(x_i, x_j\right) = \phi\left(x_i\right)^T \phi\left(x_j\right).$$

(13.5)

Substituting (13.4) and (13.5) into (13.3), we can rewrite (13.3) as

$$J_1(\alpha) = \frac{\alpha^T KUK\alpha}{\alpha^T K(I_l - U)K\alpha},$$

(13.6)

where K is an $l \times l$ symmetric matrix with $(K)_{ij} = k(x_i, x_j)$, I_l is the $l \times l$ll identity matrix, and U is an $l \times l$ block diagonal matrix. Note that $U = diag(U_1, U_2, ..., U_c)$ where U_i is a $l_i \times l_i$ matrix, the elements of which are all equal to

$$\frac{1}{l_i}.$$

We define $S_b' = KUK$ and $S_w' = K(I_l - U)K$ and respectively call them between-class matrix and within-class scatter matrix of the kernel space implicitly defined by the kernel function.

13.3.3.2 Feature Extraction Using KDCV Algorithm

The DCV (discriminative common vectors) algorithm aims at obtaining the optimal discriminant matrix W consisting of a number of discriminant vectors in the null space of the within-class scatter matrix of the original feature space. It is based on the following expression:

$$J(W) = \underset{|W^T S_w W| = 0}{\arg\max} |W^T S_b W|, \tag{13.7}$$

where S_b means the between-class scatter matrix of the original feature space. Two steps are needed for implementing the DCV algorithm. The first step is to obtain the null space of S_w. The second step is to get the optimal discriminant matrix W and the DCV. Using the DCV algorithm, we implement KDCV-based feature extraction as follows:

Step 1 Calculate the common vectors.

Let R^d denote the original sample space, V denote the non-null space of S_w', and $V^\perp$ denote the null space of S_w. Thus we obtain the following expressions: $V = span\{\beta_k \mid S_w' \beta_k \neq 0, k = 1, 2, ..., r\}$ and $V^\perp = span\{\beta_k \mid S_w' \beta_k = 0, k = r+1, r+2, ..., l\}$, where r is the rank of S_w. Indeed, β_1 β_2 . . . β_r are the eigenvectors corresponding to the nonzero eigenvalues of S_w, whereas β_{r+1} β_{r+2} . . . β_l are the eigenvectors corresponding to the zero eigenvalues of S_w'. Let $Q = [\beta_1$ β_2 . . . $\beta_r]$ and $\overline{Q} = [\beta_{r+1}$ β_{r+2} . . . $\beta_l]$. Because $R^d = V \oplus V^\perp$, every sample $\phi(x_m^i)$ can be expressed as follows:

$$\varphi(x_m^i) = \varphi(y_m^i) + \varphi(z_m^i), \tag{13.8}$$

where $\phi(y_m^i) = QQ^T \phi(x_m^i)$, $\phi(z_m^i) = \overline{Q}\,\overline{Q}^T \phi(x_m^i)$. $\phi(y_m^i)$, $\phi(z_m^i)$ respectively represent the difference vector and common vector parts of $\phi(x_m^i)$. It has been proved that all samples of the *ith* class have the same common vectors. Hereafter let $\phi(x_{com}^i)$

represent the common vector of the *ith* class instead of $\phi(z_m^i)$. Then we rewrite Eq. (13.8) and calculate $\phi(x_{com}^i)$ as follows:

$$\phi(x_{com}^i) = \phi(x_m^i) - \phi(y_m^i) = \phi(x_m^i) - QQ^T\phi(x_m^i). \tag{13.9}$$

We therefore obtain a common vectors set $A = \{\phi(x_{com}^1), \phi(x_{com}^2), ..., \phi(x_{com}^c)\}$.
Step 2 Calculate the optimal discriminant vector
S_{com}^ϕ is used to represent the total scatter matrix of A, i.e.

$$S_{com}^\phi = \sum_{i=1}^c \left(\phi(x_{com}^i) - \mu_{com}^\phi\right)\left(\phi(x_{com}^i) - \mu_{com}^\phi\right)^T, \tag{13.10}$$

where $\mu_{com}^\phi = \frac{1}{c}\sum_{i=1}^c \phi(x_{com}^i)$. The transform matrix W consisting of the optimal discriminant vectors will satisfy the following expression:

$$J(W) = \underset{|W^T S_w' W| = 0}{\arg\max} |W^T S_{com}^\phi W|, \tag{13.11}$$

where S_w' means the within-class matrix associated with S_{com}^ϕ.

Obviously, W should be composed of the eigenvectors corresponding to the nonzero eigenvalues of S_{com}^ϕ. Generally, all classes are independent of each other. Thus, all common vectors are also independent of each other and the rank of S_{com}^ϕ is $c - 1$. We can obtain nonlinear DCVs using

$$y_i = W^T\phi(x_{com}^i), i = 1, 2, ..., c. \tag{13.12}$$

Similar to DCV, y_i is also identical for the *ith* class and the feature dimension of y_i is $c - 1$. For any testing sample $\phi(x_{test})$, we transform it into a feature vector y_{test} using $y_{test} = W^T\phi(x_{test})$. The procedure presented above is called the discriminative feature extraction procedure.

13.3.3.3 Classification Using RBF

The RBF network has been widely applied to regression analysis and pattern recognition. A typical RBF network contains the following three layers: input layer, hidden layer and output layer. The neuron number of the input layer is decided by the feature vector dimension of samples, while the number of neurons in the hidden layer is adjustable. The neurons of the output layer are as many as the pattern classes. We set expected output values for the *ith* class as follows: the expected output value of the *ith* neuron is set to 1 and the expected output values of the other neurons are set to 0. The weights between the input and hidden layers are fixed at 1. The

Figure 13.5. Multi-modal biometric recognition procedure

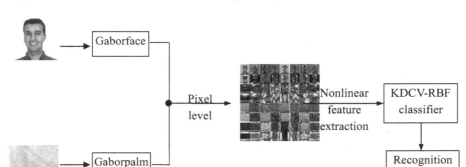

RBF network determines the classes of KDCV features, which are the derivation of the feature level fusion images. Note that a Gaussian kernel function serves as the kernel function for both the KDCV feature extraction procedure and the RBF network. Since the RBF network is used only for classifying KDCV features, we hereafter call it the KDCV-RBF classifier. Figure 13.5 briefly describes the main steps of feature extraction and classification:

Step 1 The face and palm print image sample sets X_{face} and X_{palm} are processed by the feature level fusion approach to get a fusion image sample X_{norm}. X_{norm} is a one-dimensional vector and the corresponding one-dimensional sample set is denoted by X.

Step 2 Based on X, we obtain the transform matrix W and c nonlinear DCVs using the KDCV algorithm. These nonlinear DCVs are used to construct the training sample set Y_{train}. After all testing samples are transformed by W, the testing sample set Y_{test} is obtained. The Gaussian kernel function is defined as $k(x_1, x_2) = \exp(- \| x_1 - x_2 \|^2 / 2\eta)$ where η is set as the variance of the training sample set of X.

Step 3 Respectively input Y_{train} and Y_{test} into the RBF network. The input layer, hidden layer and output layer have $c - 1$, c, and c neurons, respectively. All the c nonlinear DCVs are taken as the clustering centers and stored in the hidden neurons. The Gaussian radial basis function used here is $k(x_1, x_2) = \exp(- \| x_1 - x_2 \|^2 / 2\eta)$ with the parameter value $\eta = 10$. Note that the weights between the input and hidden layers are all 1. It is necessary to calculate only the weights' matrix W_n between the hidden and output layers. When Y_{train} is inputted into the network, G is used to denote the hidden layer values, WRBFG means the actual output values, and F is the expected output values. W_n is calculated using

$$W_n = G^+ F, \tag{13.13}$$

where G^+ denotes the pseudoinverse of G. After this, the trained RBF network is used to classify the sample set Y_{test}.

13.3.3.4 Experimental Results

In this section, two face databases (AR and FERET) and a palm print database are used to test the proposed approach. For our experiments on biometric fusion, the AR database (please refer to Section 3.4.4) and the FERET database are respectively paired with the palm print database to form two pairs of databases. The experiments compare feature level and classifier recognition approaches. Feature level approaches will use different image data and classify these data based on the KDCV–RBF classifier (here abbreviated to KDRC). Classifier approaches will use the fused Gabor-transformed images and classify them using different feature extraction and classification approaches. We implement several feature level approaches as follows: (1) Using single-mode original images respectively from the AR, FERET and palm print databases, we carry out in sequence AR-KDRC, FERET-KDRC and Palm-KDRC. (2) Instead of carrying out a Gabor transform, we use directly original images to perform feature level fusion of the two pairs of databases (i.e. AR and palm print, and FERET and palm print) and then classify the fusion results by using the RBF network. The corresponding implementation processes based on the above two pairs of databases are called ARPalm-Originalfusion-KDRC and FERETPalm-Originalfusion-KDRC, respectively. (3) We perform Gabor transform and feature level fusion in sequence. Two corresponding implementation processes based on the two pairs of databases are respectively called ARPalm-Gaborfusion-KDRC and FERETPalm-Gaborfusion-KDRC.

Several classifier approaches are implemented as follows: (1) We carry out AR-Palm-Gaborfusion-KDNC and FERETPalm-Gaborfusion-KDNC for two pairs of databases using the KDCV and NN classifier (abbreviated to KDNC). (2) Employing the DCV and NN classifier (DNC), we implement ARPalm-Gaborfusion-DNC and FERETPalm-Gaborfusion-DNC. (3) Using the Kernel PCA and NN classifier (KPNC), we carry out ARPalm-Gaborfusion-KPNC and FERETPalm-Gaborfusion-KPNC. (4) Using the KDRC classifier, we implement ARPalm-Gaborfusion-KDRC and FERETPalm-Gaborfusion-KDRC which will be presented latter.

To classify the sample features obtained using the DCV algorithm (Cevikalp, Neamtu, Wilkes, & Barkana, 2005), we use the NN (nearest neighbor) classification based on the Euclidean distance. In implementing the Kernel PCA (KPCA) (Scholkopf, Smola, & Muller, 1998), we use the same Gaussian kernel function as the one used in KDCV feature extraction.

For the AR face database, the images of the 119 individuals participating in the two image capturing sessions were selected and used in our experiment for a total number of 3094 (=119×26) samples. Every image is resized to be 60×60. The FERET database employed in our experiment includes 2200 facial images generated from 200 individuals (each having 11 images) (Phillips, Wechsler, Huang, & Rauss,1998). They are the images named with two-character strings from "ba" to "bk". We performed a histogram equalization for the cropped images and scaled them to 60×60.

The palm print database used in the experiments is from the Hong Kong Polytechnic University. This database contains palm print images of 189 individuals. The subjects are mainly volunteers of the Hong Kong Polytechnic University. Each person provided 20 images and the obtained database has a total of 3780 (=189×20) images. For each palm of every subject, the number of the acquired images is 10. Each of original images contained 384 × 284 pixels and had a resolution of 75 dpi. We obtained the subimages with a fixed size 128×128 from the original images by using the image processing approach in (Zhang, Kong, You, & Wong, 2003). In order to reduce the computational cost, we reduced the size of each subimage to 60×60 pixels. We took these subimages as palm print image samples for the experiments. The palm was imaged under varying conditions including unfixed illumination, shift and rotation of the palm. In addition, the image may also be slightly affected by the way the hand is posed, shrunk, or stretched. Figure 13.6 shows the twenty images of one subject from the palm print database.

Figure 13.6. The twenty images of one subject from the palm print database used in this section

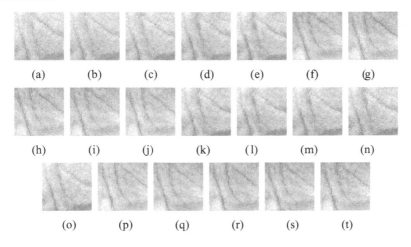

(a) (b) (c) (d) (e) (f) (g)

(h) (i) (j) (k) (l) (m) (n)

(o) (p) (q) (r) (s) (t)

13.3.3.4.1 Experiment on AR Faces and Palm Print

Note that the palm print database contains 189 classes each containing 20 samples and the AR face database has 119 classes each having 26 samples. We used the first 20 samples of each subject of the AR face database and all the pamlprint images of each of the first 119 subjects of the palm print database. We set the numbers of training samples per class to be 2 and 3, respectively, and took the remainder as

Figure 13.7. (Jing, Yao, Zhang, Yang, & Li, 2007) Random testing results on AR and palm print databases in the case where the number of training samples per class is 2

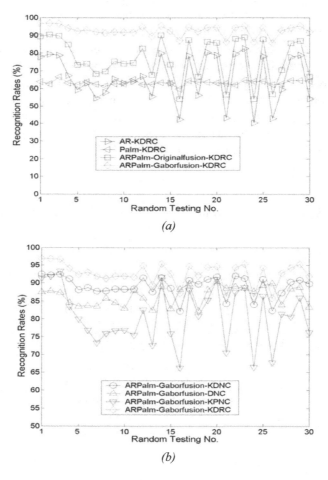

(a)

(b)

Figure 13.8. (Jing, Yao, Zhang, Yang, & Li, 2007) Random testing results on AR and palm print databases in the case where the number of training samples per class is 3

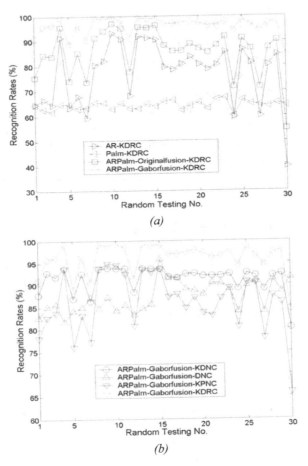

(a)

(b)

testing samples. The results of 30 random tests of different methods on two and three training samples per class will be shown in Figure 13.7 and Figure 13.8, respectively. Firstly, we set the number of training samples per class to be two so that here are 238 (=119×2) training samples and 2142 (=119×18) testing samples. From 13.7(a), we can see that the feature level fusion approaches clearly improve the recognition performance of AR-KDRC and Palm-KDRC, and ARPalm-Gaborfusion-KDRC performs best. From Figure 13.7(b), we can see that in most cases, ARPalm-Gaborfusion-KDNC outperforms ARPalm-Gaborfusion-DNC and

ARPalm-Gaborfusion-KPNC. In addition, ARPalm-Gaborfusion-KDRC obtains better recognition results than ARPalm-Gaborfusion-KDNC. Secondly, we set the number of training samples per class to be 3 so that there are 357 (=119 × 3) training samples and 2023 (=119×17) testing samples. Figure 13.8(a) shows that ARPalm-Gaborfusion-KDRC gets the best results among all the approaches. Figure 13.8(b) shows that ARPalm-Gaborfusion-KDRC performs best in almost all cases. Table 13.2 shows recognition results of all the approaches. Using a single biometric trait, AR-KDRC and Palm-KDRC obtain total average recognition rates of 71.28% and 63.81%, respectively. ARPalm-Gaborfusion-KDRC improves the total rate to 94.40% by exploiting bimodal-biometric traits and Gabor transform. Table 13.2 also shows that KDCV outperforms DCV and KPCA in extracting features of biometric traits, and that the RBF network is more suitable for classifying the KDCV features than the NN classification. The total average recognition rates of the KDRC classifier is significantly better than those of both the DNC classifier at 7.46% (=94.40%−86.94%) and the KPNC classifier at 11.04% (=94.40% − 83.36%).

13.3.3.4.2 Experiment on FERET Faces and Palm Print

Note that the FERET face database contains 200 subjects each having 11 samples and the palm print database contains 189 subjects and each subject has 20 samples. To implement fusion, we use all the 11 samples of each class of the first 189 face classes, and the first 11 samples of each class of all the 189 palm print classes. We

Table 13.2. Recognition results of different approaches on AR and palm print databases

Approaches	Number of training samples per class		Total mean values
	2	3	
	The average recognition rate (%)and the variance(%)	The average recognition rate(%) and the variance(%)	
AR-KDRC	65.67 (13.16)	76.88 (12.80)	71.28
Palm-KDRC	63.33 (1.30)	64.29 (1.57)	63.81
ARPalm-Originalfusion-KDRC	76.67 (11.68)	85.70 (9.57)	81.19
ARPalm-Gaborfusion-KDNC	89.12 (2.87)	91.35 (3.00)	90.24
ARPalm-Gaborfusion-DNC	86.54 (2.61)	87.33 (3.39)	86.94
ARPalm-Gaborfusion-KPNC	80.70 (7.94)	86.02 (6.79)	83.36
ARPalm-Gaborfusion-KDRC	92.66 (3.08)	96.14 (3.53)	94.40

Figure 13.9. Random testing results on the FERET and palm print databases in the case where 2 training samples per class

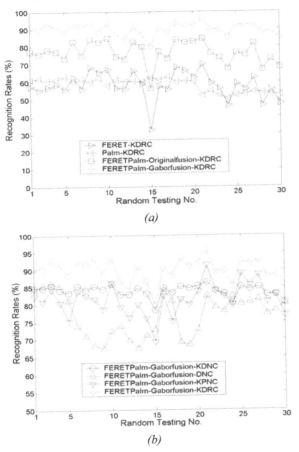

(a)

(b)

will set the numbers of training samples per class to be two and three, respectively, and the remainder is used as testing samples. When the number of training samples per class is set to be two, there are 378 (=189 × 2) training samples and 1701 (=189 × 9) testing samples in total. Figure 13.9(a) shows that feature level fusion approaches are superior to single biometric approaches, and FERETPalm-Gaborfusion-KDRC performs better than FERETPalm-Originalfusion-KDRC. Figure 13.9(b) shows that in most cases, FERETPalm-Gaborfusion-KDNC outperforms FERETPalm-Gaborfusion-DNC and FERETPalm-Gaborfusion-KPNC. In addition, FERETPalm-Gaborfusion-KDRC obtains better recognition results than

Figure 13.10. Random testing results on FERET and palm print databases in the case where 3 training samples per class

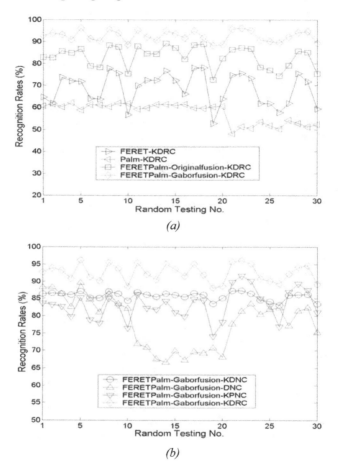

(a)

(b)

FERETPalm-Gaborfusion-KDNC in all the cases. When the number of training samples per class is set to be three, there are 567 (=189 × 3) training samples and 1512 (=189 × 8) testing samples in total. Figure 13.10(a) shows that for random tests of three training samples per class, the feature level fusion approaches outperform FERET-KDRC and Palm-KDRC, and FERETPalm-Gaborfusion-KDRC obtains the best recognition results. Figure 13.10(b) shows that for tests of three training samples per class, FERETPalm-Gaborfusion-KDRC performs best. Table 13.3 shows comparison of the average recognition results of all the approaches. Using single biometric trait, FERET-KDRC and Palm-KDRC obtain total average recognition rates of 63.35% and 57.95%, respectively. FERETPalm-Gaborfusion-KDRC improves the total rate to 91.22% by using the Gabor-based feature level fusion. Table 13.3 also shows that KDCV outperforms DCV and KPCA, and the RBF network is more suitable for classifying the KDCV features than the NN method. The total average recognition rate of the KDRC classifier is respectively 13.64% (91.22% − 77.58%=13.64%) higher and 8.95% (91.22% − 82.27%=8.95%) higher than those of both the DNC and KPNC classifiers.

13.3.3.4.3 Analysis of Experimental Results

Based on Tables 13.2 and 13.3, Figure 13.11 shows the total average recognition rates of the two groups of experiments presented above. From Figure 13.11, we can see that the total recognition rate rises from 67.32% (face recognition) and 60.88% (palm print recognition) to 92.81% (multi-modal fusion biometrics). Based on Gabor transform of two biometric traits, FacePalm-Gaborfusion-KDRC is 12.26% better than FacePalm-Originalfusion-KDRC, which uses the original biometric images. The proposed KDRC classifier improves the total recognition rates of two representative classifiers (DNC and KPNC) by 10.55% and 9.99%. These experimental results can be evaluated by using the null hypothesis statistical test based on the Bernoulli model (Beveridge, She, Draper, & Givens, 2001; Yambor, Draper, & Beveridge, 2002), which tells us that if the resulting p-value is below the desired significance level (i.e. 0.01), the null hypothesis should be rejected and the

Table 13.3. Average recognition results of the FERET and palm print databases

Methods	Number of training samples per class		Total mean values
	2	3	
	Mean values and variances (%)	Mean values and variances (%)	
FERET-KDRC	58.11 ± 7.79	68.58 ± 7.19	63.35
Palm-KDRC	58.25 ± 4.06	57.65 ± 4.54	57.95
FERETPalm-Originalfusion-KDRC	76.70 ± 6.40	83.11 ± 4.89	79.91
FERETPalm-Gaborfusion-KDNC	83.93 ± 1.72	85.77 ± 1.17	84.85
FERETPalm-Gaborfusion-DNC	76.89 ± 6.09	78.26 ± 7.24	77.58
FERETPalm-Gaborfusion-KPNC	81.40 ± 4.55	83.14 ± 4.30	82.27
FERETPalm-Gaborfusion-KDRC	89.90 ± 3.32	92.53 ± 2.46	91.22

Figure 13.11. (Jing, Yao, Zhang, Yang, & Li, 2007). Total average recognition rates of face and palm print biometric recognition

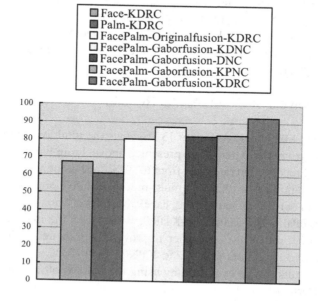

Table 13.4. Statistical analysis of the recognition performance difference of Face-Palm-Gaborfusion-KDRC and FacePalm-Gaborfusion-KDNC

Involved databases	Number of training samples per class	Number of significant differences
AR and Palm print	2	27
	3	30
FERET and Palm print	2	28
	3	30

performance difference between two algorithms are considered to be statistically significant. Table 13.4 shows the statistical analysis of the recognition performance difference between the proposed FacePalm-Gaborfusion-KDRC approach and Face-Palm-Gaborfusion-KDNC. In Table 13.4, the item "Number of significant differences ($p < 0.01$)" means the number of statistically significant differences between the two approaches occurring at a significance level of "$p < 0.01$". It seems that in most trials, there are significant differences between FacePalm-Gaborfusion-KDRC and FacePalm-Gaborfusion-KDNC. Table 13.5 shows the total statistical difference analysis for FacePalm-Gaborfusion-KDRC and other methods. The item "Number

Table 13.5. The total performance difference between FacePalm-Gaborfusion-KDRC and other approaches

Other approaches	Involved databases	Number of significant differences (p <0.01) for 60 random tests	Average number of significant differences
Face-KDRC	AR and Palm print FERET and Palm print	60 60	60
Palm-KDRC	AR and Palm print FERET and Palm print	60 60	60
FacePalm-Originalfusion-KDRC	AR and Palm print FERET and Palm print	60 60	60
FacePalm-Gaborfusion-KDNC	AR and Palm print FERET and Palm print	57 58	57.5
FacePalm-Gaborfusion-DNC	AR and Palm print FERET and Palm print	55 59	57
FacePalm-Gaborfusion-KPNC	AR and Palm print FERET and Palm print	60 60	60

of significant differences ($p < 0.01$) for random test (60 times)" means the number of statistically significant differences existing between the two approaches while the 60 random tests, each being associated with two or three training samples per class, are conducted. Table 13.5 shows that the recognition performance of Face-Palm-Gaborfusion-KDRC has a significant difference in comparison with those of the other methods.

13.3.3.4.4 Conclusion

The proposed feature level biometric fusion approach first combines the normalized Gabor-transformed face and palm print images at the feature level and then uses KDCV-RBF (KDRC) to classify the fused biometric images. The experimental results on two large face databases (AR and FERET) and a large palm print database demonstrate that this feature level biometric fusion approach is an effective solution to the small sample biometric recognition problem. While this section provides with us a typical example of bimodal biometrics, it also allows primary characteristics of the first class of feature level fusion to be clearly shown.

13.4 FUSION OF MULTIPLE FEATURE PRESENTATIONS

A real-world object can be presented in different ways. For example, it can be described in terms of its shape or color. Different feature extraction procedures may also have different focuses and produce different descriptions. For example, some feature extraction procedures may emphasize holistic characteristics whereas some other procedures may emphasize local characteristics. This makes it possible that the feature extraction results of different feature extraction procedures are complementary. In this book the term "multiple feature presentation" is used to denote multiple feature extraction results of a same biometric trait obtained using different feature extraction procedures. This section describes a technique that first takes phase and orientation information generated from the palm print image as multiple feature presentations of the palm print and then integrates these feature presentations to perform personal authentication.

13.4.1 Extraction of Phase and Orientation Information

Personal authentication presented in this section is based on a multiple feature extraction approach to a biometric trait. This approach is mainly involved in the fusion of the phase and orientation information of the 2D Gabor transform of the biometric image. While the proposed approach extracts the phase information (called PhaseCode) of an image by using four 2-D Gabor filters with different orientations, the orientation information (called OrientationCode) of the image is also extracted. The PhaseCode and the OrientationCode are fused to make a new feature, called the Phase and Orientation Code (POC). The POC-based palm print authentication approach proposed in this paper is called the POC approach. At the matching stage, a modified Hamming distance is used to measure the similarity of two POCs. The POC is calculated by using a 2D Gabor filter as defined in (13.1).

The imaginary part of the result of the Gabor transform inherently has no DC (direct current) because of the odd symmetry, whereas the real part has DC. However, the real part can be normalized to zero DC as follows:

$$\bar{G}(x,y,\theta,u,\sigma) = G(x,y,\theta,\mu\sigma) - \frac{\sum_{i=-n}^{n}\sum_{k=-n}^{n}G(x,y,\theta,u,\sigma)}{(2n+1)^2}, \qquad (13.14)$$

where $(2n = 1)^2$ is the size of the filter. After the normalization process, these filters have no DC response. This is very helpful for reducing the influence on the filtered results of the strength of illumination. We use four Gabor filters whose orientations are 0^0, 45^0, 90^0, 135^0 to extract the POC. These filters are respectively denoted by $G_j, j = 0,1,2,3$.

Let I stand for a palm print image and suppose that I has been filtered by G_j ($j = 0,1,2,3$) as follows:

$$I_{G_j} = I * G_j, \qquad (13.15)$$

where $*$ denotes the convolution operation. The magnitude of the filtering result is formulated as

$$M_j(x,y) = \sqrt{I_{G_j}(x,y)\overline{I_{G_j}}(x,y)}, \qquad (13.16)$$

where "-" denotes complex conjugate. The orientation of the point (x,y) is calculated using the following expression:

$$O(x,y) = \arg\max_{j=0,1,2,3} M_j(x,y). \qquad (13.17)$$

$O(x,y)$ is called the OrientationCode of the point (x,y). The PhaseCode can be calculated (Kong, Zhang, & Li, 2003) using:

$$P_R(x,y) = \begin{cases} 1, & \text{if} \quad \text{Re}(I_{G_j(x,y)}(x,y)) \geq 0; \\ 0, & \text{otherwise} \end{cases}$$

$$P_I(x,y) = \begin{cases} 1, & \text{if} \quad \text{Im}(I_{G_j(x,y)}(x,y)) \geq 0; \\ 0, & \text{otherwise} \end{cases} \qquad (13.18)$$

$$\qquad (13.19)$$

$$P_I(x,y) = \begin{cases} 1, & \text{if} \quad \text{Im}(I_{G_j(x,y)}(x,y)) \geq 0; \\ 0, & \text{otherwise} \end{cases}$$

$P = (P_R, P_I, O)$ is called Phase Orientation Code (POC). Figure 13.12 shows POCs of three palm print images.

Figure 13.12. POCs of three palm print images: (a),(b), (c) denote the original palm prints; (d),(e),(f) show the real parts of the POCs; (g),(h),(i) represent the imaginary parts of the POC; (j),(k),(l) denote the OrintationCode of the POC.

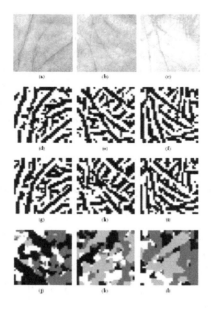

13.4.2 Similarity Measure Based on Modified Hamming Distance

We now will show that how the multiple feature representations i.e. POCs are converted into similarity measures of palm print images by using the Hamming distance. The **Hamming distance** is the number of positions in two strings of equal length for which the corresponding elements are different. For example, the Hamming distance between strings 2143896 and 2233796 is 3 and the Hamming distance between 1011101 and 1001001 is 2. The Hamming distance can be used to measure the similarity between two strings. For example, because each string of the first couple of strings (2143896 and 2233796) are 7 characters in length and there are three different elements, the percentage (7 - 3) / 7 = 57% can be used to represent the similarity between the two strings. For the second couple of strings (1011101 and 1001001), the similarity is (7 - 2) / 7 = 71%.

Here a modified Hamming distance is defined to measure the similarity of two binary matrices. A binary matrix is often used to represent an image containing an object. Because of imperfect preprocessing, there may exist some non-object pixels in the preprocessed images. Let I_1 and I_2 denote two images and suppose that M_1 and M_2 are the corresponding masks (Zhang, Kong, You, & Wong, 2003) that identify the location of the non-palm-print pixels of the two palm print images. respectively. Then the valid pixels used for matching can be represented by a binary matrix M:

$$M(i,j) = M_1(i,j) \wedge M_2(i,j).$$ (13.20)

where "$\wedge$" means the logical "AND" operator.

Let P_R and P_I denote the PhaseCode of I_1. Let O_1 denote the OrientationCode of I_1. Q_R, Q_I, and O_2 mean the PhaseCode and the OrientationCode of I_2, respectively. Then $C_1 = (P_R, P_I, O_1)$, $C_2 = (Q_R, Q_I, O_2)$ can be used to respectively represent I_1 and I_2. The binary matrixes H_R and H_I, which respectively stand for the differences between P_R and Q_R, and between P_I and Q_I, are computed as below:

$$H_R(i,j) = P_R(i,j) \quad XOR \quad Q_R(i,j).$$ (13.21)

$$H_I(i,j) = P_I(i,j) \quad XOR \quad Q_I(i,j).$$ (13.22)

The difference between O_1 and O_2 is expressed in terms of the following binary matrix H_O:

If $O_1 = O_2$, then $H_O(i,j) = 1$;

If $O_1 = O_2$, then $H_O(i,j) = 0$;

The following modified Hamming distance is used to measure the similarity $D(I_1, I_2)$ between I_1 and I_2:

$$D(I_1, I_2) = \frac{\sum_{i=1}^{N} \sum_{j=1}^{N} M(i,j) \wedge (H_R(i,j) \vee H_O(i,j))}{2 \sum_{i=1}^{N} \sum_{j=1}^{N} M(i,j)}$$
$$+ \frac{\sum_{i=1}^{N} \sum_{j=1}^{N} M(i,j) \wedge (H_I(i,j) \vee H_O(i,j))}{2 \sum_{i=1}^{N} \sum_{j=1}^{N} M(i,j)} .$$ (13.23)

where $N \times N$ is the size of the images, "$\wedge$" and "$\vee$" mean the logical "AND" and "OR", respectively. Note that $D(I_1, I_2)$ is between 0 and 1 and a large $D(I_1, I_2)$ value means that I_1 and I_2 have a great similarity.

13.4.3 Experimental Results

We tested the proposed palm print authentication approach using a database containing 7,605 palm prints collected from 392 different palms. These images were taken from the people of different ages and both sexes in the Hongkong Polytechnic University. These palm print images were captured twice, at an interval of around two months. The images in the database are of two different sizes, 384 × 284 and 768 × 568. The images of size 768 × 568 were resized to 384 × 284 pixels. Then the central 128 × 128 pixels of every obtained image were cropped to extract the POC using the preprocessing technique described in (Zhang, Kong, You, & Wong, 2003).

We performed verification experiment as follows: every sample in the database was matched against each of the remaining ones. If two palm print images from an identical palm are matched correctly, the matching result is called genuine matching; otherwise, the matching result is called impostor matching. A total of 28,914,210 matchings have been performed, of which 70,502 matching results are genuine matchings. Figure 13.13 shows the distance distributions of the genuine matching and impostor matching. It is clear that two distinct peaks are respectively associated with the two distance distributions. The peak of the distance distribution of the genuine matching is located at about 0.41, while the peak of the distance distribution of the impostor matching is located at about 0.84. Since the two peaks are widely separated and the two curves intersect very little, the Poc approach is able to authenticate palm prints with a high accuracy.

Figure 13.13. Distributions of the genuine and imposter matching distances

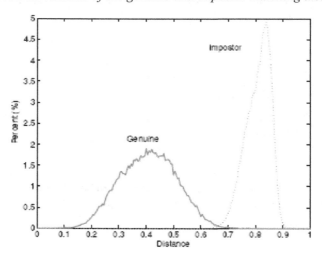

Figure 13.14. ROC curves and the ERR of the Sobel algorithm, the PhaseCode method and the POC approach with the log scale

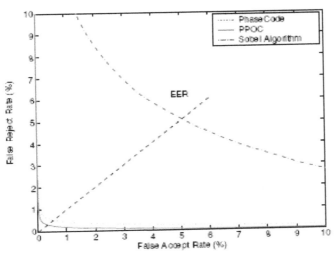

Figure 13.14 presents the receiver operating characteristic (ROC) curve of the Poc approach. Experiments of the Sobel algorithm (Han, Chen, Lin, & Fan, 2003) and the improved PalmCode (Zhang, Kong, You, & Wong, 2003) on this database, i.e. the PhaseCode method (Kong & Zhang, 2004), were also implemented and their ROC curves are also shown in Figure 13.14. The equal error rates (EERs) of each approach is listed in Table 13.6. According to Figure 13.14 and Table 13.6, we know that the Poc approach and PhaseCode method perform much better than the Sobel algorithm. The EERs of the Poc approach and PhaseCode method are 0.31% and 0.56%, respectively. From Figure 13.15 which shows the ROC curves of the Poc approach and PhaseCode method with the log scale, we can see that when the FRR is 2%, the FARs of the Poc approach and the PhaseCode method are about 0.0036% and 0.0078%, respectively.

Table 13.6. Matching distances between two POCs on the palm print images (a),(b), (c) in Figure 13.12

	(a)	(b)	(c)
(a)	0	0.8339	0.8226
(b)	0.8339	0	0.7989
(c)	0.8226	0.7989	0

Figure 13.15. ROC curves of the POC approach and the PhaseCode method with the log scale

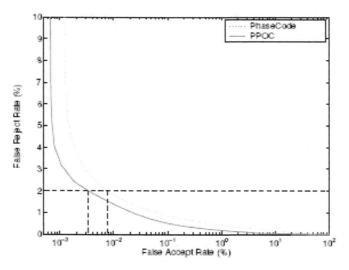

Table 13.7. The EERs of the Sobel algorithm, the PhaseCode method and the POC approach

Approach	POC	Sobel Algorithm	PhaseCode
ERR value (%)	0.31	5.0	0.56

13.4.4 Conclusion

The POC approach is an improvement of the PhaseCode method. The POC approach uses four 2D Gabor filters to calculate the phase and the orientation information, which are then combined to obtain a new feature, i.e. phase and orientation code (POC). Palm print identification or verification can be performed by the Poc approach based on a modified Hamming distance. The experimental results on a palm print database show that the Poc approach is powerful for palm print authentication. The Poc approach and the PalmCode approach perform much better than the Sobel-based approach. The EER of the Poc approach decreased from 0.56% of the PhaseCode method to 0.31% and when the FRR is 2%, the FARs of the POC approach has decreased from 0.0078% of the PhaseCode method to 0.0036%.

13.5 COMMENTS

Among the three classes of information fusion, feature level fusion is able to convey the richest information. However, the fact there are only a little number of literatures on feature level fusion shows that fusion at the feature level has probably not received the amount of attention it deserves. Feature level fusion may encounter two potential problems. First, it might be difficult to perform a combination at the feature level when the relationship between the feature spaces of different biometric traits is unknown and the feature representations are not compatible. Second, it is possible that the feature values of a certain individual biometric trait may not be accessible because of their proprietary nature or because the user does not have this biometric trait.

REFERENCES

Beveridge, J. R., She, K., Draper, B., & Givens, G. H. (2001). Parametric and non-parametric methods for the statistical evaluation of human ID algorithms. *Proc. of the Third Workshop Empirical Evaluation of Computer Vision Systems.*

Cevikalp, H., Neamtu, M., Wilkes, M., & Barkana, A. (2005). Discriminative common vectors for face recognition. *IEEE Trans. Pattern Anal. Mach. Intell.,* 27(1), 4-13.

Chang, K., Bowyer, K. W., & Sarkar, S. (2003). Comparison and combination of ear and face images in appearance-based biometrics. *IEEE Trans. Pattern Anal. Machine Intell.,* 25(9), 1600-1165.

Chetty, G., & Wagner, M. (2008). Robust face-voice based speaker identity verification using multilevel fusion. *Image and Vision Computing,* 26, 1249-1260.

Choi, K., Choi, H., & Kim, J. (2005). Fingerprint mosaicking by rolling and sliding. *Proceedings of Audio- and Video-based Biometric Person Authentication* (AVBPA), Rye Brook, NY (pp. 260–269).

Gunatilaka, A. H., & Baertlein, B. A. (2001). Feature-level and decision-level fusion of noncoincidently sampled sensors for land mine detection. *IEEE Trans. Pattern Anal. Machine Intell.,* 23(6), 577-589.

Gunes, H., & Piccardi, M. (2005). Affect recognition from face and body: early fusion vs. late fusion. *Proc. of 2005 IEEE International Conference on Systems, Man and Cybernetics* (pp. 3437-3443).

Han, C., Chen, H., Lin, C., & Fan, K. (2003). Personal authentication using palmprint features. *Pattern Recognition, 36*(2), 371-381.

Jain, A. K., Ross, A., & Prabhakar, S. (2004). An introduction to biometric Recognition. *IEEE Trans. Circuits and Systems for Video Technology, Special Issue on Image- and Video-Based Biometrics, 14*(1), 4-20.

Jing, X. Y., Yao, Y. F., Zhang, D., Yang, J. Y., & Li, M. (2007). Face and palmprint pixel level fusion and Kernel DCV-RBF classifier for small sample biometric recognition. *Pattern Recognition, 40*, 3209-3224.

Kober, R., Harz, U., & Schiffers, J. (1997). Fusion of visual and acoustic signals for command-word recognition. *Proc. of International Conference on Acoustics, Speech and Signal Processing* (pp. 1495–1497).

Kong, W., & Zhang, D. (2004). Feature-level fusion for effective palmprint authentication. *Proc. of International Conference on Biometric Authentication* (pp. 761-767).

Kong, A., Zhang, D., & Kamel, M. (2006). Palmprint identification using feature-level fusion. *Pattern Recognition, 39*, 478-487.

Kong, W. K., Zhang, D., & Li W. (2003). Palmprint feature extraction using 2-D Gabor filters. *Pattern Recognition, 36*(10), 2339-2347.

Kor, S., & Tiwary, U. (2004). Feature level fusion of multimodal medical images in lifting wavelet transform domain. *26th Annual International Conference of the IEEE Engineering in Medicine and Biology Society*, (IEMBS '04),*1*, 1479 -1482.

Kumar, A., & Zhang, D. (2006). Personal recognition using hand shape and texture. *IEEE Transactions on Image Processing, 15*(8), 2454 – 2461.

Liu, X., Ma, L., & Mathew, J. (2006). Machinery fault diagnosis based on feature level fuzzy integral data fusion techniques. *2006 IEEE International Conference on Industrial Informatics* (pp. 857–862).

Liu, Z., & Liu, C. (2007). Fusion of the complementary Discrete Cosine Features in the YIQ color space for face recognition. *Computer Vision and Image Understanding*, doi:10.1016/j.cviu.2007.12.002.

Liu, W., Meng, H., Hong, W., Wang, L., & Song, J. (2007). A new method for dimensionality reduction based on multivariate feature fusion. *IEEE International Conference on Integration Technology, 2007 (ICIT '07)* (pp. 108–111).

Patnaik, D. (2006). Biomedical image fusion using wavelet transforms and SOFM neural network. *IEEE International Conference on Industrial Technology 2006 (ICIT2006)* (pp.1189–1194).

Phillips, P. J., Wechsler, H., Huang, J., & Rauss, P. (1998). The FERET database and evaluation procedure for face-recognition algorithms. *Image Vision Comput.*, *16*(5), 295-306.

Rahman, M. M., Desai, B. C., & Bhattacharya, P. (2006). A feature level fusion in similarity matching to content-based image retrieval. *Proceedings of the 9th International Conference on Information Fusion* (pp. 10-13).

Ratha, N., Connell, J., & Bolle, R. (1998). Image mosaicing for rolled fingerprint construction. *Proceedings of 14th International Conference on Pattern Recognition, Brisbane* (pp. 1651–1653).

Rattani, A., KisKu, D. R., Bicego, M., & Tistarelli, M. (2006). Robust feature-level multibiometric classification. *2006 Biometrics Symposium: Special Session on Research at the Biometric Consortium Conference* (pp.1–6).

Rattani, A., Kisku, D. R., Bicego, M., & Tistarelli, M. (2007). Feature level fusion of face and fingerprint biometrics. *First IEEE International Conference on Biometrics: Theory, Applications, and Systems (BTAS 2007)* (pp.1–6).

Ross, A., & Govindarajan, R. (2005). Feature level fusion using hand and face biometrics. *Proc. of SPIE Conference on Biometric Technology for Human Identification II* (pp. 196-204).

Ross, A., & Jain, A. (2003). Information fusion in biometrics. *Pattern Recognition Letters*, *24*(13), 2115-2125.

Scholkopf, B., Smola, A,. & Muller, K. (1998). Nonlinear component analysis as a Kernel eigenvalue problem. *Neural Comput.*, *10*(5), 1299-1319.

Sim, T., Zhang, S., Janakiraman, R., & Kumar, S. (2007). Continuous verification using multimodal biometrics. *IEEE Trans. Pattern Analysis and Machine Intelligence*, *29*(4), 687-700.

Singh, R., Vatsa, M., Ross, A., & Noore, A. (2005). Performance enhancement of 2d face recognition via mosaicing. *Proceedings of Fourth IEEE Workshop on Automatic Identification Advanced Technologies (AuotID)*, Buffalo, USA (pp. 63–68).

Son, B., & Lee, Y. (2005). Biometric authentication system using reduced joint feature vector of iris and face. *Lecture Notes in Computer Science, 3546/2005*, 1611-3349.

Wang, J., Yau, W., Suwandy, A., & Sung, E. (2008). Person recognition by fusing palmprint and palm vein images based on "Laplacianpalm" representation. *Pattern Recognition, 41* (2008), 1514 – 1527.

Wender, S., & Dietmayer, K. C. J. (2007). A feature level fusion approach for object classification. *2007 IEEE Intelligent Vehicles Symposium* (pp.1132–1137).

Xu, Y., Yang, J. Y., & Jin, Z. (2003). Theory analysis on FSLDA and ULDA. *Pattern Recognition, 36*(12), 3031-3033.

Xu, Y., Yang, J. Y., Lu, J. F., & Yu, D. J. (2004). An efficient renovation on kernel Fisher discriminant analysis and face recognition experiments. *Pattern Recognition, 37*(10), 2091-2094.

Yambor, W., Draper, B., & Beveridge, R. (2002). *Empirical evaluation methods in computer vision.* Singapore World Scientific Press.

Zhang, D., Kong, W. K., You, J., & Wong, M. (2003). Online palmprint identification. *IEEE Trans. Pattern Anal. Mach. Intell., 25*(9), 1041-1050.

Zhou, X., & Bhanu, B. (2008). Feature fusion of side face and gait for video-based human identification. *Pattern Recognition, 41,* 778–795.

Chapter XIV
Matching Score Level Fusion

ABSTRACT

With this chapter we aims at describing several basic aspects of matching score level fusion. Section 14.1 provides a description of basic characteristics of matching score fusion in the form of introduction. Section 14.2 shows a number of matching score fusion rules. Section 14.3 surveys several typical normalization procedures of raw matching scores. Section 14.4 gives an example of matching score level fusion method. Finally, Section 14.5 provides several brief comments on matching score fusion.

14.1 INTRODUCTION

Matching score level fusion is the most commonly used biometric information fusion strategy because matching scores are easily available and because they retain sufficient information to distinguish genuine matching from impostor matching. Generally, a multi-biometric system based on the matching score level fusion works as follows: each subsystem of the multi-biometric system exploits one biometric trait to produce a matching score. Then these matching scores are normalized and integrated to obtain the final matching score or final decision for personal authentication. Studies on the basis and potential of score level fusion are very helpful for us to understand and implement fusion at the score level. For example, based on the likelihood ratio test Nandakumar, Chen, Dass and Jain (2008) proposed a framework for the optimal combination of matching scores. Their study showed that when finite Gaussian mixture model was used to model the distributions of genuine and impostor match scores, the matching score level fusion could produce good performance. Toh Kim, and Lee (2008b) studied the issue of optimizing the ROC performance of the multimodal biometric system using the matching score fusion strategy. Jain, Nandakumar, and Ross (2005) provided us with comprehensive descriptions of various score normalization rules. Snelick, Uludag, Mink, Indovina and Jain (2005) and Poh and Bengio (2006) presented the performances of matching score level fusion algorithms and systems obtained using elaborate evaluation.

A number of studies (Dass, Nandakumar, & Jain, 2005; Kittler, Hatef, Duin, & Matas, 1998; Poh & Bengio, 2006; Ross & Jain, 2003; Schmid, Ketkar, Singh, & Cukic, 2006; Snelick Uludag, Mink, Indovina, & Jain, 2005; Vielhauer & Scheidat, 2005) have demonstrated that the matching score level fusion strategy can lead to a higher accuracy than the single biometric system. A variety of cases of matching score fusion have also been proposed (Brunelli & Falavigna, 1995; Doddington, Liggett, Martin, Przybocki, & Reynolds, 1998; Islam, Mangayyagari, & Sankar, 2007; Kumar & Zhang, 2004; Scheidat, Vielhauer, & Dittmann, 2005; Tsalakanidou, Malassiotis, & Strintzis, 2007; Tulyakov & Govindaraju, 2005; Yan & Bowyer, 2005). For example, Ribaric and Fratric (2005) acquired images containing both fingerprints and palm prints and then used the extracted eigenpalm and eigenfinger features to perform matching score level fusion. By conducting experiments on a population approaching 1,000 individuals, Snelick, Uludag, Mink, Indovina and Jain (2005) demonstrated that the multimodal fingerprint and face biometric system, which combines the two biometric traits at the matching score level, was significantly more accurate than any individual biometric systems.

In the context of verification, fusion at the matching score level can be carried out using three distinct approaches. The first approach treats fusion as a classification problem (Ma, Cukic, & Singh, 2005) whereas the second approach treats fusion as a combination problem. The third approach, namely the density-based approach, treats fusion at the matching score level as a density-based score fusion problem, which is based on the likelihood ratio test and explicit estimation of genuine and impostor match score densities (Griffin, 2004). In the first approach, the matching score outputs of the individual biometric traits are first concatenated to form a feature vector. This feature vector is then classified into one of two classes: genuine user or impostor. This is also referred to as classifier-based score fusion (Nandakumar, Chen, Dass and Jain, 2008). Examples of matching score level fusion using the first approach include fusion of face and speech data (Yacoub, Abdeljaoued, & Mayoraz, 1999), fusion of face and iris recognition (Wang, Tan, & Jain, 2003), fusion of face and voice (Verlinde & Cholet, 1999), fusion of visual facial and acoustic features (Chatzis, Bors, and Pitas, 1999), and fingerprint authentication (Jain, Prabhakar, & Chen, 1999; Jain, Hong, & Bolle, 1997), etc. Note that the first approach suffers from the following issues: The first issue is the unbalanced training set. That is, genuine match scores available for training are much fewer than available impostor scores, since the numbers of available genuine match scores and impostor scores are $O(n)$ and $O(n)^2$, respectively, where n is the number of users. The second issue is that selecting and training a classifier that gives the optimal performance may be difficult. In the second approach, the individual matching scores are combined to generate the final matching score which is then used to make the final decision. In the following of this chapter, if there is no clear specification, the term 'matching score fusion' refers to fusion using the second approach mentioned above. The density-based approach has the following advantage: If the score densities can be estimated accurately, it is able to achieve optimal performance at any desired FAR. A comparison of eight biometric fusion techniques conducted by NIST showed that Product of Likelihood Ratios was most accurate (Ulery, Hicklin, Watson, Fellner, & Hallinan, 2006). However, it also appeared that Product of Likelihood Ratios was most complex to implement.

Generally a normalization step is used to normalize the matching scores generated from different biometric traits and then the normalized scores are integrated to obtain the final matching score. One reason that the normalization step is adopted is the matching scores of multiple biometric traits may not be homogeneous. For example, it is possible that while a biometric trait yields a distance measure, another biometric trait produces a similarity measure. In this case, it is obviously not suitable to directly integrate two matching scores generated from the two biometric traits. Another reason for using the normalization step is that the matching scores of different biometric traits may have different numerical scales (ranges). For instance, if the first biometric trait yields scores in the range [10, 100] and the score from the second biometric trait is in the range [0,1], directly fusing the scores without any normalization will dramatically eliminate the contribution of the second biometric trait. The third reason is that the matching scores produced by different subsystems of a multi-biometric system may follow different statistical distributions. Due to these reasons, a normalization procedure is essential to transform the matching scores of individual biometric traits into a common domain prior to combining them.

Generally, a normalization procedure applied to raw matching scores has the following two purposes: to convert the raw matching scores into ones that are of the same kind of measurement, such as similarity or dissimilarity, and to make the obtained matching scores of different biometric traits have a common range. A good normalization procedure should be robust and effective. Robustness means insensitivity to the presence of outliers. Effectiveness refers to the proximity of the obtained estimate to the optimal estimate when the distribution of the data is known. A variety of normalization procedures have been proposed for matching score level fusion (Snelick, Uludag, Mink, Indovina, & Jain, 2005). The normalized matching scores will be further integrated to produce the final matching score for personal authentication by using different approaches.

A number of fusion rules have been proposed for matching score level fusion. It is likely that Simple-Sum, Min-Score and Max-Score are the most common matching score level fusion rules. These rules appear to be not only simple but also effective. In addition, Kittler, Hatef, Duin and Matas (1998) have tested several fusion rules for the combination of face and voice, including sum, product, minimum, median, and maximum rules. They also showed that the sum rule was not significantly affected by the probability estimation errors. Dass, Nandakumar and Jain (2005) combined the matching scores of multi-biometric traits based on generalized density estimation. Jain and Ross (2002) and Brunelli and Falavigna (1995) respectively proposed their user weighted fusion approaches, which assign different weights to individual biometric traits. Lucey, Chen, Sridharan, and Chandran (2005), Chibelushi, Deravi, and Mason (2002) and Dupont and Luettin (2000) exploited an exponential weighting on the acoustic and visual a posteriori probability estimates to perform audio-visual speech and speaker recognition. Toh, Kim, and Lee (2008a) conducted biometric score fusion based on total error rate minimization. M. Montague and J. A. Aslam (2001) proposed the relevance score normalization scheme. Fernandez, Veldhuis, and Bazen (2006), Nandakumar, Chen, Jain, and Dass (2006) and Fierrez-Aguilar, Ortega-Garcia, Gonzalez-Rodriguez, and Bigun (2005) proposed to design score normalization schemes that exploit quality information.

As presented above, 'matching score fusion' has two key points, the normalization procedure and the fusion approach using a certain fusion rule. In general, the main steps of 'matching score fusion' can be described as follows:

- **Step 1.** Raw matching scores of different biometric traits are converted into the same kind of measurement.
- **Step2.** The matching scores obtained using Step 1 are normalized by using the normalization procedure.
- **Step3.** The normalized matching scores are integrated to obtain the final matching score or decision by using the fusion rule.
- **Step4.** Personal authentication is performed based on the final matching score or decision.

14.2 MATCHING SCORE FUSION RULES

Suppose that R biometric traits can be used for personal authentication and each biometric trait produces a matching score. If these matching scores have been normalized by the normalization procedure, they can be integrated. For the kth user, let $S_{k1}, S_{k2}, ..., S_{kR}$ denote the normalized matching scores of his (her) R biometric traits. The final matching score of the kth user can be obtained using the rules shown in Sections 14.2.1 and 14.2.2.

14.2.1 General Matching Score Fusion Rules

As presented in Section 14.1, matching score fusion rules integrate normalized matching scores of a user to produce the final matching score. In this subsection we present some widely used matching score fusion rules. These rules integrate multiple normalized matching scores to produce the final scalar matching score.

Simple-Sum rule: The Simple-Sum rule takes the sum of the R matching scores of the kth user as the final matching score S_k of this user. S_k is calculated as follows:

$$S_k = \sum_{i=1}^{R} S_{ki}. \tag{14.1}$$

Product rule: The Product rule regards the multiplication result of the R matching scores of the kth user as the final matching score of this user, which is shown as follows:

$$S_k = \prod_{i=1,2,...,R} S_{ki} \tag{14.2}$$

In the case where the matching score means the a postpriori probability, the product rule is essentially subject to the hypothesis that different biometric traits are independent of each other, which ensures that the combinatorial postpriori probability of multiple biometric traits equals the product of their respective postpriori probabilities.

Min-Score rule: The Min-Score rule selects the minimum score from the R matching scores of the kth user as the final matching score of this user. This rule is expressed as follows:

$$S_k = \min(S_{k1}, S_{k2}, ..., S_{kR}). \tag{14.3}$$

Max-Score rule: The Max-Score rule selects the maximum score from the R matching scores of the kth user as the final matching score of this user. This rule is shown as follows:

$$S_k = \max(S_{k1}, S_{k2}, ..., S_{kR}). \tag{14.4}$$

Weighted Sum rule: The Weighted Sum rule assumes that the R biometric traits have different significance in personal authentication and assigns different weights to the matching scores of different traits. The weighted sum of the R matching scores, which is shown in (14.5), is considered as the final matching score of the kth user.

$$S_k = \sum_{n=1}^{R} w_n S_{kn},$$ (14.5)

where w_n represents the weight of the matching score of the nth biometric trait of the kth user.

Weighted Product rule : Let w_n stand for the weight of the matching score of the nth biometric trait of the kth user. A Weighted Product rule can determine the final matching score of the kth user using

$$S_k = \prod_{n=1,\dots,R} S_{kn}^{w_n},$$ (14.6)

The rules presented in this section can integrate multiple matching scores representing one of the following measurements: a similarity measurement, the a postpriori probability of the sample belonging to a certain class, or a distance measurement between the sample and the registered template. The meaning of the final matching score in personal verification can be described as follows. If the integrated matching scores and the obtained final score are all probability or similarity measurements, then the higher the final score between the sample and the registered template of the claimed user is, the more likely the tested user is the genuine subject. On the other hand, if the integrated matching scores and the obtained final score are all distance measurements, then the smaller the final score between the sample and the registered template of the claimed user is, the more likely the tested user is the genuine subject. It should be pointed out that when the raw matching scores denote different measurements, they cannot be integrated directly. Instead, they should be first converted into the same kind of measurement and then be integrated.

14.2.2 Probability-Based Matching Score Fusion

Probability-based matching score fusion is also popular in the field of biometrics. We now will present several rules of probability-based matching score fusion to fuse multi-biometric data at the matching score level from the viewpoint of classification. In the context below we can find that these rules all integrate multiple biometric traits by integrating their posteriori probabilities. Note that these rules such as the probability-based Product, probability-based Max and probability-based Min rules are formally different from the general Product, Max-score and Min-score rules for fusing matching scores as presented in Section 14.2.1. Indeed, probability-based matching score fusion can be viewed as a special kind of fusion, which integrates multiple matching scores to directly obtain the final authentication decision rather than the final matching score. Probability-based matching score fusion is able to do so because what it integrates are probabilities rather than ordinary matching scores. Though probability-based matching score fusion directly produces the final authentication decision and is similar to decision level fusion at this point, we do not regard it as decision level fusion. The reason is that decision level fusion usually combines multiple decisions to obtain the final decision whereas what probability-based matching score fusion integrates are probabilities, a special kind of matching score, rather than decisions.

Suppose that the biometric identification problem has m possible classes $\omega_1, \omega_2, ..., \omega_m$ and the multi-biometric system consists of R subsystems each exploiting one biometric trait. Let x_i, $i = 1, 2, ..., R$ be the vector representing the ith biometric trait. If $p(\omega_k)$ and $p(x_i | \omega_k)$ respectively denote the a prior probability and the conditional probability of x_i given ω_k, we can describe probability-based matching score fusion rules as follows.

14.2.2.1 Probability-Based Product Rule

The following rule to combine probabilities of multiple biometric traits is called the probability-based product rule (Kittler, Hatef, Duin, & Matas, 1998):

Assign $z \rightarrow \omega_j$, if

$$p^{-(R-1)}(\omega_j) \prod_i p(\omega_j | x_i) = \max_k p^{-(R-1)}(\omega_k) \prod_i p(\omega_k | x_i). \tag{14.7}$$

For a given sample represented by $x_1, x_2, ..., x_R$, this rule computes the product

$$p^{-(R-1)}(\omega_k) \prod_i p(\omega_k | x_i)$$

with respect to each class ω_k and then classifies the sample into the class that has the maximum product value. Note that though both the probability-based Product rule and the general Product rule as defined in (14.2) produce the final score based on the idea that the final score and the normalized matching scores has a relation of product, they are formally different. This is because the probability-based Product rule is established on the basis of a more specific knowledge background as presented in the end of this section. The underlying rationale of (14.7) will be also briefly shown in the end of this section.

14.2.2.2 Probability-Based Sum Rule

The probability-based Sum rule combines probabilities of multiple biometric traits to carry out classification for a sample denoted by $x_1, x_2, ..., x_R$ as follows:

$$(1-R)p(\omega_j) + \sum_{i=1}^{R} p(\omega_j \mid x_i) = \max_k ((1-R)p(\omega_k) + \sum_{i=1}^{R} p(\omega_k \mid x_i)).$$

$$(14.8)$$

Indeed, the probability-based Sum rule first adds the sum of the a postpriori probabilities with respect to each class of every biometric trait of a user to the corresponding prior probabilities multiplied by $(1-R)$. Then this rule classifies the user into the class that has the maximum adding result.

14.2.2.3 Probability-Based Max Rule

The probability-based Max rule can be presented as follows:
   Assign $z \to \omega_j$, if

$$(1-R)p(\omega_j) + R \max_{i=1,...,R} p(\omega_j \mid x_i) = \max_{k=1,...,m} [(1-R)p(\omega_k) + R \max_{i=1,...,R} p(\omega_k \mid x_i)].$$

$$(14.9)$$

14.2.2.4 Probability-Based Min Rule

The probability-based Min rule combines probabilities of multiple biometric traits to perform classification as allows:

   Assign $z \to \omega_j$, if

$$p^{-(R-1)}(\omega_j) \min_{i=1,...,R} p(\omega_j \mid x_i) = \max_{k=1,...,m} (p^{-(R-1)}(\omega_k) \min_{i=1,...,R} p(\omega_k \mid x_i)). \qquad (14.10)$$

14.2.2.5 Probability-Based Median Rule

According to the probability-based Median rule, probabilities of multiple biometric traits should be combined for classification in the following way:
   Assign $z \to \omega_j$, if

$$median(p(\omega_j \mid x_i)) = \max_{k=1,...,m} median_{i=1,2,...R}(p(\omega_k \mid x_i)),$$ (14.11)

where *median* denotes the median of the a posteriori probabilities.

Note that it has been demonstrated that the above probability-based rules to combine different biometric traits all can be explained from the point of view of Bayesian statistics (Kittler, Hatef, Duin, & Matas, 1998). For example, the condition that the representations $x_1, x_2,...,x_R$ for different biometric traits of a sample are conditionally independent, can allow the probability-based Product rule to be produced. Another example is that under the condition that the a posteriori probabilities of $x_1, x_2,...,x_R$ do not deviate dramatically from the prior probabilities, we are easy to obtain the probability-based Sum rule.

We now will briefly show that how the probability-based Product rule can be generated from the Bayesian decision theory. Indeed, if we apply the Bayesian decision theory to the pattern recognition problem, we will classify a pattern z described by vectors $x_1, x_2,..., x_R$ using the following decision:

Assign $z \to \omega_j$ if

$$p(\omega_j \mid x_1, x_2,...,x_R) = \max_k p(\omega_k \mid x_1, x_2,...,x_R).$$ (14.12)

$p(\omega_k \mid x_1, x_2,...,x_R)$ can be evaluated using

$$p(\omega_k \mid x_1, x_2,...,x_R) = \frac{p(x_1, x_2,...,x_R \mid \omega_k)p(\omega_k)}{p(x_1, x_2,...,x_R)}.$$ (14.13)

(14.13) also shows that for given $x_1, x_2,...,x_R$, $p(x_1, x_2,...,x_R)$ has the same effect on the value of the $p(\omega_k \mid x_1, x_2,...,x_R)$. Therefore, rule (14.12) is equivalent to the following rule:

Assign $z \to \omega_j$ if

$$p(x_1, x_2,...,x_R \mid \omega_j)p(\omega_j) = \max_k p(x_1, x_2,...,x_R \mid \omega_k)p(\omega_k).$$ 14.14)

Suppose that the representations $x_1, x_2,...,x_R$ are conditionally independent, then we get

$$p(x_1, x_2,...,x_R \mid \omega_k) = \prod_i p(x_i \mid \omega_k),$$ (14.15)

Combining (14.14) and (14.15), we obtain the following rule:

Assign $z \rightarrow \omega_j$ if

$$p(\omega_j)\prod_i p(x_i \mid \omega_j) = \max_k p(\omega_k)\prod_i p(x_i \mid \omega_k). \qquad (14.16)$$

We also know that $p(x_i \mid \omega_k)p(\omega_k) = p(\omega_k \mid x_i)p(x_i)$. This allows rule (14.16) to become

Assign $z \rightarrow \omega_j$ if

$$(\prod_i p(x_i))p^{-(R-1)}(\omega_j)\prod_i p(\omega_j \mid x_i) = \max_k(\prod_i p(x_i))p^{-(R-1)}(\omega_k)\prod_i p(\omega_k \mid x_i).$$

$$(14.17)$$

Because (14.17) shows that for given $x_1, x_2, ..., x_R$, $\prod_i p(x_i)$

has no influence on the classification decision, we can eliminate it from this rule and obtain (14.7).

As presented early, probability-based matching score fusion is a special kind of matching score fusion. Indeed, we can consider that probability-based matching score fusion implicitly implements the following two procedures: the first procedure of integrating probabilities of multiple biometric traits and the second procedure of using the integrated probabilities and the Bayesian decision theory for final decision-making. This, therefore, makes probability-based matching score fusion formally different from ordinary matching score fusion, which usually integrates matching scores of multiple biometric traits to produce the final matching score and no authentication decision will be made.

14.3 NORMALIZATION PROCEDURES OF MATCHING SCORES

As presented in Section 14.1, normalization of matching scores is very critical for 'matching score fusion'. This subsection focuses on some popular score normalization procedures.

Min-Max normalization procedure, which is best suited for the case where the bounds of the matching score of each biometric trait is known, is one of the simplest score normalization procedures. This procedure maps raw scores to the [0, 1] range using (14.18). The quantities max(S) and min(S) denote the upper and lower bounds of the score range, respectively.

$$S_k' = \frac{S_k - min(S)}{max(S) - min(S)}. \tag{14.18}$$

Z-score normalization procedure aims at transforming the raw matching score to a distribution having mean of 0 and standard deviation of 1. The transformation is defined as follows:

$$S_k' = \frac{S_k - mean(S)}{std(S)}, \tag{14.19}$$

where *mean(S)* and *std(S)* are respectively used to denote the arithmetic mean and standard deviation operators. It should be pointed out that because both the mean and standard deviation are sensitive to outliers, this procedure is not robust. As a result, the Z-score normalization procedure does not guarantee that the normalized scores have a common numerical range.

Tanh normalization procedure maps the raw matching scores to the (0, 1) range using the following equation:

$$S_k' = \frac{1}{2}[tanh(0.01\frac{S - mean(S)}{std(S)}) + 1], \tag{14.20}$$

where *mean(S)* and *std(S)* also denote the arithmetic mean and standard deviation operators, respectively.

Median and median absolute deviation normalization procedure normalizes raw matching scores as follows:

$$S_k' = \frac{S_k - median(S)}{median(|S_k - median(S)|)}, \tag{14.21}$$

where *median(S)* stands for the median value of *S*. Indeed, the term 'median' means the middle of a distribution. That is, half the scores are above the median and the other half are below the median. The median is less sensitive to extreme scores than the arithmetic mean and this makes it be a better measure. This procedure is insensitive to outliers and it is therefore more robust than the Z-score normalization procedure.

Before we discuss the next normalization procedure, we analyze the error of personal authentication using a single biometric trait. The errors caused by individual biometric traits stem from the overlap of the genuine and impostor score distributions. This overlap region can be partially described by its center c and its width w. The next normalization procedure (logistic normalization) is able to decrease the effect of the overlap and to increase the separation of the genuine and impostor distributions, while it still maps the scores to the [0,1] range.

Logistic normalization procedure uses a logistic function to normalize raw matching scores. This logistic function is defined as

$$S'_k = \frac{1}{1 + A \cdot e^{-BS_{mm}}}, \tag{14.22}$$

where S_{mm} denotes the normalized matching score obtained using the Min-Max normalization procedure. Note that the constants A and B are respectively calculated using

$$A = \frac{1}{\Delta} - 1 \text{ and } B = \frac{\ln A}{c}.$$

Figure 14.1. Illustration of the logistic normalization procedure

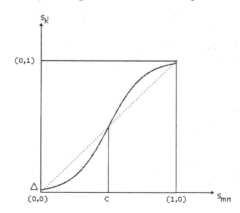

Figure 14.2. Illustration of the Quadric-Line-Quadric procedure

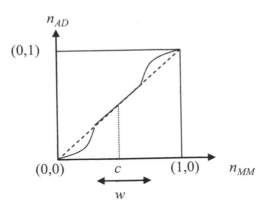

The constant Δ is selected to be a small value. This specification results in the inflection point of the logistic function occurring at c, i.e. the center of the overlap region. A logistic normalization function defined as in (14.22) is shown in Figure 14.1.

Quadric-Line-Quadric procedure leaves the overlap zone, with center c and width w, of the genuine and impostor score distributions unchanged and transforms the other regions using two quadratic functions. This procedure is formulated as (14.23) and illustrated as Figure 14.2.

$$S_k' = \begin{cases} \dfrac{1}{c-w/2}S_{nm}^2, & (S_{nm} \leq c-w/2) \\[2mm] S_{nm}, & (c-w/2) < S_{nm} < (c+w/2) \\[2mm] (c+w/2)+\sqrt{(1-c-w/2)(S_{nm}-c-w/2)}, & otherwise \end{cases}$$

(14.23)

where S_{nm} still denotes the normalized matching score obtained using the Min-Max normalization procedure.

Jain, Nandakumar and Ross (2005) studied the performance of different normalization techniques and fusion rules in the context of a multimodal biometric system based on the face, fingerprint and hand-geometry traits of a user. Their experiments on a database of 100 users indicate that the applications of the min–max, z-score, and tanh normalization rules followed by a simple sum scheme of score fusion obtain better recognition performance than other methods. However, experiments also show that the min–max and z-score normalization techniques were sensitive to outliers in the data.

14.4 EXEMPLIFICATION: INFORMATION FUSION OF FACE AND PALM PRINT

This section presents a scheme for fusing face and palm print information to conduct personal authentication. The used information fusion strategy is the first approach of the matching score level fusion, which considers the matching score outputs of the individual biometric traits as a feature vector and then personal authentication is performed on the basis of this feature vector. The proposed scheme also uses the claimed identity of users as a feature for fusion. The experimental results show that the facial and palm print images can be simultaneously acquired by using a pair of digital cameras and can be integrated to obtain a high accuracy of personal authentication. This section also analyzes and evaluates the performance of a personal authentication system using two-class separation criterion functions. The scheme proposed in this section may also be applicable to other multi-biometric systems.

14.4.1 Introduction

This section investigates a bimodal biometric system using face and palm print. Face has highest user acceptance and its acquisition is most convenient to users (Prabhakar, Pankanti, & Jain, 2003). Face and palm print images can be conveniently acquired from a digital camera. One of the important features that is only available in personal authentication, but not in recognition, is the claimed user identity. The claimed user identity is unique for every user and can be used to restrict the decision space, i.e. range of matching scores, in user authentication. The claimed user identity can be suitably coded and then used as a feature to classify the genuine and impostor matching scores and is investigated in this section.

14.4.2 Proposed System and Method

The block diagram of the proposed bimodal biometric authentication system is shown in Figure 14.3. The acquired grey-level images from the palm print and face are presented to the system. The matching scores generated from each of the two biometric traits are used as inputs of a neural network classifier. Because each user has its claimed identity, the claimed user identity is also used as a feature to neural

Figure 14.3. Personal authentication using face and palm print

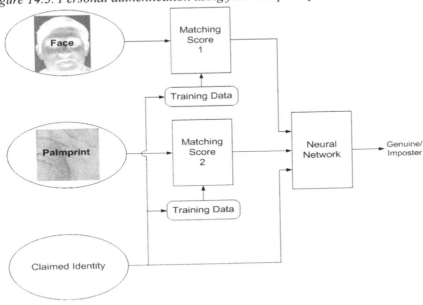

network classifier. The trained neural network classifies the user as a genuine user or impostor.

14.4.2.1 Computation of Face Matching Scores

We use the eigenface (Turk & Pentland, 1991) algorithm, a popular appearance based face representation algorithm to transform face images into lower-dimensional data. Original face images acquired from all the subjects are of size $M \times N$ and each image can be represented by a one-dimensional vector of MN dimension using row ordering. Principal component analysis (PCA) is applied to the normalized set of such training vectors to produce a set of orthogonal vectors, also known as eigenfaces. Note that the projection is in the form of a vector. The projection of a face image on eigenfaces is used as features of the face image.

The matching score for features (x_q) of each test face image is obtained by calculating the similarity between the features (x_q) of the claimed identity and features (x_c) of a training sample as follows.

$$\eta_1 = \frac{x_q^T x_c}{\|x_q\| \cdot \|x_c\|},$$ (14.24)

14.4.2.2 Computation of Palm Print Matching Scores

Palm print contains several complex features, e.g. minutiae, principal lines, wrinkles and texture. The palm print matching approach used in this work is same as detailed in (Kumar, Wong, Shen, & Jain, 2003). Four directional spatial masks are used to capture line features from each of the palm print images. The combined directional map is generated from voting of the resultant four images. The standard deviation of pixels, from each of the 24×24 pixel overlapping block with 25% overlap, in the combined image is used to form the feature vector. The palm print matching scores are generated by computing the similarity measure η_2, similar to (14.24), between the feature vectors from a testing image and those stored during the training phase.

14.4.2.3 Neural Networks-Based Classification

The matching scores from the face and palm print are used as inputs to train a feed-forward neural (FFN) network. We also use the claimed identity of every user as an input of the FFN. A three-layer FFN with P_l neurons in the *lth* ($l = 1,2,...,Q$) layer is based on the following architecture (Kumar, 2003):

$$\varphi_j^l = \sum_{i=1}^{P_{l-1}} w_{ij}^{l-1,l} y_i^{l-1}, y_i^{l-1} = g(\varphi_i^{l-1}),$$ (14.25)

where the sum of weighted inputs for the *jth*($j = 1,2,...,P_l$) neuron in the *lth*($l = 1,2,...,Q$) layer is represented by φ_j^l. The weights from the *ith* neuron at the ($l = 1$)*th* layer to the *jth* neuron in the *lth* layer are denoted by $w_{ij}^{l-1,l}$ and y_j^l is the output for the *jth* neuron in the *lth* layer. The values -1 and 1, corresponding to 'impostor' and 'genuine' responses, were given to the FFN during training as the correct output responses for expected classification during the training. As defined as in (14.26), the hyperbolic tangent sigmoid activation function is empirically selected for first two layers, while a linear activation function is chosen for third layer.

$$\begin{cases} g(\varphi_j^l) = \tanh(\varphi_j^l), & l = 1,2 \\ g(\varphi_j^3) = a(\varphi_j^3) \end{cases}.$$ (14.26)

The back-propagation training algorithm is used for minimizing the target function T_e defined by:

$$T_e = \frac{1}{KP_Q}\sum_{k=1}^{K}\sum_{j=1}^{P_Q}(y_{jk}^Q - o_{jk})^2, \qquad (14.27)$$

where k is an index for input-output pair and $(y_{jk}^Q - o_{jk})^2$ is the squared difference between the actual output value at the *jth* output layer neuron for pair k and the target output value. The FFN uses Levenberg-Marquardt algorithm (Masters, 1995) and a constant learning rate to update the connection weights $w_{ij}^{l-1,l}$.

14.4.3 Experiment and Results

The proposed method was investigated on the ORL face database (please refer to Section 3.2.3) from 40 subjects with 10 images per subject. The hand images from 40 subjects, with 10 images per subject, were acquired by using a digital camera. Each of the subjects for palm print and face were randomly paired to obtain a bimodal set for every subject. For the palm print image, a 300×300 region of interest was automatically segmented and the 144-dimensional feature vector was extracted as detailed in Kumar, Wong, Shen and Jain (2003). The eigenface algorithm was applied to produce 40-dimensional feature vector for every face image. The matching scores for face and palm print were computed by using similarity measure (14.24). The first four images samples, from face and palm print, were used for training and rest six were for testing. Then genuine and impostor matching scores from the training samples were used to train the 18/5/1 FFN. The learning rate was fixed at 0.01. Because a neural network cannot guarantee that the obtained training error is global, the FFN was trained 10 times with the same parameters and the result with the smallest of training errors of all the results are reported. The trained neural network was used to test 240 (40×6) genuine and 9360 (40×39×6) impostor matching scores from the test data. The claimed user identity was also used as an input component of FFN. The experimental results are shown in Table 14.1. From Table 14.1, we know that the total error is 1.5% (=0.7%+0.8%). However, if the claimed user identity was not exploited as an input component of the FFN, the total minimum error obtained by the FFN would be 2.8 %. In order to ascertain the improvement (or degradation) in the separation of the FFN outputs on the genuine and impostor, the performance indices using three objective functions (Kumar & Pang, 2002), were considered.

Table 14.1. Experimental results of personal authentication using face and palm print

	FAR	FRR
Face	3.0	10
Palm print	3.8	3.2
Experimental results using face and palm print	0.7	0.8

Table 14.2. Performance indices of personal authentication using face and palm print

	J_1	J_2	J_3	EER
Face	3.85(1.05)	2.11(0.00)	4.42(2.34)	8.33%(8.69%)
Palm print	4.38(1.03)	2.61(0.00)	8.61(3.71)	3.65%(4.32%)
Experiment using face and palm print	4.84(4.78)	3.04(2.99)	35.57(23.78)	0.84%(2.09%)

$$J_1 = \frac{\mu_g}{\mu_i}, \quad J_2 = \frac{(\mu_g - \mu_i)^2}{\mu_g \mu_i}, \quad J_3 = \frac{(\mu_g - \mu_i)^2}{\sigma_g^2 + \sigma_i^2} \qquad (14.28)$$

where μ_g and μ_i represent the means of the FFN outputs on the genuine and imposter class, respectively, and σ_g, σ_i are the standard deviations of the FFN outputs on the genuine and imposter class. Note that J_1 and J_2 do not account for the variance of the FFN outputs whereas J_3 simultaneously account for the mean and variance of the FFN outputs. These indices were computed from the test data and are displayed in Table 14.2. The bracketed entries in this table show the respective indices when the claimed identity of user is not used as an input component of the FFN. These entries can be used to interpret the performance increase when the claimed user identity is used as an input component of the FFN. Table 14.2 also shows the equal error rate (EER) for each of the corresponding cases.

14.4.4 Conclusions

Palm print and face images can be simultaneously acquired and used to perform personal authentication. The experimental result shows that the proposed bimodal system can achieve a higher accuracy than the single biometric system using palm print or face images. J_3 appears to be an effective performance index for evaluating the improvement in performance of the multi-biometric system. The experimental result also shows that the claimed user identity has significant effect in improving performance of the biometric system. This improvement is attributed to the fact that the FFN classifier uses the claimed user identity to reduce the uncertain range of the output value for the corresponding user.

14.5 COMMENTS

Fusion at the matching score level is the most popular fusion strategy in the field of multi-biometrics. The performance of this fusion strategy can be seen in numerous studies. The application presented in Section 14.3 uses the second approach of matching score fusion. Note that besides different biometric traits can be fused at the matching score level; matching score level fusion may be also performed for two distinct kinds of features generated from the same biometric trait such as the shape and texture features of tongue-print (Zhang, Liu, Yan, & Shi, 2007). There are some preferred normalization procedures and fusion rules. For example, a variety of applications has shown the satisfactory performance of the simple sum rule in increasing the system accuracy. Studies on Min-max and z-score, two extensively applied normalization procedures, showed that they could work well in a large portion of real-world cases. It is also known that some normalization schemes will work well if the scores follow a specific distribution. For example, z-score normalization is optimal if the scores of all the biometric traits follow the Gaussian distribution. However, no matching score fusion rule or normalization procedure can work well under all circumstances. In this sense, it is worthwhile to explore the possibility of determining and applying different normalization techniques or score fusion rules to matching scores of different biometric traits. It is also considered that setting different weights for the matching scores of different biometric traits (Griffin, 2004; Kumar, Wong, , Shen, & Jain, 2003) allows the multi-biometric system to perform better than the systems that assign the same set of weights to all the biometric traits.

REFERENCES

Brunelli, R., & Falavigna, D. (1995). Person identification using multiple cues. *IEEE Trans. Patt. Anal. Machine Intell.*, *12*(10), 955-966.

Chatzis, V., Bors, A. G., & Pitas, I. (1999). Multimodal decision-level fusion for person authentication. *IEEE Trans. Systems, Man, and Cybernetics, Part A: Systems and Humans*, *29*(6), 674-681.

Chibelushi, C. C., Deravi, F., & Mason, J. S. D. (2002). A review of speech-based bimodal recognition. *IEEE Trans. Multimedia*, *4*(1), 23-37.

Dass, S. C., Nandakumar, K., & Jain, A. K. (2005). A principled approach to score level fusion in multimodal biometric systems. *Proc. of Audio- and Video-based Biometric Person Authentication (AVBPA)* (pp.1049-1058).

Doddington, G., Liggett, W., Martin, A., Przybocki, M., & Reynolds, D. (1998). Sheeps, goats, lambs and wolves: A statistical analysis of speaker performance in the NIST 1998 speaker recognition evaluation. *Proceedings of the 5th International Conference on Spoken Language Processing,* Sydney, Australia.

Dupont, S., & Luettin, J. (2000). Audio-visual speech modeling for continuous speech recognition. *IEEE Trans. Multimedia*, *2*(3), 141-151.

Fernandez, F. A., Veldhuis, R., & Bazen, A. M. (2006). On the relation between biometric quality and user-dependent score distributions in fingerprint verification. *Proc. of the Second International Workshop on Multimodal User Authentication,* Toulouse, France, May 2006.

Fierrez-Aguilar, J., Ortega-Garcia, J., Gonzalez-Rodriguez, J., & Bigun, J. (2005). Discriminative multimodal biometric authentication based on quality measures. *Pattern Recognition*, *38*(5), 777-779.

Griffin, P. (2004). Optimal biometric fusion for identity verification. (Identix Corporate Research Center, Tech. Rep. RDNJ-03). New Jersey.

Islam, T., Mangayyagari, S., & Sankar, R. (2007). Enhanced speaker recognition based on score level fusion of AHS and HMM. *Proceedings of IEEE SoutheastCon.* (pp. 14–19).

Jain, A. K., Hong, L., & Bolle, R. (1997). On-line fingerprint verification. *IEEE Trans. Patt. Anal. Machine Intell.*, *19*(4), 302-314.

Jain, A. K., Nandakumar, K., & Ross, A. (2005). Score normalization in multimodal biometric systems. *Pattern Recognition*, *38*(12), 2270-2285.

Jain, A. K., Prabhakar, S., & Chen, S. (1999). Combining multiple matchers for a high security fingerprint verification system. *Pattern Recognition Letters*, *20*(11-13), 1371-1379.

Jain, A. K., & Ross, A. (2002). Learning use-specific parameters in a multibiometric system. *Proc. of International Conference on Image Processing (ICIP)*, (pp. 22-25).

Kittler, J., Hatef, M., Duin, R. P. W., & Matas, J. (1998). On combining classifiers. *IEEE Trans. Patt. Anal. Machine Intell.*, *20*(3), 226-239.

Kumar, A. (2003). Neural network based detection of local textile defects. *Pattern Recognition*, *36*(7), 1645-1659.

Kumar, A., & Pang, G. (2002). Defect detection in textured materials using optimized filters. *IEEE Trans. Systems, Man, and Cybernetics: Part B, Cybernetics*, *32*(5), 553-570.

Kumar, A., Wong, D. C. M., Shen, H., & Jain, A. K. (2003). Personal verification using palmprint and hand geometry biometric. *Proceedings of Audio—and Video—based Biometrie Person Authentication* (pp. 668-678).

Kumar, A., & Zhang, D. (2004). Palmprint authentication using multiple classifiers. *Proc. SPIE Symposium on Defense & Security - Biometric Technology for Human Identification* (pp. 20-29).

Lucey, S., Chen, T., Sridharan, S., & Chandran, V. (2005). Integration strategies for audio-visual speech processing: applied to text-dependent speaker recognition. *IEEE Trans. Multimedia, 7*(3), 495-506.

Ma, Y, Cukic, B., & Singh, H. (2005). A classification approach to multibiometric score fusion. *Proc. Fifth Int'l Conf. Audio Video-Based Biometric Person Authentication* (pp. 484-493).

Masters, T. (1995). *Advanced algorithms for neural networks: A C++ source book.* New York: John Wiley & Sons, Inc.

Montague, M., & Aslam, J. A. (2001). Relevance score normalization for metasearch. *Proc of Tenth International Conference on Information and Knowledge Management* (pp. 427-433).

Nandakumar, K., Chen, Y., Dass, S. C., & Jain, A. K. (2008). Likelihood ratio-based biometric score fusion. *IEEE Trans. Patt. Anal. Machine Intell.*, *30*(2), 342-347.

Nandakumar, K., Chen, Y., Jain, A. K., & Dass, S. (2006). Quality-based score level fusion in multibiometric systems. *Proc. Int'l Conf. Pattern Recognition* (pp. 473-476).

Poh, N., & Bengio, S. (2006). Database, protocol and tools for evaluating score-level fusion algorithms in biometric authentication. *Pattern Recognition, 39*(2), 223-233.

Prabhakar, S., Pankanti, S., & Jain, A. K. (2003). Biometric recognition: security and privacy concerns. *IEEE Spectrum, 1*(2), 33-42.

Ribaric, S., & Fratric, I. (2005). A biometric identification system based on eigenpalm and eigenfinger features. *IEEE Trans. Patt. Anal. Machine Intell., 27*(11), 1698-1709.

Ross, A., & Jain, A. K. (2003). Information fusion in biometrics. *Pattern Recognition Letters, 24*(13), 2115-2125.

Scheidat, T., Vielhauer, C., & Dittmann, J. (2005). Distance-level fusion strategies for online signature verification. *Proc. IEEE Int. Conf. on Multimedia and Expo (ICME)* (pp. 1294-1297).

Schmid, N. A., Ketkar, M., Singh, H., & Cukic, B. (2006). Performance analysis of iris-Based identification system at the matching score level. *IEEE Trans. Information Forensics and Security, 1*(2), 154-168.

Snelick, R., Uludag, U., Mink, A., Indovina, M., & Jain, A. (2005). Large-scale evaluation of multimodal biometric authentication using state-of-the-art systems. *IEEE Trans. Patt. Anal. Machine Intell., 27*(3), 450-455.

Tsalakanidou, F., Malassiotis, S., & Strintzis, A. (2007). A 3D face and hand biometric system for robust user-friendly authentication. *Pattern Recognition Letters, 28*(16), 2238-2249.

Toh, K. A., Kim, J., & Lee, S. (2008a). Biometric scores fusion based on total error rate minimization. *Pattern Recognition , 41*(3), 1066-1082.

Toh, K. A., Kim, J., & Lee, S. (2008b). Maximizing area under ROC curve for biometric scores fusion. *Pattern Recognition, 41*(11), 3373-3392.

Tulyakov, S., & Govindaraju, V. (2005). Combining matching scores in identification model. *Proc. of Eighth International Conference on Document Analysis and Recognition* (pp. 1151-1155).

Turk, M. A., & Pentland, A. P., (1991). Eigenfaces for recognition. *J. Cognitive Neuroscience, 3*(1), 71-76.

Ulery, B., Hicklin, A. R., Watson, C., Fellner, W., & Hallinan, P. (2006). Studies of biometric fusion(NIST). Gaithersburg, MD: National Institute of Standards and Technology.

Verlinde, P., & Cholet, G. (1999). Comparing decision fusion paradigms using k-NN based classifiers, decision trees and logistic regression in a multi-modal identity verification application. *Proc. of Second International Conference on AVBPA* (pp. 188-193).

Vielhauer, C., & Scheidat, T. (2005). Multimodal biometrics for voice and handwriting. *Proceedings of the 9th International Conference on Communications and Multimedia Security* (pp. 191-199).

Wang, Y., Tan, T., & Jain, A. K. (2003). Combining face and iris biometrics for identity verification. *Proc. of Fourth International Conference on AVBPA* (pp. 805-813).

Yacoub, S. B., Abdeljaoued, Y., & Mayoraz, E. (1999). Fusion of face and speech data for identity verification. *IEEE Trans. Neural Networks*, *10*(5), 1065-1075.

Yan, P., & Bowyer, K. W. (2005). Multi—Biometrics 2D and 3D ear recognition. *Proceedings of Audio—and Video—based Biometrie Person Authentication* (pp. 503-512).

Zhang, D., Liu, Z., Yan, J., & Shi, P. (2007). Tongue-Print: A novel biometrics pattern. *Proceedings of the International conference on Biometrics* (pp.1174-1183).

Chapter XV
Decision Level Fusion

ABSTRACT

With this chapter, we first present a variety of decision level fusion rules and classifier selection approaches, and then show a case study of face recognition based on decision level fusion, and finally offer a summary of three levels of biometric fusion technologies. In a multi-biometric system, classifier selection techniques may be associated with the decision level fusion as follows: classifier selection is first carried out to select a number of classifiers from all classifier candidates. Then the selected classifiers make their own decisions and the decision level fusion rule is used to integrate the multiple decisions to produce the final decision. As a result, in this chapter, we also introduce classifier selection by showing a classifier selection approach based on correlation analysis. This chapter is organized as follows. Section 15.1 provides an introduction to decision level fusion. Section 15.2 presents several simple and popular decision level fusion rules such as the AND, OR, RANDOM, Voting rules, as well as the weighted majority decision rule. Section 15.3 introduces a classifier selection approach based on correlations between classifiers. Section 15.4 presents a case study of group decision-based face recognition. Finally, Section 15.5 offers some comments on three levels of biometric fusion.

15.1 INTRODUCTION

Though the term 'decision level fusion' has appeared widely in the biometric literature, it is not used only in the field of biometrics. Indeed, as an information fusion strategy, decision level fusion also has been widely applied in a number of areas such as multisensor data fusion (Hall & Llinas, 1997), multispectral image fusion and geoscience data fusion (Jeon & Landgrebe, 1999; Fauvel, Chanussot, & Benediktsson, 2006). We would like to regard 'decision level fusion' as a term of information science rather than a term of biometrics. In some cases on multi-biometrics, the term 'symbol level fusion' (Tien, 2003; Gee & Abidi, 2000; Dop, 1999) is also used to represent decision level fusion. The decision level fusion strategy integrates biometric information in a simple and straightforward way in comparison with feature level fusion, which usually directly integrates different biometric traits at the feature level, and matching score level fusion which usually requires that before fusion the matching scores of different biometric subsystems be normalized. A system using the decision level fusion strategy integrates different biometric data at a later stage than the multi-biometric system using feature level fusion or matching score level fusion strategies. The multi-biometric system using the decision level fusion strategy can be described as follows: The system consists of a number of biometric subsystems each of which uses a biometric trait and makes the authentication decision independently. The decision level fusion strategy is then used to combine the decisions of the biometric subsystems to produce the final decision.

Various decision level fusion methods such as Boolean conjunctions, weighted decision methods, classical inference, Bayesian inference, and Dempster–Shafer method (Jain, Lin, Pankanti, & Bolle, 1997), voting (Zuev & Ivanon, 1996) have been proposed. Prabhakar and Jain (2002) combined classifier selection and decision level fusion techniques to perform fingerprint verification. Hong and Jain (1998) integrated faces and fingerprints at the decision level. Chatzis, Bors, and Pitas (1999) used fuzzy clustering algorithms to implement decision level fusion. Osadciw, Varshney and Veeramachaneni (2003) proposed a Bayesian framework to perform decision fusion based on multiple biometric sensors. In addition, modified KNN approach (Teoh, Samad, & Hussain, 2002), decision trees and logistic regression (Verlinde & Cholet, 1999) were also used to fuse multiple biometric traits at the decision level. More studies on decision level fusion such as fusion of iris and face, fusion of 3D data can be found in (Wang, Tan, & Jain, 2003; Gökberk & Akarun, 2006; Li, Zhao, Ao, & Lei, 2005; Gokberk, Salah, & Akarun, 2005; Freedman, 1994; Teoh, Samad, & Hussain, 2004; Niu, Han, Yang, & Tan, 2007). It should be noted that the theoretical framework described by Kittler, Hatef, Duin and Matas (1998) is able to derive a number of real rules for combining classifiers. Roli, Kittler, Fumera, and Muntoni (2002) classified the decision fusion strategies into two main classes: fixed and trained rules. Fusion strategies such as majority voting and the sum rule are recognized as fixed rules. These strategies might allow combination of different systems with similar performance to perform well. Some techniques such as weighted averaging and behavior knowledge space are examples of trained rules, which may allow combination of systems with different performance to improve authentication performance.

With this chapter, we mainly analyze and discuss a variety of decision fusion rules, classifier selection approaches, and a case study of face recognition based on decision fusion. In the following section, we will present some simple and popular decision fusion rules such as the AND, OR, RANDOM, Voting rules. Also, we will present weighted majority decision rule and classification combination based on the confusion matrix with sufficient description.

15.2 RULES AND METHODS OF DECISION LEVEL FUSION

Here we briefly introduce some typical rules and methods proposed for decision level fusion.

AND rule: This rule allows a user to be accepted as a genuine user only if all of the decisions of different subsystems using different biometric traits provide positive authentication results. Usually the method using this rule produces a low false acceptance rate whereas it also results in a high false rejection rate. This can be shown as follows: suppose that a multi-biometric system using the 'AND' rule consists of two biometric subsystems each exploiting one of two single biometric traits and the two biometric traits are independent of each other. If the false accept rate and false reject rate of the first subsystem are respectively FAR_1 and FRR_1 and the two rates of the second subsystem are respectively FAR_2 and FRR_2, we can consider that the false accept and false reject rates of the multi-biometric system are $FAR_1 * FAR_2$ and FRR_2, respectively. Because FAR_1, FRR_1, FAR_2 and FRR_2 are all smaller than 1, the multi-biometric system has a lower false accept rate than both of the two subsystems, whereas the multi-biometric system has a higher false reject rate than both of the two subsystems.

OR rule: This rule means that a user will be treated as a genuine user by a multi-biometric system if either of his/her multiple biometric traits is accepted by the system. Generally, this rule produces a lower false rejection rate and a higher false acceptance than each of the biometric subsystems. For the case where there are two independent biometric traits, we can consider that the false reject and false accept rates of the multi-biometric system using the 'OR' rule are $FRR_1 * FRR_2$ and $FAR_1 + FAR_2 - FAR_1 * FAR_2$, respectively. Here FAR_1 and FRR_1 are still the false accept rate and false reject rate of the first biometric subsystem, respectively. FAR_2 and FRR_2 are also the false accept rate and false reject rate of the second biometric subsystem, respectively. This implies that the multi-biometric system has a lower false reject rate than both of the two subsystems, whereas it has a higher false accept rate than both of the two subsystems.

RANDOM rule: This rule allows a biometric trait to be randomly chosen to perform personal authentication. This very simplistic idea can make it harder for intruders to spoof the system. Moreover it comes without the inconvenience of a multilevel data acquisition for each authentication attempt.

Voting: When voting techniques are used, the global decision rule is obtained simply by fusing the decisions made by subsystems using different biometric traits. Majority voting is a popular voting method. In this method, the class voted by most of the subsystems will be regarded as the result of a fusion decision. If no class won more than half of the votes, the input may be rejected. The method is simple and easy to realize.

Rank Method: This kind of method is used to fuse information of multiple biometric traits in the case where the classifiers produce a ranked list of class labels. The Borda count method is a widely used rank-based fusion scheme. This method can be used for single-winner elections in which each voter rank-orders all the candidates. The Borda count method calculates the combined ranking by summing the class ranks as assigned by the individual voters. The candidate with the maximum ranking score will be accepted as the winner. More specifically, we describe the Borda Count method for an election as follows: Each candidate gets 1 point for each last place vote received, 2 points for each next-to-last point vote, etc., all the way up to N points for each first place vote (where N is the number of candidates/alternatives). The candidate with the largest point total wins the election. If the Borda Count method is applied to a 4 candidate election, each 4th place vote is worth 1 point, each 3rd place vote is worth 2 points, each 2nd place vote is worth 3 points, and each 1st place vote is worth 4 points.

Note that in the Borda Count Method for multi-biometric verification, there are only two candidates, i.e. 'genuine user' and 'imposter'. Therefore, there are only two point numbers, 1 and 2. Each subsystem of a multi-biometric system actually acts as a voter. A tested biometric trait is classified into one candidate ('genuine user' or 'imposter') that has the maximum sum of points.

15.2.6 Weighted Majority Decision Fusion Rule

15.2.6.1 Idea of Weighted Majority Decision Fusion

If there are p available biometric traits, decision level fusion for multi-biometric can be viewed as an issue to make an optimum final decision u_0 under the condition that the decisions $\{u_1, \cdots, u_p\}$ respectively for all single biometric traits are all given. Note that u_1 is made by using only the first biometric trait, u_2 is made by using only the second biometric trait, etc., all the way up to u_p. $\{u_1, \cdots, u_p\}$ are called local decisions. It should be pointed out that among $u_1, \cdots, u_p$ some decisions may be identical. We can determine a decision fusion method based on a cost function. The idea to design the cost function is as follows (Jeon & Landgrebe, 1999): among the local decisions $\{u_1, \cdots, u_p\}$, some of the decisions are more dependable in terms of reliability than the others. Therefore, it would be desirable if the final decision u_0 is as consistent as possible with those reliable local decisions. To implement the idea of emphasizing reliable local decisions among $\{u_1, \cdots, u_p\}$, we can define the following cost function:

$$J(u_0; u_1, \ldots, u_p, \omega_j) = \sum_{k=1}^{p} J(u_0; u_k, \omega_j), \qquad (15.1)$$

where ω_j is the genuine class of the user of the multi-biometric system, $J(u_0; u_k, \omega_j)$ is a cost function associated with the *kth* biometric traits. Indeed, $J(u_0; u_k, \omega_j)$ shows the cost given to an action of selecting u_0 based on the local decision u_k. Eq.(15.1) regards the sum of all the local costs as the actual cost of the action of selecting u_0 based on $\{u_1, \cdots, u_p\}$.

We can determine the final decision based on a cost function $J(u_0; u_k, \omega_j)$ satisfying

$$J(u_0; u_k, \omega_j) = J(u_0; u_k) = 1 - C_k(u_k)\delta(u_0, u_k), \qquad (15.2)$$

where $0 \leq C_k(u_k) \leq 1$. The value of $\delta(u_0, u_k)$ is

$$\delta(u_0, u_k) = \begin{cases} 1 & u_0 = u_k \\ 0 & othrwise. \end{cases}$$

According to (15.2), we know that the cost of selecting the local decision u_k as the final decision u_0 is $1 - C_k(u_k)$, whereas the cost in other cases is one. $C_k(u_k)$, therefore, can control relative importance of consistency between u_0 and u_k. We can select appropriate values for $C_k(u_k)$ in such a way that the less reliable the decision u_k is, the less effect on making the final decision it has.

If we combine Eq.(15.1) and Eq.(15.2), we can know that $J(u_0; u_1, \ldots, u_p, \omega_j) = p - \sum_{k=1}^{p} C_k(u_k)\delta(u_0, u_k)$. Based on $E\{J(u_0; u_1, \ldots, u_p, \omega_j)\} = P(u_1, \ldots, u_p)J(u_0; u_1, \ldots, u_p, \omega_j))$, we can obtain the following equation representing the expected cost (Jeon & Landgrebe, 1999):

$$E\{J(u_0; u_1, \ldots, u_p, \omega_j)\} = P(u_1, \ldots, u_p)(p - \sum_{k=1}^{p} C_k(u_k)\delta(u_0, u_k)). \qquad (15.3)$$

where $P(u_1,...,u_p)$ is the joint probability of $u_1,...,u_p$.

It is clear that Eq.(15.3) will be minimized if

$$\sum_{k=}^{p} C_k(u_k)\delta(u_0,u_k)$$

is maximized with regard to the final decision u_0. Therefore, we define that the optimum final decision u_0 for multi-biometric should maximize

$$\sum_{k=}^{p} C_k(u_k)\delta(u_0,u_k).$$

The rationale to do so can be partially illustrated by the following case: if all $C_k(u_k)$ are equal to 1,

$$\sum_{k=}^{p} C_k(u_k)\delta(u_0,u_k)$$

will has the maximum value only if u_0 is the same as the majority of all the local decisions. More specifically, in a case of personal verification where more than half of the local decisions accept the person as the genuine user,

$$\sum_{k=}^{p} C_k(u_k)\delta(u_0,u_k)$$

will be maximized only if u_0 also takes the 'accept' decision. In a case of personal identification,

$$\sum_{k=}^{p} C_k(u_k)\delta(u_0,u_k)$$

will be maximized only if u_0 takes the same classification decision as the majority of $u_1,\cdots,u_p$. Therefore, we can conclude that if all $C_k(u_k)$ are equal to 1, the decision fusion rule on the basis of the maximization of the expected cost as shown in Eq. (15.3) will be identical to majority voting. As for other $C_k(u_k)$, a decision u_k with a large weight $C_k(u_k)$ has great effect on the final decision. This is why the decision fusion rule presented above is called as the 'weighted majority rule'.

15.2.6.2 How to Set the Weight

Though we show that maximization of

$$\sum_{k=}^{p} C_k(u_k)\delta(u_0,u_k)$$

can be regarded as the goal of the optimum final decision, how to set the weight $C_k(u_k)$ is still not answered. We now will address this issue. We can assign a large cost to the fusion rule when it fails to follow a local decision of large reliability. Because the decision made by different biometric traits have different reliabilities, we use $rel(k,u_k), k = 1,2,...,p$ to denote the reliability of the decision u_k made by using the *kth* biometric trait. We use $REL(k), k = 1,2,...,p$ to represent the reliability of the *kth* biometric trait as a whole.

Because the decision fusion presented in this paper is devoted to authentication, we may assume that a biometric trait with higher authentication accuracy is more reliable than the others. A simple way to set $REL(k), k = 1,2,...,p$ is to let it be directly associated with the authentication accuracy of the *kth* biometric trait.

As for $rel(k), k = 1,2,...,p$, we can specify that it should be also large for a reliable local decision and consequently the final decision is affected as much as possible by this reliable local decision. Hence, We define that

$$rel(k,u_k = \omega_j) = P(x_k \in \omega_j \mid u_k = \omega_j), k = 1,2,...,p \qquad (15.4)$$

where x_k stands for the sample of the *kth* biometric trait. Indeed, Eq.(15.4) takes that the probability that the local decision u_k is correct as the reliability of u_k. Eq.(15.4) also implies that the higher the probability of the local decision u_k being correct is, more strongly u_k influences the final decision of x_k.

In order to associate the reliability measures of the biometric trait and the local decision with the weight $C_k(u_k)$ of the weighted majority decision fusion rule, we can simply define that

$$C_k(u_k) = rel(k,u_k) \cdot REL(k), k = 1,2,...,p. \qquad (15.5)$$

15.2.7 Decision Combination Based on the Confusion Matrix

If classifiers are of mutual independency, we can evaluate the error of each classifier using the confusion matrix and combine classifiers based on confusion matrices (Congalton, 1991). For a multiple class recognition problem with M classes, the error for the *kth* classifier e_k can be represented by a two-dimensional confusion matrix as shown in Eq.(15.6).

$$PT_k = \begin{bmatrix} n_{11}^k & n_{12}^k \dots n_{1M}^k \\ n_{21}^k & n_{22}^k \dots n_{2M}^k \\ \cdot & \\ \cdot & \\ \cdot & \\ n_{M1}^k & n_{M2}^k \dots n_{MM}^k \end{bmatrix}, k = 1,\dots,K \qquad (15.6)$$

where n_{ij}^k denotes the number of the samples from the *ith* class while classified into the *jth* class by the *kth* classifier.

The confusion matrix can be clearly illustrated in the case of two-class classification. In this case, the confusion matrix is a 2 by 2 matrix, which contains information about actual class and predicted class by classification decisions of the classifier. If the four entries of the confusion matrix are a, b, c, d, respectively, then the meanings of these entries are shown in Table 15.1.

a is the number of correct predictions that the sample is from the negative class; b is the number of incorrect predictions that the sample is from the positive class; c is the number of incorrect predictions that the sample is from the negative class, and d is the number of correct predictions that the sample is from the positive class.

The definition of accuracy, which is shown in Eq.(15.7), is helpful to show the classification performance of a classifier for the two-class classification problem.

The accuracy (AC) is defined as the proportion of the total number of predictions that were correct.

$$AC = \frac{a+d}{a+b+c+d}. \qquad (15.7)$$

Note that the accuracy determined using Eq.(15.7) may not be an adequate performance measure when the number of negative or positive cases is much greater

Table 15.1. Meanings of the entries in the confusion matrix of a two-class classifier

		Predicted class by the classification decision	
		Negative class	Positive class
Actual class	Negative class	a	b
	Positive class	c	d

than the number of the other cases. For example, suppose there are 500 cases, 490 of which are negative cases and 10 of which is positive cases. If the system classifies them all as negative, the accuracy would be 98%, even though the classifier missed all positive cases. However, the following definitions can be used to provide more measure for the classifier performance.

The precision (*P*) is defined as the proportion of the predicted positive cases that were correct.

$$P = \frac{d}{b+d}.$$

The recall or true positive rate (*TP*) is defined as the proportion of actual positive cases that were correctly classified.

$$TP = \frac{d}{c+d}.$$

The false negative rate (*FN*) is defined as the proportion of actual positives cases that were incorrectly classified.

$$FN = \frac{c}{c+d}.$$

The false positive rate (*FP*) is defined as the proportion of actual negatives cases that were incorrectly classified.

$$FP = \frac{b}{a+b}.$$

The true negative rate (*TN*) is defined as the proportion of actual negatives cases that were classified correctly.

$$TN = \frac{a}{a+b}.$$

We can evaluate belief measure of recognition for each classifier on the basis of the confusion matrix as follows:

$$Bel(x \in c_i \mid e_k(x)) = P(x \in c_i \mid e_k(x) = j), \tag{15.8}$$

$$P(x \in c_i \mid e_k(x) = j) = n_{ij}^{(k)} \Big/ \sum_{i=1}^{M} n_{ij}^{(k)}$$

where $n_{ij}^{(k)}$ denotes the number of the samples from the *ith* class while classified into the *jth* class by the *kth* classifier, $i,j = 1,2,...,M$. e_k stands for the *kth* classifier. $e_k(x)$

$= j$ means that the *kth* classifier classifies the sample x into the *jth* class. Indeed, the belief measure $Bel(x \in c_i \mid e_k(x))$ is used to denote the conditional probability that x is from the *ith* class (i.e. $x \in c_i$) under the condition that the event $e_k(x) = j$ occurs.

Combining the belief measures of all classifiers, we obtain the following final belief measure of the multiple classifier system (Chen, Wang, & Chi, 1997):

$$Bel(i) = \frac{\prod_{k=1}^{K} P(x \in c_i \mid e_k(x) = j_k)}{\sum_{i=1}^{M} \prod_{k=1}^{K} P(x \in c_i \mid e_k(x) = j_k)}. \tag{15.9}$$

The final classification decision can be made as follows: if

$$Bel(k) = \max_{i=1,2,\ldots,M} Bel(i),$$

then the sample is classified into the *kth* class. The belief of the final classification decision is $Bel(k) = \max_{i=1,2,\ldots,M} Bel(i)$.

Note that one of the limitations of the decision combination based on the confusion matrix is that it requires mutual independencies among multiple classifiers which do not usually hold in real-world applications (Gee & Abidi, 2000).

15.3 SELECTING CLASSIFIERS BASED ON CORRELATIONS BETWEEN CLASSIFIERS

In a number of cases, multiple available decisions are made by different classifiers. In these cases, decision fusion is directly associated with the classifier selection problem. The reason to select classifiers for multi-classifier-based decision fusion is that the combination of different classifiers can result in different fusion performance. A proper set of classifiers should be robust and be able to generate the best fusion performance. Among a number of available selection methods such as Q statistic, generalized diversity and agreement (Kuncheva, Whitaker, Shipp, & Duin, 2003; Partridge & Krzanowski, 1997; Petrakos & Benediktsson, 2001), the degree of correlation is an index of agreement of classifiers. It is commonly admitted that the dependency among classifiers can affect the fusion results. Goebel, Wilson and Sirohey (1995) selected classifiers according to the correlation degree of n different classifiers defined as follows:

$$\rho_n = \frac{nN^f}{N - N^f - N^c + nN^f}, \tag{15.10}$$

where N^f stands for the number of samples that are misclassified by all classifiers, N^c denotes those samples that are classified correctly by all classifiers and N is the total number of the classified samples.

Generally, a smaller correlation degree p can lead to better performance of classifier fusion because the independent classifiers can give more effective information.

We can select a set of classifiers using the following steps:

Step 1: *Select an appropriate performance measure as the initial evaluation criterion, such as the ratio of number of samples classified correctly to the total samples;*
Step 2: *Find the best classifier as the first classifier of the set of classifiers;*
Step 3: *Calculate the correlation degree between the first classifier and the other classifiers using Eq. (15.10);*
Step 4: *Select the classifier having the "low correlation" and add it to the set of classifiers.*
Step 5: *Repeat Steps 3 and 4. Classifier selection is not terminated until a sufficient number of classifiers have been selected. Then the optimal sequence of classifiers can be obtained.*

15.4 A CASE STUDY OF GROUP DECISION-BASED FACE RECOGNITION

Among the various face feature extraction methods (Chellappa, Wilson, & Sirohey, 1995), the algebraic feature method is a kind of effective method to represent the face feature. The singular value (SV) feature is a commonly used algebraic feature. It was used by (Hong & Yang, 1991; Cheng & Yang, 1992) for face image classification and obtained promising experimental results. However, they adopted the face samples with small variations and do not preprocess the image. Hence, when the samples have more changes in expression, pose and illumination, the SV feature can't obtain the ideal result. Therefore, in order to improve its classification performance, we design a new algorithm based on a group decision-making approach. We first preprocess the face images by employing the orthogonal wavelet transform, respectively extract the SV features of four sub-images, and then perform classification for each sub-image using the conventional nearest neighbor classifier. We design a real-time classifier combination algorithm, termed Group Decision-Making (GDM), to combine the four classification procedures of the four sub-images. We also compare the combination result of our algorithm with the classification result of the SV feature of the original image, and the combination result of the conventional mark-counting method.

15.4.1 Singular Feature Extraction

Wavelet transforms have been widely applied in the field of the image processing. As a powerful tool of signal analysis and processing, a wavelet transform decomposes a signal into different frequency bands. The bandwidth of the filters is not variant in the logarithmic scale. This is similar with a model of human vision, which also has the attribute of logarithmic variation. An image signal may be regarded as a kind of nonlinear and non-smooth signal.

An orthogonal wavelet transform can not only keep the original information of an image but also has the attribute of unique decomposition and decorrelation. We select a normal orthogonal wavelet base, namely Daubechies wavelet base, to perform discrete wavelet transform for a face image of 64×64 pixels. Figure 15.1 shows an original image and the resultant image of the wavelet decomposition. Note that the resultant image are indeed four subimages, namely left-up one, right-up one, left-down one and right-down one, which are respectively approximation, horizontal, vertical, and diagonal detailed subimages.

An algebraic feature of an image extracted by an algebraic transform or matrix decomposition is an intrinsic feature of the image. As a kind of algebraic feature, SV features have the following attributes (Hong & Yang, 1991): (1) they are not sensitive to the variation of image noise and illumination. (2) They are invariable to image translation and an image mirror transform.

We first extract the SV feature from the original image of 64×64 pixels and obtain 64-dimensional feature vector. We use the conventional nearest neighbor classifier to classify the obtained feature. Then we respectively apply the above procedure to the four subimages generated from a wavelet transform. Consequently we obtain four groups of classification results.

15.4.2 Group Decision and Combination of Classification Results

We design a group decision-making approach for effectively combining different classifiers (Jing, Zhang, & Yang, 2003). Generally, a group decision-making ap-

Figure 15.1. Original image and four wavelet subimages

proach is applied in the decision problem of M schemes and N principles (Bryson, 1996). We will gradually introduce the relational concepts and algorithm.

First, we take the Shannon entropy as the divisibility measurement of classification results. This requires us to give the estimate of the posterior probability. When the number of training samples is small and we use the nearest neighbor classifier, the posterior probability can be approximately evaluated by the similar value between the training sample and the testing sample. Generally the smaller their distance, the larger their similarity. Assume that c is the class number, d_i is the distance between the ith class and the testing sample, and u_i is the estimation of posterior probability. The object function is defined as follows:

$$J = \sum_{i=1}^{c} u_i^m * d_i^2 \text{ and } \sum_{i=1}^{c} u_i = 1 \qquad (15.11)$$

where m is the fuzzy index, $m > 1$. Solving the above equation to obtain the maximum value of J, we have

$$u_i = (\frac{1}{d_i^2})^{\frac{1}{m-1}} \Big/ \sum_{j=1}^{c} (\frac{1}{d_j^2})^{\frac{1}{m-1}} \qquad (15.12)$$

If $m = 2$, Eq.(15.12) will be rewritten

$$u_i = (\frac{1}{d_i^2}) \Big/ \sum_{j=1}^{c} (\frac{1}{d_j^2}). \qquad (15.13)$$

After computing u_i using Eq.(15.12), we can calculate the Shannon entropy value.

The similarity between classifiers should also be evaluated. Let x, y be two c-dimensional classification result vectors. We can use $s(x,y) = 1 - \sin(x,y)$ to stand for the similarity of two vectors. We present several definitions as follows.

Definition 15.1 Suppose that x, y are c-dimensional vectors, then

$$\cos(x, y) = \frac{x^{\mathrm{T}} y}{\| x \| \cdot \| y \|}, \sin(x, y) = \sqrt{1 - \cos^2(x, y)}, s(x, y) = 1 - \sin(x, y),$$

$$(15.14)$$

We call a similarity measurement between x and y. It is clear that .

Definition 15.2 Suppose that x^d $(d=1,2,\cdots,M)$ is the classification result corresponding to the dth decision-maker and h^d is the entropy value of the dth decision-maker. The individual consistency index of the dth decision-maker is defined as follows:

$$I^d = \left(\sum_{r=1,r\neq d}^{M} s\left(x^d,x^r\right) \middle/ (M-1) \right) * \left(1/h^d\right) \tag{15.15}$$

Clearly, measures the average similarity between an individual and the group divisibility. Definition **15.2** tells us that the larger is, the more representative the dth decision-maker is for the group.

Definition 15.3 The combination result of group decisions is defined as

$$x^G = \sum_{d=1}^{M} s(I^d,x^d) \middle/ \sum_{d=1}^{M} I^d.$$

Definition 15.4 The group consistency index is formulated as follows:

$$I^G = \sum_{d=1}^{M} s(x^G,x^d) \middle/ M \tag{15.16}$$

Definition 15.5 If $I^G \geq \alpha$, we say that the group is consistent in level α; otherwise we say it is inconsistent in level α. The proper value of α can be determined according to the specific details of the application.

The key idea of our approach is as follows: first, under the constraint of $I^G \geq \alpha$, find a consistent decision for the whole group. This means either using all classifiers that can provide a commonly supported opinion, or selecting part of them which can provide an opinion for the majority. Second, perform linear classifers combination according to I^d $(d=1,2,\cdots,M)$. The concrete algorithm of group decisiom-making is described in the following.

Step 1. We compute

I^d $(d=1,2,\cdots,M)$ using Definition 15.2 and sort them in descending order.

Step 2. Evaluate the group decision-making using

$$x^G = (\sum_{d=1}^{M} I^d \cdot x^d) \middle/ \sum_{d=1}^{M} I^d. \tag{15.17}$$

Step 2. Calculate I^G using Eq.(15.16). If $I^G \geq \alpha$, then x^G is regarded as the result of group decision-making; otherwise, go to Step 3.

Step 3. If $I^G \geq \alpha$, assume that the sort result in Step 1 is $I = (I^1, I^2, \cdots, I^M)$. Define that $t^d = I^d / I^{d(L)}$, where $I^{d(L)}$ is the average value of all the components of I ranking behind I^d, i.e.

$$I^{d(L)} = \left(I^{d+1} + I^{d+2} + \cdots + I^M \right) \big/ (M - d).$$ (15.18)

Let

$$T = \max_d \left\{ t^d \right\} = \max_d \left\{ I^d / I^{d(L)} \right\}.$$ (15.19)

The first k classifiers are selected to form a sub-group that plays the dominant role in the whole group. Repeat Step 1 using this new group which has k available classifiers. The final solution of x^G is the result of group decision-making.

15.4.3. Experiment Results

We conducted an experiment using the NUST603 face databases (Jin, Yang, Hu, & Lou, 2001) of Nanjing University of Science and Technology, China. The face images of this database are from 18 persons each providing 12 captured images of 64×64 pixels. There are significant changes in both expression and pose, and small changes in illumination and the relative distance between the camera and person.

The group consistency level α is set to 0.8. In other words, the similarity value between the vectors is 0.8. Table 15.1 shows the results, including those for the original images, four group subimages, the Borda count method, and the group decision-making approach of setting the group consistency level α or not.

From Table 15.2, we learn that combining the four group classification results can effectively improve the classification performance of the SV feature, using either of two combination methods. The maximum improvement in accuracy obtained using group decision-making is 12.6%. Moreover, the group decision-making approach can obtain better combination results than the conventional Borda count method. In particular, the group decision-making approach setting the group consistency level α obtains a maximum improvement in accuracy of 7.3% in comparison with the Borda count method.

Table 15.2. Recognition results of different approaches. I, I1, I2, I3 and I4 respectively stand for right recognition rates of original image, approximation, horizontal, vertical, and diagonal detailed subimages. B, G1 and G2 respectively denote the Borda count method, the group decision-making approach, with and without setting the group consistency level α.

Different sample sets				Recognition rate (%)							
				I	Four subimages				B	G	
					I1	I2	I3	I4		G1	G2
Training sample number per class	4	Test class number	12	78.5	77.6	61.8	67.4	58.3	81.3	84.7	85.4
			14	74.7	73.2	58.3	60.7	56.0	79.2	81.6	82.7
			16	71.8	71.1	56.3	60.2	54.7	79.7	82.8	84.4
			18	70.5	69.4	52.8	58.3	48.2	75.5	80.1	81.2
	5	Test class number	12	80.7	80.1	65.3	68.0	59.7	81.9	84.0	86.8
			14	75.6	74.4	61.3	60.1	58.9	78.6	82.1	83.9
			16	73.4	72.9	60.4	59.4	57.3	82.3	81.9	83.4
			18	71.1	69.9	54.2	56.9	55.0	78.2	79.2	79.6
	6	Test class number	12	82.6	81.8	65.2	70.8	59.9	84.6	88.2	90.3
			14	77.2	76.8	60.1	63.7	60.1	79.6	84.5	86.9
			16	75.4	74.0	60.7	62.5	59.9	81.8	84.4	86.8
			18	75.0	71.3	54.5	58.8	56.3	77.8	80.1	81.9

15.5 COMMENTS ON BIOMETRIC FUSION AT THE THREE LEVELS

In this and the previous two chapters, we have presented three categories of multi-biometric fusion strategies i.e. feature level fusion, matching score level fusion and decision level fusion. A number of studies have shown the effectiveness and power of the multi-biometric system using these fusion strategies. The advantages of decision level fusion include easy implementation and a simple way to directly fuse decisions of different biometric subsystems. However, unlike feature level and matching score level fusion, decision level fusion does not allow information of multiple biometric traits to be fully exploited. Indeed, decision fusion for verification fuses only the "accept" or "reject" decisions associated with different biometric traits and decision fusion for identification fuses only the class label decisions associated with different biometric traits. It is commonly considered that fusion at the decision level does not has the same potential to improve the overall system performance as fusion at the matching score level or fusion at the feature level. Additionally, simple decision level fusion rules such 'AND' or 'OR' may have difficulties in simultaneously obtaining satisfactory FAR and FRR. Fusion at the feature level fuses multiple biometric traits at the most early stage and can enable these traits to be fully exploited for personal authentication. However, fusion at the feature level also has weaknesses. It may encounter difficulties in properly combining feature vectors that are generated from different biometric traits and are possibly non-compatible. They may also have difficulties in the cases where the user does not possess all the biometric traits, which makes fusion at the feature level not feasible. Fusion at the matching score level fuses multiple biometric traits at a later stage than fusion at the feature level and can exploit more information generated from the multiple biometric traits than fusion at the decision level. It seems that fusion at the matching score level is used most among the three fusion strategies.

Our categorization of multi-biometric technologies into three levels is not meant to imply that multiple biometric traits should be fused at only one of these three levels. Indeed, hybrid fusion technologies, such as using multiple strategies or rules (Aude, Carneiro, & Serdeira, 1999; Scheunert, Lindner, Richter, & Tatschke, 2007; McCullough, Dasarathy & Lindberg, 1996), have received more and more research interests and achieved encouraging results. Some new methods such as semantic fusion (Oermann, Scheidat, & Vielhauer, 2006), fuzzy theory (Lau, Ma, & Meng, 2004) are also being exploited for personal authentication in the field of biometric research. Evidential reasoning (Reddy, 2007) has also been introduced into the multimodal fusion of human computer interaction. Adaptive multi-biometrics is also an attractive example of new methods in the field of biometrics. An adaptive multi-biometric system will adaptively determine the weights for different biometric traits or adaptively select the most suitable biometric traits to conduct a varying multi-biometric implementation with various environments or conditions (Hui, Meng, & Mak, 2007). Moreover, adaptive multimodal biometrics (Veeramachaneni, Osadciw, & Varshney, 2005) can adaptively determine the decision fusion rule and even threshold values for decision-making. Chatzis, Bors and Pitas (1999) showed the advantage of using the unimodal reliability information for fusing multimodal biometrics. The fuzzy clustering algorithm can also be used for fusing multi-biometric traits at the decision level (Chatzis, Bors and Pitas 1999). Soft computing for biometrics (Franke, Ruiz-del-Solar, & Köppen, 2002) might provide the multi-biometric system with new available biometric information. It is considered that since soft computing has the ability to consider variations and uncertainty in data, it is suitable for biometric measurements that do not have an absolute "ground truth". Existing approaches to and techniques for multi-biometric fusion also include multivariate polynomial model, byperbolic functions and neural networks (Toh, Yau, & Jiang, 2004; Toh & Yau, 2004).

REFERENCES

Aude, E., Carneiro, G., & Serdeira, H. (1999). CONTROLAB MUFA: a multi-level fusion architecture for intelligent navigation of a telerobot. *Proc. IEEE International Conference on Robotics and Automation* (pp. 465-472).

Bryson, N. (1996). Group decision-making and the analytic hierarchy process: exploring the consensus-relevant information bontent. *Computers & Operations Research, 23*(1), 27-35.

Chatzis, V., Bors, A. G., & Pitas, I. (1999). Multimodal decision-level fusion for person authentication. *IEEE Trans. System, Man, and Cybernetics, part A, 29*(6), 674-680.

Chellappa, R., Wilson, C., & Sirohey, S. (1995). Human and machine recognition of faces: a survey. *Proceedings of the IEEE, 83*(5), 705-740.

Chen, K., Wang, L., & Chi, H. (1997). Methods of combining multiple classifiers with different features and their applications to text-independent speaker identification. *International Journal of Pattern Recognition and Artificial Intelligence, 11*(3), 417-445.

Cheng, Y. Q., & Yang, J. Y. (1992). Aircraft identification based on the algebraic method. *SPIE* (pp. 298-305).

Congalton, R. G. (1991). A review of assessing the accuracy of classifications of remotely sensed data. *Remote Sensing of Environment, 37*(1), 35-46.

Dop, E. V. (1999). *Multi-sensor object recognition: The case of electronics recycling.* Ph.D thesis, University of Twente, Holland.

Fauvel, M., Chanussot, J., & Benediktsson, J. A. (2006). Decision fusion for the classification of urban remote sensing images. *IEEE Trans. Geoscience and Remote Sensing, 44*(10), 2828-2838.

Franke, K., Ruiz-del-Solar, J., & Köppen, M. (2002). Soft biometrics: Soft computing for biometric applications. *International Journal of Fuzzy Systems, 4*(2), 665-672.

Freedman, D. D. (1994). Overview of decision level fusion techniques for identification and their application. *Proc of the American Control Conference* (pp.1299-1303).

Gee, L. A., & Abidi, M. A. (2000). Multisensor fusion for decision-based control cues. *Proc. of SPIE on Signal Processing, Sensor Fusion, and Target Recognition IX* (pp. 249-257).

Goebel, K., Yan, W. Z., & Cheetham, W. (2002). A method to calculate classifier correlation for decision fusion. *Proc. of Decision and Control* (pp. 135-140).

Gökberk, B., & Akarun, L. (2006). Comparative analysis of decision-level fusion algorithms for 3D face recognition. *Proc. of International Conference on Pattern Recognition (ICPR)* (pp. 1018-1021).

Gokberk, B., Salah, A. A., & Akarun, L. (2005). Rank-based decision fusion for 3D shape-based face recognition. *Proc. of Audio- and Video-based Biometric Person Authentication* (pp. 1019-1028).

Hall, D. L., & Llinas, J. (1997). An Introduction to Multisensor Data Fusion. *Proceedings of the IEEE*, 85(1), 6-23.

Hong, L., & Jain, A. K. (1998). Integrating faces and fingerprints for personal identification. *IEEE Trans. Pattern Anal. Machine Intell.*, 20(12), 1295-1307.

Hong, Z. Q., & Yang, J. Y. (1991). Algebraic feature extraction of image for recognition. *Pattern Recognition*, 24(2), 211-219.

Hui, H. P., Meng, H. M., & Mak, M. W. (2007). Adaptive weight estimation in multi-biometric verification using fuzzy logic decision fusion. *Proceedings of the IEEE International Conference on Acoustics, Speech and Signal Processing* (pp. 501-504).

Jain, A. K., Lin, H., Pankanti, S., & Bolle, R. (1997). An identity-authentication system using fingerprints. *Proceedings of the IEEE*, 85(9), 1365-1388.

Jeon, B., & Landgrebe, D. A. (1999). Decision fusion approach for multitemporal classification. *IEEE Trans. Geoscience and Remote Sensing*, 37(3), 1227-1233.

Jin, Z., Yang, J. Y., Hu, Z., & Lou, Z. (2001). Face recognition based on the uncorrelated discriminant transformation. *Pattern Recognition*, 34(7), 1405-1416.

Jing, X. Y., Zhang, D., & Yang, J. Y. (2003). Face recognition based on a group decision-making combination approach. *Pattern Recognition*, 36(7), 1675-1678.

Kittler, J., Hatef, M., Duin, R. P. W., & Matas, J. (1998). On Combining Classifiers. *IEEE Trans. Pattern Analysis and Machine Intelligence*, 20(3), 226-239.

Kuncheva, L. I., Whitaker, C. J., Shipp, C. A., & Duin, R. P. W. (2003). Limits on the majority vote accuracy in classifier fusion. *Pattern Analysis and Applications*, 6(1), 22-31.

Lau, C. W., Ma, B., & Meng, H. M.. (2004). Fuzzy logic decision fusion in a multimodal biometric system. *Proceedings of the 8th International Conference on Spoken Language Processing (ICSLP)* (pp. 108-115).

Li, S. Z., Zhao, C., Ao, M., & Lei, Z. (2005). Learning to fuse 3D+2D based face recognition at both feature and decision levels. *IEEE International Workshop on Analysis and Modeling of Faces and Gestures* (pp. 44-54).

McCullough, C. L., Dasarathy, B. V., & Lindberg, P. C. (1996). Multi-level sensor fusion for improved, target discrimination. *Proceedings of the 35th IEEE Conference on Decision and Control* (pp. 3674-3675).

Niu, G., Han, T., Yang, B. -S., & Tan, A. C. C. (2007). Multi-agent decision fusion for motor fault diagnosis. *Mechanical Systems and Signal Processing, 21*(3), 1285-1299.

Osadciw, L. A., Varshney, P. K., & Veeramachaneni, K. (2003). Optimum fusion rules for multimodal biometrics. *Multisensor Surveillance Systems: A Fusion Perspective*, Boston: Kluwer Academic Publishers.

Partridge, D., & Krzanowski, W. (1997). Software diversity: practical statistics for its measurement arid exploitation. *Information and Software Technology, 39*(10), 707-717.

Petrakos, M., & Benediktsson, J. A. (2001). The effect of classifier agreement on the accuracy of the combined classifier in decision level fusion. *IEEE Trans. Geoscience and Remote Sensing, 39*(11), 2539-2546.

Prabhakar, S., & Jain, A. K. (2002). Decision-level fusion in fingerprint verification. *Pattern Recognition, 35*(4), 861-874.

Oermann, A., Scheidat, T., Vielhauer, C., et al. (2006). Semantic fusion for biometric user authentication as multimodal signal processing. *Proceedings of international workshop Multimedia content representation, classification and security (MRCS)* (pp. 546-553).

Reddy, B. S. (2007). *Evidential reasoning for multimodal fusion in human computer interaction.* A thesis presented to the University of Waterloo, Ontario, Canada.

Roli, F., Kittler, J., Fumera, G., & Muntoni, D. (2002). An experimental comparison of classifier fusion rules for multimodal personal identity verification systems. *Proc. of the Third International Workshop on Multiple Classifier Systems* (pp. 325-335).

Scheunert, U., Lindner, P., Richter, E., & Tatschke, T. (2007). Early and multi level fusion for reliable automotive safety systems. *Proc. 2007 IEEE Intelligent Vehicles Symposium* (pp. 196-201).

Teoh, A. B. J., Samad, S. A., & Hussain, A. (2002). Decision fusion comparison for a biometric verification system using face and speech. *Malaysian Journal of Computer Science, 15*(2), 17-27.

Teoh, A. B. J., Samad, S. A., & Hussain, A. (2004). Nearest neighbourhood clas-sifiers in a bimodal biometric verification system fusion decision scheme. *Journal of Research and Practice in Information Technology, 36*(1), 47-62.

Tien, J. M. (2003). Toward a decision informatics paradigm: a real-time information based approach to decision making. *IEEE Trans. SMC-C, 33*(1), 102-113.

Toh, K. A., & Yau, W. Y. (2004). Combination of hyperbolic functions for multi-modal Biometrics Data Fusion. *IEEE Trans. Systems, Man, and Cybernetics, Part B, 34*(2), 1196-1209.

Toh, K. A., Yau, W. Y., & Jiang, X. (2004). A reduced multivariate polynomial model for multimodal biometrics and classifiers fusion. *IEEE Trans. Circuits and Systems for Video Technology (Special Issue on Image- and Video-Based Biomet-rics), 14*(2), 224-233.

Veeramachaneni, K., Osadciw, L. A., & Varshney, P. K. (2005). An adaptive multimodal biometric management algorithm. *IEEE Trans. Systems, Man, and Cybernetics, Part C, 35*(3), 344-356.

Verlinde, P., & Cholet, G. (1999). Comparing decision fusion paradigms using k-NN based classifiers, decision trees and logistic regression in a multi-modal identity verification application. *Proc. of 2nd Int'l Conf. on Audio- and Video-based Person Authentication* (pp. 188-193).

Wang, Y., Tan, T., & Jain, A. K. (2003). Combining face and iris biometrics for identity verification. *Proc.of International Conference on Audio and Video-Based Biometric Person Authentication (AVBPA)* (pp. 805-813).

Zuev, Y. A., & Ivanon, S. (1996). The voting as a way to increase the decision re-liability. *Proc. Foundations of Information/Decision Fusion with Applications to Engineering Problems* (pp. 206-210).

Chapter XVI
Book Summary

ABSTRACT

With the title "Advanced Pattern Recognition Technologies with Applications to Biometrics" this book mainly focuses on two kinds of advanced biometric recognition technologies, biometric discrimination techniques and multi-biometrics. Biometric discrimination techniques are presented in Parts I and II, while multi-biometrics is described in Part III. While the methods and algorithms described in Parts I and II are very suitable for biometrics as they take into account characteristics of biometric applications such as high dimensionality and small sample size, Part III mainly introduces three kinds of biometric fusion techniques that respectively fuse biometric information at the feature level, matching score level and decision level as well as their applications cases. This chapter summarizes the book from a holistic viewpoint. Section 16.1 summarizes the contents of the book and indicates the relationship between different chapters in each part. Section 16.2 reveals that how the methods and algorithms described in different parts can be applied to different data forms of biometric traits. Section 16.3 provides comments on the development of multi-biometrics.

16.1 CONTENT SUMMARY

In this section we summarize the contents of all the three parts and indicate the themes of different parts, respectively. While Part I explores several advanced biometric discrimination technologies such as orthogonal discriminant analysis, parameterized discriminant analysis, and maximum scatter difference discriminant analysis, this part is indeed focused on biometrics with the small sample size (SSS) characteristic. In Chapter IV, by defining the three SSS strategies (SSS Strategy one, SSS Strategy two and SSS Strategy three) for solving the SSS problem using discriminant analysis, we provide clear and detailed description on how a discriminant analysis technique should be properly applied to biometrics with the SSS characteristic. On the other hand, in Chapter V and Chapter VI we develop novel discriminant analysis methods applicable to biometrics with the SSS characteristic. In Chapter V, we address biometric issues with the SSS characteristic by developing two weighted discriminant analysis methods respectively on the basis of the nullspace and the range space of the within-class scatter matrix. In Chapter VI, we address biometric issues with the SSS characteristic by proposing the maximum scatter difference discriminant analysis method. The most advantage of this method is that when applied to biometrics the nature of the method allows the SSS problem to be automatically avoided. This excellent property of the method also allows one to use discriminant analysis for biometrics with ease.

Part II mainly presents tensor-based biometric discrimination technologies, tensor independent component analysis, tensor non-negative factorization, tensor canonical correlation analysis and tensor partial least squares as well as their applications to biometrics. These techniques allow ideas of conventional methods and algorithms such as the idea of conventional linear discriminant analysis (LDA) methods to be applied to new data forms such as two-dimensional matrices. For example, whereas conventional LDA is just applicable to one-dimensional vector, tensor-based discriminant analysis method enables the discriminant analysis methodology to be directly applied to two-dimensional matrix data. Indeed, a number of tensor-based methods and algorithms described in Part II can be viewed as improvements to conventional methods and algorithms that are workable for only sample data in the form of vectors as shown in Part I. In addition, when we describe well-known two-dimensional PCA and LDA respectively from the points of view of tensor PCA and LDA, we provide readers with a more easy way to understand tensor methods.

Part III primarily presents multi-biometric technologies including feature level fusion, matching score level fusion and decision level fusion technologies and applications examples of these technologies. Fundamental concepts and definitions of multi-biometrics such as multi-biometric technology taxonomies are also presented in this part. One of the relationships between this part and the previous two parts is as follows: The methods presented in Parts I and II can serve as feature extraction methods of multi-biometrics and then the multi-biometric system can implement the verification or recognition task by integrating the multi-biometric technologies with the feature extraction result. On the other hand, Part III is also different from Parts I and II as follows: Part III primarily emphasizes technical aspects of multi-biometrics, whereas Parts I and II mainly focus on theoretical aspects of foundation of biometrics, presenting different discriminant analysis methods and algorithms applicable to biometrics.

16.2 METHOD APPLICABILITY

Biometric data has three typical representation forms: the vector form, the two-dimensional image form and the 3D matrix form. This book also has the potential to provide us with three types of biometric discriminant methods applicable to biometric traits with different representation forms. The methods presented in Part I are suited to biometric data in the vector form. This type of methods is referred to as one-dimensional biometric method. Part II provides a type of methods that is applicable to the two-dimensional image form and is referred to as two-dimensional biometric method. These methods include two-dimensional LPP, two-dimensional PCA and LDA as well as GLRAM, and so on. From Part II, we know that it is also possible for the tensor-based methods to provide us with a tool to directly analyze and exploit biometric data in the 3D matrix form. This novel type of analysis techniques for 3D biometric data can be referred to as three-dimensional biometric method.

The three types of biometric methods mentioned above have different characteristics. For the two-dimensional biometric method, aside the low computational complexity, it also has the advantage of being able to avoid the SSS problem. This is because the two-dimensional biometric method first directly exploits the two-dimensional biometric data i.e. "biometric image" to produce the so-called total covariance matrix, between-class scatter matrix, the between-class scatter matrix, and so on. Because the dimensionality of these matrices is usually smaller than the number of biometric samples, they are nonsingular matrices. As a result, the SSS problem does not exist when one solve the certain equation consisting of these nonsingular matrices. In contrast, a conventional feature extraction method usually has a high computational complexity and suffers from the SSS problem. This is because the conventional feature extraction method requires that the biometric sample usually in the form of "biometric image" be converted into one-dimensional vector in advance. Consequently, the corresponding total covariance matrix, between-class scatter matrix, the between-class scatter matrix have a very high dimensionality that is larger then the number of biometric samples. A conventional feature extraction method thus encounters the SSS problem. In this sense, the methods and algorithms in Part II can well address the high dimensionality characteristic of biometrics.

The methods and technologies presented in different parts of this book have different merits. Our one-dimensional biometric methods presented in Part I not only can deal with the SSS problem well but also can obtain a high accuracy. Our two- dimensional biometric methods presented in Part II can be directly and efficiently applied to biometric data in the form of two-dimensional matrices and there is no need to in advance convert the data into the one-dimensional form. As for the three-dimensional biometric method, it has the following characteristic: It allows us to directly extract features for 3D biometric samples. This indeed provides us with an effective way to directly exploiting 3D data for performing personal authentication.

16. 3 COMMENTS ON MULTI-BIOMETRICS DEVELOPMENT

16.3.1 Issues and Challenge

Though a number of biometric and multi-biometric systems have been applied in the real world, there are still challenge and issues. For example, the following several issues deserve further investigations. First, it is usually considered that multimodal biometric traits are independent of each other and multiple biometric traits allows more information to be exploited by the biometric system, which indeed has been taken as the base for the multimodal biometric system to produce better performance than the single biometric system. However, for a certain multi-biometric system, such as a multi-biometric system of fusing multiple feature extraction algorithms or multiple classifiers using only a single biometric trait, it is likely that the fused data are not independent. For this type of system, the following issues should be considered: what is the rationale for a multi-biometric system using dependent biometric information? How to design a fusion algorithm to properly exploit the dependent biometric information? Second, if the multi-biometric system is applied in the case of a large user population identification system, there are often more than tens or hundreds of millions of subject images already enrolled in the matcher databases and the system has to process more than hundreds of thousands of identification requests. In this kind of case, to establish a multi-biometric system that can meet the following three requirements will be also a challenge task: a quite high accuracy; low need of staffing levels to properly operate the system; the system is efficient enough to serve as an on-line application.

Real-world applications of multi-biometrics should also pay attention to the following issues:

A. Harsh Environments

In the real world, multi-biometrics may be applied in unfavourable climates or online or mobile environments. In this kind of environment, the possibility of biometric trait acquisition failure or the acquisition of low-quality biometric traits makes biometric-based personal authentication more challenging. Therefore, harsh environments require that the multi-biometric system have high reliability and stability.

Some special challenges and threats to privacy also arise in the case of network based biometric applications, as the multiple biometric traits may be simultaneously exposed through the network. A multi-biometric system may reduce threats to privacy and provide high feasibility by adopting the following recommendations: both location information and device characteristics should be protected; ease of use of the mobile identity management tools and simplified languages and interfaces for non-experts should be enhanced; the verifiable link between the user and his digital identity has to be ensured (Please refer to: swami.jrc.es/pages/Conference2006.htm). Other challenges may be encountered in real-world applications of multi-biometrics include continuous verification necessary for high-security environments in which the protected resource needs to be continuously monitored for unauthorized use (Janakiraman, Kumar, Zhang, & Sim, 2005; Kumar, Sim, Janakiraman, & Zhang, 2005; Sim, Zhang, Janakiraman, & Kumar, 2007), performance prediction of the fusion system given the characteristics of the individual sensors (Wang & Bhanu, 2006), etc.

B. Tradeoff between Security and Convenience

Requiring high-quality biometric trait acquisition can improve system security. Rigorous acceptance thresholds can also improve security against spoofing because it reduces the acceptance error. But these means might also reduce the convenience of the system. In addition, though the use of more multiple biometric traits can make systems highly accurate, acquisition of the biometric traits is also more inconvenient for the user and takes a longer time than the acquisition of the single biometric traits. As a result, the system must make a proper tradeoff between security and convenience.

C. Choice of Biometric Traits and Fusion Strategies

Usually a choice-based combination of biometric traits produces better performance than arbitrary combination of biometric traits. In addition, appropriate fusion strategies are also of significance for integrating multiple biometric traits, because different fusion strategies have their own advantages and disadvantages and are suited to different situations.

D. Tradeoff between Cost and System Performance

For multi-biometric systems, high performance requirements usually mean higher system costs including device costs. Therefore, multi-biometric systems with a high performance to cost ratio are an important goal.

E. Other Negative Factors

Cultural and race background may also affect degree of user acceptance of the biometric application. Even if in the case where "users are unhappy with interactions that impose a high physical or mental workload, or require them to perform actions they find distasteful" (SASSE, 2007, p.79), the application may also be somewhat influenced.

16.3.2 Development and Trend of Biometrics

16.3.2.1 Requirements of Large-Scale Applications

Note that early biometric applications usually store and use biometric data locally. Nowadays, large scale distributed biometric applications, which use biometric data nationally or internationally, have become more and more common. The biometric applications operate in more variable and even unpredictable environments and involve more demographically diverse and larger biometric datasets. It seems that the future requirements of large-scale identity systems for government use will pay more emphasis on robustness, scalability, and interoperability (Nadel, 2007).

16.3.2.2 High-Resolution and the 3D Biometrics

High-resolution biometrics and 3D biometrics are two significant and recently-developed biometric techniques. Typical high-resolution biometric systems include high-resolution finger identification system and signature authentication system, and so on. The fact that a high-resolution signature authentication system is capable of documenting a large number of levels such as up to 512 different levels of pressure and a quite high reading resolution (please refer to web site: http://www. wacom-asia.com/press/20070427.html) allows the system to capture much more signature information than a low-resolution system. A high-resolution fingerprint identification system allows fingerprints to be authenticated at three different levels i.e. pattern level, minutia point level, as well as the pore and ridge contour level (Jain, Chen, & Demirkus, 2006, 2007). A 1,000 dpi fingerprint scan can simultaneously capture information at these three levels. The algorithm is another key point of this kind of system. The algorithm developed for the high-resolution biometrics should be able to adequately exploit the much information provided by the system. The high-resolution system cooperating with a fine algorithm dedicated to the high-resolution data is able to produce a higher authentication accuracy than the low-resolution system.

3D biometric techniques acquire 3D-image data of biometric traits (Gökberk & Akarun, 2006; Gokberk, Dutagaci, Akarun, & Sankur, 2007; Gokberk, Salah, & Akarun, 2005; Li, Zhao, Ao, & Lei, 2005; Sala, Zappa, & Cigada, 2006; Woodard, Faltemier, Yan, Flynn, & Bowyer, 2006) and the corresponding systems are therefore called 3D biometric systems. Examples of 3D biometrics include 3D face (Gökberk & Akarun; Gokberk, Dutagaci, Akarun, & Sankur; Gokberk, Salah, & Akarun; Li et al.; Sala, Zappa, & Cigada) and 3D fingerprint. While the high-resolution and the 3D biometric systems promise higher accuracy, they also suffer from some problems. First, they usually involve a high device cost. Second, since the system retains a large quantity of information from the subject, it is necessary for the system to have a large memory and a high computation performance.

16.3.2.3 Cancelable Biometrics and Biometric Key Generation

Issues relating to identity theft, privacy, and cancelable biometrics also attract increasing attention of the researchers in the field of biometrics (Bolle, Connel, & Ratha, 2002; Uludag, Pankanti, Prabhakar, & Jain, 2004). Usually a real-world biometric system captures and stores a large-scale of biometric data in a database. When the identity theft issue occurs in the biometric system, serious issues may be caused. This is because unlike secret passwords or physical tokens, biometric data in the traditional biometric system cannot be refreshed or reissued.

The technique of cancelable biometrics can enable biometric data to be "refreshed" and "reused". Cancelable biometrics stores a transformed version of the biometric data and it is able to provide a higher level of privacy by allowing multiple templates to be generated from the same biometric data (Jin & Connie, 2006). Different sets of the template can also been stored in different databases. Maltoni,, Maio, Jain, and Prabhakar (2003) presented the following three principal objectives of cancellable biometrics:

i.   **Diversity:** No same cancellable template can be used in two different applications.
ii. **Reusability:** Straightforward revocation and reissue in the event of compromise.
iii **One-way transformation:** Non-invertibility of template computation to prevent recovery of biometric data. Besides that, the formulation should not deteriorate the recognition performance for sure.

The goal of "diversity" and "reusability" mentioned above requires that different application use different biometric templates. The biometric system can achieve this goal in the following way. During enrollment the biometric system stores only the transformed version of the original biometric sample rather than the biometric sample itself. Here the transform means a change in the representation of an entity, where the transformed version may comprise exactly the same information as in the previous one or may reflect a loss or augmentation of information contained in the original representation. During authentication, the biometric system would convert the received biometric sample using the same transform and the biometric matching would be carried out in the transformed space. As different applications can use different transforms (or different parameters of the same transform), the template issued for a specific application can only be used by that application. If a biometric template is ever compromised, a new one can be issued by using a different transform. Because such a template does not reveal a user's biometric information, it is called cancelable biometrics (Ratha, Connell, & Bolle, 2001) or a private template (Davida, Frankel, & Matt, 1998).

Differing from cancelable biometrics, the method of biometric key generation attempts to consolidate the system security by integrating biometric information into a cryptosystem (Uludag et al., 2004). It is possible that such a solution is more secure than cancelable biometrics because of the following factors: The generation process integrates a private key into the user biometric information in a nice way and consequently both the cryptographic key and biometric information in the template are inaccessible to the attacker and the cryptographic key will be released to the corresponding application upon valid presentation of the user biometric template. Moreover, since the system does not have to perform the biometric matching at all, it is no need to access biometric information in the template. The method of biometric key generation can be exploited for digital content protection, copyright protection and other similar tasks.

Biometric key generation is also different from traditional cryptosystems. The traditional cryptosystems such as AES (advanced encryption standard) (National Institute of Standards and Technology, 2001) accept only identical keys designed for encryption and decryption. Differing from this, specific biometric representations from a subject may vary dramatically. As a result, it is necessary for researchers to address the issue of producing perfect encryption/decryption performance which expects that the decrypted message is identical to the encrypted message, given the imperfect biometric authentication technology (Uludag et al., 2004).

REFERENCES

Advanced encryption standard (2001). *Federal information processing standards publication 197*. National Institute of Standards and Technology (online available: http://csrc.nist.gov/publications/fips/fips197/fips-197.pdf).

Bolle, R. M., Connel, J. H., & Ratha, N. K. (2002). Biometric perils and patches. *Pattern Recognition*, 35 (12), 2727–2738.

Davida, G. I., Frankel, Y., & Matt, B. J. (1998). On enabling secure applications through off-line biometric identification. *Proc. 1998 IEEE Symp. Privacy and Security* (pp. 148–157).

Gökberk, B., & Akarun, L. (2006). Comparative analysis of decision-level fusion algorithms for 3D face recognition. *Proc. of 18th International Conference on Pattern Recognition* (pp. 1018-1021).

Gokberk, B., Dutagaci, H., Akarun, L., & Sankur, B. (2007). Representation plurality and decision level fusion for 3D face recognition. *IEEE Trans. System Man and Cybernetics*, accepted.

Gokberk, B., Salah, A. A., & Akarun, L. (2005). Rank-based decision fusion for 3D shape-based face recognition. *Proceedings of the International Conference on Audio- and Video-Based Biometric Person Authentication* (pp. 1019-1028).

Jain, A., Chen, Y., & Demirkus., M. (2006). Pores and ridges: fingerprint matching using level 3 features". *Proc.of 18th International Conference on Pattern Recognition (ICPR)* (pp. 477-480).

Jain, A., Chen, Y., & Demirkus., M. (2007). Pores and ridges: high-resolution fingerprint matching using level 3 features. *IEEE Trans. Pattern Anal. Machine Intell.*, 29(1), 15-27.

Janakiraman, R., Kumar, S., Zhang, S., & Sim, T. (2005). Using continuous face verification to improve desktop security. *Proc. IEEE Workshop Applications of Computer Vision* (pp. 501-507).

Jin, A. T. B., & Connie, T. (2006). Remarks on BioHashing based cancelable biometrics in verification system. *Neuro Computing*, 69, 2461–2464.

Kumar, S., Sim, T., Janakiraman, R., & Zhang, S. (2005). Using continous biometrics verification to protect interactive login sessions. *Proc. 21st Ann. Conf. Computer Security Applications* (pp. 441-450).

Li, S. Z., Zhao, C., Ao, M., & Lei, Z. (2005). 3D+2D Face recognition by fusion at both feature and decision levels. *Proceedings of IEEE International Workshop on Analysis and Modeling of Faces and Gestures*, Beijing, Oct. 16.

Maltoni, D., Maio, D., Jain, A. K., Prabhakar, S. (2003). Handbook of fingerprint recognition. New York: Springer (pp. 301-307).

Nadel, L. (2007). Biometric identification: a holistic perspective. *SPIE Defense and Security Symposium Biometric Technology for Human Identification IV*, April 10, 2007.

Ratha, N., Connell, J., & Bolle, R. (2001). Enhancing security and privacy in bio-metrics-based authentication systems. *IBM Syst. J.*, 40(3), 614–634).

Sala, R., Zappa, E., & Cigada, A. (2006). Personal identification through 3D bio-metric measurements based on stereoscopic image pairs. *Proc. of the 2006 IEEE International Workshop on Measurement Systems for Homeland Security, Contra-band Detection and Personal Safety* (pp. 10-13).

SASSE, M. A. (2007). Red-eye blink, bendy shuffle, and the yuck factor - A user experience of biometric airport systems. *IEEE Security & Privacy*, 5(3), 78-81.

Sim, T., Zhang, S., Janakiraman, R., & Kumar, S. (2007). Continuous verification using multimodal biometrics. *IEEE Trans. Pattern Analysis and Machine Intel-ligence*, 29(4), 687-700.

Uludag, U., Pankanti, S., Prabhakar, S., & Jain, A. K. (2004). Biometric cryptosys-tems: issues and challenges. *Proc. IEEE* (Vol. 92, No. 6, pp. 948–960).

Wang, R., & Bhanu, B. (2006). Performance Prediction for Multimodal Biomet-rics. *Proceedings of the International Conference on Pattern Recognition* (pp. 586-589).

Woodard, D. L., Faltemier, T. C., Yan, P., Flynn, P. J., & Bowyer, K. W. (2006). A comparison of 3D biometric modalities. *Proc. of Conference on Computer Vision and Pattern Recognition Worksho*p *(CVPRW'06)* (2006).

Glossary

Preface

PCA, or K-L transform: principal component analysis
LDA: Fisher linear discriminant analysis
ICA: independent component analysis
CCA: canonical correlation analysis
PLS: partial least squares
KPCA: kernel principal component analysis
KFD: kernel Fisher discriminant
LMLP: large margin linear projection
OFD: orthogonalized Fisher discriminant
FDS: Fisher discriminant with Schur decomposition
MMSD: multiple maximum scatter difference
DCV: discriminant based on coefficients of variances
NIST: National Institute of Science and Technology
BSSR1: Biometric Scores Set - Release 1
SSS: small sample size
MNMSE: minimum norm minimum squared-error
MSE: minimum squared-error

Chapter I

AFIS: Automated Fingerprint Identification System
ATMs: Automated Teller Machines
DNA: Deoxyribonucleic acid
BSSR1: Biometric Scores Set - Release 1

OCR: optical character recognition
NMF: non-negative matrix factorization
CKFD: complete kernel Fisher discriminant
KDDA: kernel direct discriminant analysis
ISOMAP: isometric feature mapping
LLE: locally linear embedding
2DPCA: two-Dimensional PCA
GLRAM: generalized low rank approximation of matrices
LMLP: large margin linear projection

Chapter II

FDC: Fisher discriminant criterion
MSE: minimum squared-error
LSVM: linear Support Vector Machine
FLD: Fisher linear discriminant
FSD: Foley-Sammon discriminant
MSD: maximum scatter difference
N-LDA: nullspace LDA
D-LDA: direct LDA
C-LDA: complete LDA

Chapter III

FDC: Fisher discriminant criterion
2DPCA: two-dimensional principal component analysis
FSD: Foley-Sammon discriminant
MSD: maximum scatter difference
U-LDA: uncorrelated linear discriminant analysis
OCS: orthogonal complementary space

Chapter IV

OCD: orthogonal component discriminant
EFLD: extended Fisher linear discriminant
EFSD: extended FSD
EOCD: extended OCD

Chapter V

PD-LDA: parameterized direct linear discriminant analysis
WN-LDA: weighted nullspace LDA
NN: nearest neighbor
ARR: average recognition rate
WLDA-RWS: weighted linear discriminant analysis in the range of the within-class scatter
LDA-RWS: LDA in the range of the within-class scatter matrix

Chapter VI

FLD: Fisher linear discriminant
K-L: Karhunen-Loève
CV: coefficient of variation
MCV: minimum coefficient of variance

Chapter VII

SVD: singular value decomposition
CP: CANDECOMP-PARAFAC

Chapter VIII

No

Chapter IX

FOSDV: Foley-Sammon optimal discriminant vectors
UDV: uncorrelated discriminant vectors
2D: two-dimensional
UIDA: uncorrelated image discriminant analysis
LM: Liu's method
DRM: direct recognition method
UK: University of Essex
NHDLDA: non-iterative HDLDA

Chapter X

VQ: vector quantization
L2 distance: Euclidean distance
PCA I: vertically cantered PCA
PCA II: horizontally cantered PCA
MICA: multilinear independent components analysis
NF: non-negative factorization

Chapter XI

SVM: support vector machines
MHKS: modified HK algorithm
MatMHKS: matrix-based MHKS
FLS-SVM: fuzzy LS-SVM
STL: supervised tensor learning
MPM: minimax probability machines
TMPM: tensor MPM
DPLS: discriminant partial least squares
HK: Ho-Kashyap
LP: linear programming
LFP: linear fractional programming
QP: quadratic programming
QCQP: quadratically constrained quadratic programming
SOCP: the second-order cone programming
SDP: semidefinite programming
GP: geometric programming
LPM: linear programming machine
DML: distance metric learning
2DPLS: 2D partial least squares

Chapter XII

FRR: false reject rate
FAR: false accept rate
FMR: false match rate
FNMR: false non-match rate
FTAR: failure to acquire rate

FTER: failure to enrol rate
ROC: receiver operating characteristic
EER: equal error rate
INCITS: InterNational Committee for Information Technology Standards
ITI: Information Technology Industry Council
FRVT 2002: 2002 Face Recognition Vendor Test

Chapter XIII

KDCV: kernel discriminative common vectors
RBF: radial base function
DCV: discriminative common vectors
KDRC: KDCV–RBF classifier
KDNC: KDCV and NN classifier
DNC: DCV and NN classifier
POC: phase and orientation code
DC: direct current

Chapter XIV

FFN: feed-forward neural network

Chapter XV

AC: accuracy
P: precision
TP: recall or true positive rate
FN: false negative rate
FP: false positive rate
TN: true negative rate
SV: singular value
GDM: group decision-making

Chapter XVI

AES: advanced encryption standard

About the Authors

David Zhang graduated in computer science from Peking University (1974). He received his MSc in computer science in 1982 and PhD in 1985 from the Harbin Institute of Technology (HIT). From 1986 to 1988, he was a postdoctoral fellow at Tsinghua University and then an associate professor at the Academia Sinica, Beijing. In 1994, he received his second PhD in electrical and computer engineering from the University of Waterloo, Ontario, Canada. Currently, he is a chair professor at the Hong Kong Polytechnic University, where he is the founding director of the Biometrics Technology Centre (UGC/CRC) supported by the Hong Kong SAR government in 1998. He also serves as visiting chair professor in Tsinghua University, and adjunct professor at Shanghai Jiao Tong University, Beihang University, HIT and the University of Waterloo. He is the founder and editor-in-chief of the *International Journal of Image and Graphics* (IJIG); book editor of the Springer International Series on Biometrics (SISB); organizer of the International Conference on Biometrics 2004 and 2006 (ICBA 2004 and ICB 2006); associate editor of more than 10 international journals, including *IEEE Transactions on SMC-A/SMC-C/Pattern Recognition*; chair of IEEE/CIS Technical Committee on Intelligent System Application; and the author of more than 10 books and 160 journal papers. Professor Zhang is a Croucher senior research fellow, distinguished speaker of the IEEE Computer Society, and fellow of the International Association of Pattern Recognition (IAPR).

Fengxi Song graduated in applied mathematics from the Anhui University (1984). He earned his MSc in applied mathematics from the Changsha Institute of Technology (1987) and PhD in pattern recognition from the Nanjing University of Science and Technology (2004). From 2005 to 2007, he was a postdoctoral fellow at ShenZhen Graduate School, Harbin Institute of Technology. Currently, he is a professor at New Star Research Institute of Applied Technology in Hefei City, China. He is the author of more than 30 scientific papers in pattern recognition and computer vision. He is a reviewer of several international journals such as *IEEE Transactions and Pattern Recognition*. His research interests include pattern recognition, computer vision, image processing, and text categorization.

Yong Xu was born in Sichuan, China, in 1972. He received his BS and MS degree at Air Force Institute of Meteorology (China) in 1994 and 1997, respectively. He then received his PhD in pattern recognition and intelligence system at the Nanjing University of Science and Technology (NUST) in 2005. From May 2005 to April 2007, he worked at Shenzhen graduate school, Harbin Institute of Technology (HIT) as a postdoctoral research fellow. Now he is an associate professor at Shenzhen graduate school, HIT. He also acts as a research assistant researcher at the Hong Kong Polytechnic University from August 2007 to June 2008. He has published more than 40 scientific papers. He is an associate editor of the *International Journal of Image and Graphics*, a reviewer of several international journals such as *IEEE Transactions on Systems, Man, and Cybernetics*, *International Journal of Pattern Recognition and Artificial Intelligence and Neurocomputing*. His current interests include pattern recognition, biometrics, machine learning and image processing.

Zhizheng Liang graduated in Department of Automation from TianJin University of Technology and Education in 1999. He received his MSc in Department of Automation in Shandong University in 2001 and got his PhD in pattern and intelligent system from Shanghai Jiaotong University, P.R.China in 2005. From 2005 to 2007, he is a postdoctoral researcher at Shenzhen Graduate School in Harbin Institute of Technology. Currently, he is a research fellow at City University of Hong Kong. His current interests include image processing, pattern recognition and machine learning.

Index

N

normalization step 307
Nullspace LDA 87
nullspace linear discriminant analysis
        14, 78, 89, 103

O

one-dimensional biometric methods 351
optimal projection direction
        26, 31, 34, 43, 44, 45
optimization model 26, 27, 31, 35, 36,
        44, 58, 59, 60, 64, 67, 96, 109,
        122, 123, 124, 125, 177
orthogonal discriminant analysis 14, 15,
        28, 58, 60, 70, 72, 75, 349

P

palm print recognition 6, 12, 15, 291
pattern recognition 1, 5, 13, 25, 27,
        28, 32, 37, 55, 56, 60, 61, 78,
        107, 119, 132, 228, 250, 251,
        282, 313
performance indices 321
performance to cost ratio 354
personal authentication 2, 3, 6, 7, 8, 11,
        254, 255, 262, 266, 271, 274,
        275, 276, 294, 305, 308, 310,
        316, 318, 322, 331, 344, 352,
        353
Principal component analysis 150, 319

R

recognition technologies 1, 5, 8, 12, 349

S

Schur decomposition 14, 58, 65, 66, 67
single biometrics 256, 257

small sample size problem 14, 15, 17,
        28, 56, 76, 104, 105, 132, 228,
        250, 276
SSS problem 13, 60, 61, 350, 351
support vector machine
        17, 26, 32, 55, 227, 251

T

tensor 9, 10, 12, 13, 14, 16, 20, 110,
        133, 135, 136, 137, 138, 139,
        140, 141, 142, 143, 144, 145,
        146, 147, 148, 149, 150, 151,
        153, 159, 160, 161, 168, 169,
        170, 171, 186, 188, 190, 197,
        198, 199, 200, 202, 204, 205,
        212, 213, 218, 219, 220, 223,
        224, 226, 227, 236, 237, 238,
        244, 249, 250, 252, 350, 351

U

uncorrelated linear discriminant analysis
        37, 41, 126

V

verification 2, 5, 8, 9, 17, 25, 257,
        258, 259, 262, 265, 266, 267,
        268, 269, 270, 271, 273, 275,
        298, 300, 301, 303, 306, 310,
        324, 325, 326, 327, 329, 331,
        333, 343, 346, 347, 348, 350,
        353, 357, 358

W

within-class scatter matrix 11, 14, 28,
        34, 35, 45, 47, 48, 49, 50, 51,
        55, 59, 60, 61, 62, 78, 79, 82,
        87, 89, 95, 97, 103, 107, 108,
        109, 114, 120, 176, 280, 281,
        350